THE PATHOPHYSIOLOGY of the MICROCIRCULATION

Nicholas A. Mortillaro
Aubrey E. Taylor

CRC

CRC Press
Boca Raton Ann Arbor London Tokyo

Library of Congress Cataloging-in-Publication Data

The Pathophysiology of the microcirculation / edited by Nicholas A. Mortillaro and Aubrey E. Taylor.
p. cm.
Includes bibliographical references and index.
ISBN 0-8493-4547-2
1. Microcirculation disorders—Pathophysiology. I. Mortillaro, Nicholas A. II. Taylor, Aubrey E.
[DNLM: 1. Microcirculation—physiopathology. WG 104 P297 1994]
RC700.M53P38 1994
616.1′3—dc20
DNLM / DLC
for Library of Congress 93-43112
CIP

International Standard Book Number 0-8493-4547-2
Library of Congress Card Number 93-43112
Printed in the United States of America 2 3 4 5 6 7 8 9 0
Printed on acid-free paper

FOREWORD

When I first learned that this book was in preparation, I immediately felt a twinge of delight even before knowing its specific content. The reason was simple: the book covers an area of circulatory physiology that is developing extremely rapidly and that badly needs a coordinated synthesis of many new ideas. But, even more important, the two editors, as well as their chosen authors, have all been central figures in the basic research and development of imaginative approaches to still unclear concepts of microcirculatory function.

In the last twenty years, new avenues of microvascular research have abounded, helping us to understand many previously misunderstood mechanisms of local blood flow control. This has been especially true for control of blood flow to match the local metabolic needs of each tissue. And equally important is new knowledge that helps to explain the distribution of vascular resistance control between small and large blood vessels. Unfortunately, though, microvascular research has taken many directions in numerous laboratories, and the results have been published in widely dispersed individual articles in almost equally as many journals. This present book edited by Drs. Mortillaro and Taylor is one of the few attempts to provide a synthesis of this field in both normal and pathological conditions.

Each time that I have studied more about this book during its development, my enthusiasm has increased. The reader will certainly appreciate my reaction if it is his intent to gain a deeper, coordinated understanding of microcirculatory function.

Arthur C. Guyton, M.D.
Professor Emeritus
Department of Physiology and Biophysics
School of Medicine
University of Mississippi Medical Center
Jackson, Mississippi

To our families — wives, children, and grandchildren.

THE EDITORS

Nicholas A. Mortillaro is a Professor in the Department of Physiology at the University of South Alabama College of Medicine. Originally educated in electronic engineering at the New Jersey Institute of Technology, where he received both a B.S.E.E. and M.S.E.E., he later earned a Ph.D. in physiology studying under Dr. Leif Horn at the University of Medicine and Dentistry of New Jersey. He was a National Institute of Health Postdoctoral Fellow at the University of Mississippi School of Medicine in the Department of Physiology and Biophysics under Dr. Aubrey E. Taylor. He is a long-standing member of the American Physiological Society, the American Microcirculatory Society, the North American Lymphology Society, and the American Gastroenterological Association. He has served both on the membership and the annual meetings committees of the Microcirculatory Society. He has served on various National Institutes of Health study sections and has been a field reviewer for various scientific journals, including *American Journal of Physiology, Journal of Investigative Dermatology, Journal of Applied Physiology, Journal of Orthopedic Research, Gastroenterology*, and *Microvascular Research.*

He is the editor/author of *The Physiology and Pharmacology of the Microcirculation*, in two volumes. His primary research interest and publications have been in the area of the microcirculation of the splanchnic bed with an emphasis on local blood flow, flow distribution, and fluid exchange dynamics associated with the small intestine.

Aubrey E. Taylor is Professor and Chairman of the Department of Physiology, University of South Alabama College of Medicine. He received his Ph.D. under Dr. Arthur C. Guyton and did his postdoctoral at Harvard Medical School in the Biophysical Laboratory under Dr. Peter Curran. He is a past president of the American Physiological Society, the Microcirculatory Society, and the North American Lymphology Society. He is a past council member of Federation of American Societies for Experimental Biology and vice president of the International Society of Pathophysiology. He serves as a section editor of *Journal of Applied Physiology*, has served for the past few years as a special editor for the *Journal of Critical Care Medicine*, and is on the editorial boards for several major journals. He has served as a member and chairman of numerous National Institutes of Health, American Heart Association, and American Thoracic Society study sections. Dr. Taylor has been the recipient of the Landis Award from the Microcirculatory Society, the Wiggers Award from the American Physiological Society circulation section, the Dickson-Richardson Award from the American Heart Association, and the Cecil Drinker Award from the North American Lymphology Society. He has been elected to fellowships in the American Association for the Advancement of Science and the Royal Society of Medicine. In 1989, he was recognized as the Scientist of the Year in the State of Alabama.

His major research interest contributions have been in the microvascular exchange of solute and water with special emphasis on macromolecular exchange and mechanisms associated with edema in lungs, skeletal muscle and the GI tracts. He is the author of over 600 publications, including four books.

PREFACE

The ultimate expression of the cardiovascular system is found at the level of the microvascular system where the interactions of circulatory function, nutritional requirements and the removal of the products of metabolism are coupled via the microvascular's regulation of tissue perfusion, blood-tissue exchange and regional blood volume. At any given moment, both intrinsic (local) and extrinsic (nervous and humoral) factors, acting directly or indirectly, exert control over the three basic components of the microcirculation, i.e., arterioles (resistance vessels), capillaries (exchange vessels) and venules (capacitance vessels). The modulation of blood flow through a microvascular bed is accomplished through the regulation of arteriolar diameter, while flow distribution, and hence tissue exchange, is regulated by the binary state of precapillary sphincters located at the origin of each capillary, e.g., opened/closed, on/off; thus, in this manner, the important exchange parameters of capillary-to-cell diffusion distances and capillary surface area available for exchange are regulated. Finally, the terminus of the microvascular tree are the venules acting as capacitance vessels and are the major site within the microcirculation where blood volume is stored and available for recruitment.

Beginning with Chapter 1, the general structure of the normal microvascular system with a special emphasis on those characteristics of blood vessel segments collectively comprising that system is discussed. With the coronary circulation used as the model, Chapter 2 explores the molecular and cellular mechanisms and their control that contribute to new vascular development and restructuring, that is, the phenomenon of angiogenesis. In Chapter 3 the angiogenic mechanisms and control as it relates to vascular and nonvascular tumors is examined. In Chapter 4 the importance of the microcirculation in the genesis of hypertension is presented with a discussion of the mechanisms of vascular resistance and reactivity as contributors of hypertension. Chapter 5 reviews the microvascular response of key organ systems during shock. A section is devoted to exploring the new microvascular problem associated with AIDS. Focusing on the intestine, Chapter 6 explores the evidence on the possible role of reactive oxygen metabolites and granulocytes in ischemia/reperfusion induced microvascular dysfunction. Chapter 7 explores the mechanisms of hyperglycemia-induced development of diabetic vascular disease and the pathogenesis of diabetic microangiopathy. The role of the vascular endothelium induced inflammatory and immunologic injury through the action of cytokines produced by circulating leukocytes is examined in Chapter 8. Chapter 9 describes the process involved in edema formation associated with thermal (burn) and smoke inhalation injury. The structural and functional changes in the microcirculation associated with the aging process is presented in Chapter 10. The discussion of these changes focuses on the cutaneous, skeletal muscle, myocardial, conjunctival, and cerebral circulation.

Chapter 11 of the book concludes with a presentation of the putative biological effects of environmental factors on the microcirculation. The discussion emphasizes the target-organ specificity associated with the cardiac, cerebral, gastrointestinal, hepatic, integument, pulmonary, renal and skeletal microcirculation.

We wish to thank all participants for their excellent and timely authoring of the chapters. A special thanks to Monique Power, Managing Editor of Life Science at CRC Press, for her most helpful and pleasant demeanor, and patience, during the preparation and production of the book.

Nicholas A. Mortillaro, Ph.D., Professor
Aubrey E. Taylor, Ph.D., Professor and Chairman
Department of Physiology, College of Medicine
University of South Alabama, Mobile, Alabama

TABLE OF CONTENTS

CONTRIBUTORS

Russell C. Bowes, B.S.
Graduate Student, Doctoral Candidate
Departments of Veterinary Physiology and Pharmacology and Medical Physiology
Texas A&M University
College Station, Texas

Charles S. Cox, Jr., M.D.
Postdoctoral Fellow
Department of Surgery
University of Texas Medical Branch
Galveston, Texas
Postdoctoral Fellow
Shriners Burns Institute
Galveston, Texas

Linda E. Czisny, D.V.M.
Research Associate
Department of Medical Physiology
Texas A&M University
College Station, Texas

David J. Dzielak, Ph.D.
Associate Professor
Departments of Surgery (Research) and Physiology and Biophysics
School of Medicine
University of Mississippi
Jackson, Mississippi

Thomas E. Emerson, Jr., Ph.D.
Research Fellow
Department of Preclinical Cardiovascular Pharmacology
Miles, Inc.
Pharmaceutical Division
West Haven, Connecticut

Susan P. Fuselier, D.V.M.
Research Associate
Department of Physiology and Biophysics
Louisiana State University Medical Center
Shreveport, Louisiana

D. Neil Granger, Ph.D.
Professor and Head
Department of Physiology and Biophysics
Louisiana State University Medical Center
Shreveport, Louisiana

Harris J. Granger, Ph.D.
Professor and Head
Department of Medical Physiology
Director
Microcirculation Research Institute
Texas A&M University
College Station, Texas

Joey P. Granger, Ph.D.
Professor
Department of Physiology and Biophysics
School of Medicine
University of Mississippi
Jackson, Mississippi

James R. Hawker, Jr., Ph.D
Research Associate
Department of Medical Physiology
Texas A&M University
College Station, Texas

David N. Herndon, M.D.
Professor — Jesse H. Jones Distinguished Chair in Surgery
Department of Surgery
University of Texas Medical Branch
Chief of Staff
Shriners Burns Institute
Galveston, Texas

Robert L. Hester, Ph.D.
Associate Professor
Department of Physiology and Biophysics
School of Medicine
University of Mississippi
Jackson, Mississippi

CONTRIBUTORS (*continued*)

Michael A. Hill, Ph.D.
Assistant Professor
Department of Physiology
Eastern Virginia Medical School
Norfolk, Virginia

Lerner B. Hinshaw, Ph.D., FCCM
Professor and Member
Department of Free Radical Biology and Aging Research
Oklahoma Medical Research Foundation
George Lynn Cross Research Professor
Department of Physiology
University of Oklahoma
Oklahoma City, Oklahoma

Sarah N. Jerome, B.S.
Graduate Student, Doctoral Candidate
Department of Physiology and Biophysics
Louisiana State University Medical Center
Shreveport, Louisiana

Ronald J. Korthuis, Ph.D.
Associate Professor
Department of Physiology and Biophysics
Louisiana State University Medical Center
Shreveport, Louisiana

Margaret A. Krasovich, M.S.
Advanced Research Specialist
Department of Anatomy
College of Medicine
University of Arizona
Tucson, Arizona

Paul Kubes, Ph.D.
Assistant Professor
Department of Physiology
Gastrointestinal Research Group
University of Calgary Health Science Center
Calgary, Alberta, Canada

Peter Kvietys, Ph.D.
Professor
Department of Physiology and Biophysics
Louisiana State University Medical Center
Shreveport, Louisiana

Christopher W. Lentz, M.D.
Resident
Department of Surgery
Medical College of Wisconsin
Milwaukee, Wisconsin
Research Fellow
Department of Anesthesia Research
Shriners Burns Institute
Galveston, Texas

Robert S. McCuskey, Ph.D.
Professor and Head
Department of Anatomy
College of Medicine
University of Arizona
Tucson, Arizona

Cynthia J. Meininger, Ph.D.
Assistant Research Scientist
Department of Medical Physiology
Texas A&M University
College Station, Texas

Roberto F. Nicosia, M.D., Ph.D.
Associate Professor
Department of Pathology
Medical College of Pennsylvania
Philadelphia, Pennsylvania

Giuseppe G. Pietra, M.D.
Professor
Department of Pathology and Laboratory Medicine
School of Medicine
Director, Division of Anatomic Pathology
University Hospital
University of Pennsylvania
Philadelphia, Pennsylvania

CONTRIBUTORS (*continued*)

Russell L. Prewitt, Ph.D.
Professor
Department of Physiology
Eastern Virginia Medical School
Norfolk, Virginia

Kenneth S. Ramos, Ph.D.
Associate Professor
Departments of Veterinary Physiology and Pharmacology and Medical Physiology
Texas A&M University
College Station, Texas

Daniel R. Richardson, Ph.D.
Professor
Department of Physiology
and
Sanders-Brown Center on Aging
University of Kentucky
Lexington, Kentucky

Daniel L. Traber, Ph.D.
Professor
Departments of Anesthesiology and Physiology and Biophysics
University of Texas Medical Branch
Chief of Anesthesia Research and Coordinator of Research
Shriners Burns Institute
Galveston, Texas

Lillian D. Traber, R.N.
Laboratory Supervisor
Department of Anesthesia Research
Shriners Burns Institute
Galveston, Texas

Donna H. Wang, M.D.
Research Assistant Professor
Department of Internal Medicine
University of Texas Medical Branch
Galveston, Texas

David C. Zawieja, Ph.D.
Assistant Professor
Department of Medical Physiology
Texas A&M University
College Station, Texas

Marina Ziche, M.D.
Senior Research Scientist
Department of Preclinical and Clinical Pharmacology
University of Florence
Florence, Italy

Chapter 1

Anatomy of the Microvascular System

Robert S. McCuskey and Margaret A. Krasovich

CONTENTS

I. INTRODUCTION

Sustaining an optimal microcirculation is a requirement for the maintenance and survival of virtually all vertebrate cells, tissues, and organs. Failure to maintain an optimal microcirculation results in tissue hypoxia or anoxia, lack of nutrition, the accumulation of metabolic products, and cellular death. As a result, the lack of oxygen delivery to the vital cells and tissues of organs is one of the major and fundamental causes of death. This chapter will review briefly some of the basic principles of the dynamic morphology of the microvascular system during health while subsequent chapters will discuss its pathophysiology.

II. DEFINITIONS AND BASIC CONCEPTS

The term "microvascular system" has been introduced into the literature as a generic term that includes all blood vessels, their contents, and associated structures which are visible only by microscopic examination, i.e., blood vessels smaller than 300 μm.[1-3] The use of the term "microcirculation" should be restricted only to the blood flowing within these vessels. Unfortunately, the term, microcirculation, frequently is used incorrectly in the literature to refer to the vessels as well as the flow within them.[1-3]

A. GENERAL CHARACTERISTICS OF THE MICROVASCULAR SYSTEM

The structure of the microvascular system reflects its functions which include circulating the blood within tissues and organs bringing the blood in close proximity to the cells of organs, and providing a semipermeable membrane for the transit of select substances between the blood and cells of the organs. Close apposition is assured between the blood and cells of organs by circulating the blood through vessels whose internal diameters are about the size of a single red blood cell (8 μm). In addition, these vessels are arranged in a pattern whereby nearly every parenchymatous cell of an organ abuts a blood vessel. Not only is close proximity assured but these vessels provide an enormous surface area thereby providing a favorable condition for the transit of an adequate volume of sub-

0-8493-4547-2/94/$0.00+$.50

stances through the walls of the vessels. An appreciation of the area that is available for transit is provided by realizing that there are about 2000 capillaries in 1 mm^2 of skeletal muscle, and in a 70-kg man, 6300 m^2 of surface area potentially are available for transit. The transit is controlled by the response of endothelium, a semipermeable membrane which lines all blood vessels. In short, endothelium characterizes the vascular system just as the neuron characterizes the nervous system. The extent of the microvascular system may be appreciated by the fact that it constitutes more than 99% of the vessels of the cardiovascular system.

The majority of the microvascular system consists of arterioles, capillaries, and venules. In addition, there are sinusoids in some organs (liver, spleen, and bone marrow) which function as capillaries but usually have a diameter larger than capillaries.

Finally, there are two types of vessels that shunt blood from arterioles to venules. The first are arterio-venous anastomoses which are structurally similar to arterioles. The second are thoroughfare or preferential channels which are found most frequently in connective tissue and skeletal muscle. These vessels are structurally similar to capillaries and function like them, but have blood flowing through them continuously.

B. GENERAL STRUCTURES OF THE MICROVASCULATURE

All vessels have four characteristics which pertain to (1) their spatial arrangement in organs and tissues, (2) their longitudinal configuration, (3) the arrangement of their internal structure, and (4) their cellular components. Several of these characteristics often are extensively modified depending upon the site of vessels in the body and because of such modification it is desirable to know both the general structural plan of vessels and the nature of the variations in the major organs because of the importance of these organs for body function. In short, vessels are only "typical" for a specific organ.

The spatial arrangement of vessels in an organ is related to its functions and is reflected in the complexity of its vascular pattern and number of vessels per unit area. In general, the vascularity of an organ is directly proportional to its metabolic activity. As examples, this principle is illustrated in the liver, pancreas, mesenteries, skeletal muscle, and kidney.

The liver has a dual flow blood supply with its exchange vessels (sinusoids) receiving blood from branches of both the hepatic arterioles and portal venules. In addition, each hepatic parenchymal cell is surrounded, at least on two sides, by sinusoids so that the maximum distance between blood and a parenchymatous cell is about half the distance of a liver cell.[4-6] In contrast, the metabolic activity of mesenteries is considerably less and the vascular pattern is simple and capillaries are separated by many tens of microns.[7-10] Other striking differences are seen in the pancreas where capillaries abut several sides of each endocrine cell in the islets, whereas in the exocrine tissue the number of capillaries is dramatically reduced and only the base of each acinar cell is in contact with a capillary.[11] The longitudinal arrangement of capillaries in parallel with skeletal muscle fibers[10] contrasts strikingly with the tortuous loops found in the renal glomerulus.[12]

Thus, the microvasculature of the liver, pancreas, kidney, spleen, lung, etc., all differ from each other and that of other organs. Such differences probably are significant and must be considered in the final analysis of blood flow in each organ or tissue.[13] However, only limited attempts[14] have been made to evaluate the functional significance of these differences in health and disease especially as they are related to adequate oxygenation of the tissues and cells involved.[15]

There are three types of longitudinal configurations of vessels. The arterial and venous vessels are cone shaped, with a taper about 1 to 2° per branch toward the capillary vessels.[8,16] Capillaries are cylindrical.[8,9,16-18] Thus, the greatest resistance to flow is in the arterial system as the blood flows into vessels having an ever decreasing bore and taper while the opposite occurs in the venous system as their bore and taper increase in the normal direction of flow.[16]

Thus, while there are many structural and functional similarities between the microvascular beds of various organs and tissues, enough dissimilarities exist that extrapolation of data from one site to another frequently is impossible. As a result, to date, no totally adequate unified nomenclature has been developed to further classify most of these vessels although certain morphological and functional sub-classifications have been suggested. Nevertheless, a few generalizations about the vessels that comprise the microvascular system can be made.

III. MORPHOLOGY OF MICROVASCULAR SEGMENTS

The basic morphology of all vessels is similar throughout the vascular system, including the microvasculature. All blood vessels have three coats or tunics: an internal one, the *tunica intima*; an intermediate one, the *tunica media*, and an external one, the *tunica adventitia*. All vessels, including capillaries, have three tunics; but the ratio to each other is frequently different. Each tunic is characterized by a predominant function and cell; the intima by the endothelial cell and transvascular exchange, the media by the smooth muscle and control of vessel diameter, and the adventitia by connective tissue, nerves, and blood vessels that provide protection and nourishment to a vessel.

A. ARTERIOLES

Arterioles are afferent vessels that supply the capillary bed (Figures 1–3). As indicated above, such vessels are tapered and have a lumen with a decreasing bore as the capillaries are approached.[19,20]

The tunica intima consists of an endothelial cell lining and its associated basal lamina.[8,16,17,21] The structural details of endothelium are contained below in the section on capillaries. External to the endothelial lining, the subendothelial connective tissue and

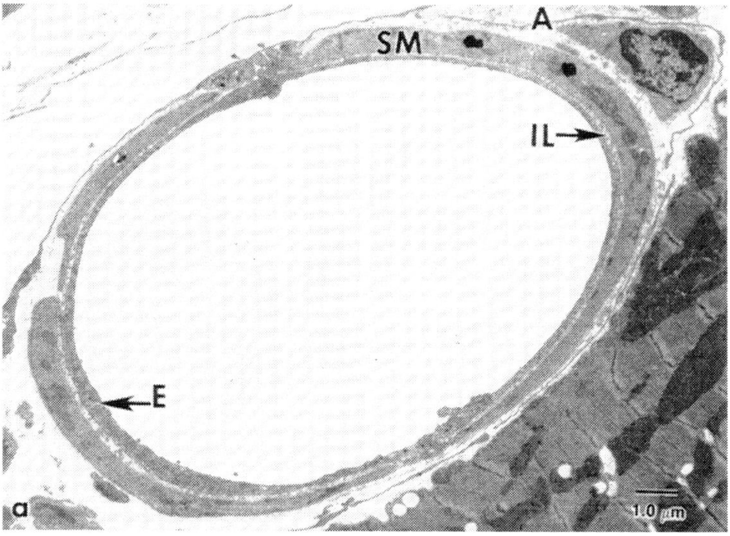

Figure 1-1 Arterioles in (**a**) dilated and (**b**) contracted states. Note the reduced thickness and smoothed contour of the endothelium (E) concomitant with dilation (a). Smooth muscle (SM); connective tissue of the adventitia (A), containing unmyelinated nerves (N); internal elastic lamella (IL).

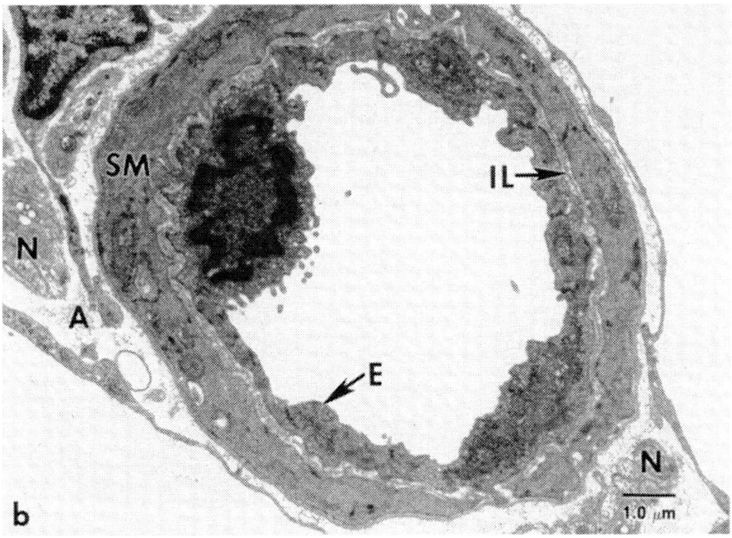

Figure 1-1 (Continued).

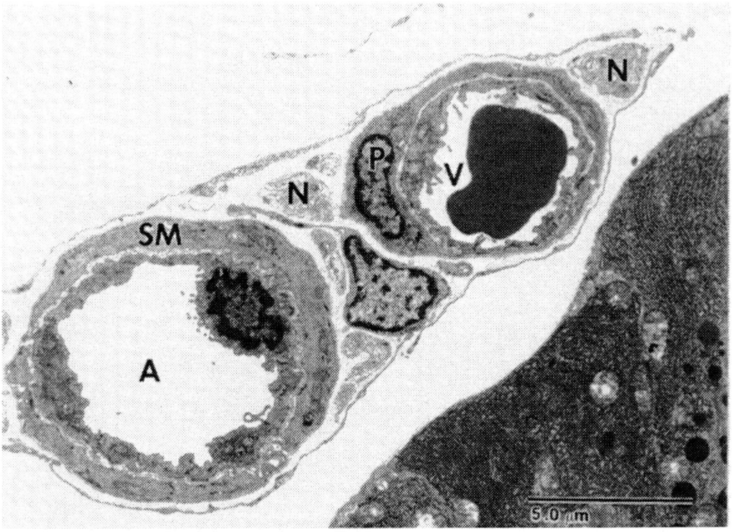

Figure 1-2 Arteriole (A), unmyelinated nerves (N), and pericytic venule (V) in the acinar pancreas. Note the incomplete investment of the venular wall by the pericyte (P) in contrast to the arteriole with a complete investment of smooth muscle (SM).

external elastic lamella is thin and discontinuous. In vessels smaller than 50 μm, it gradually disappears (Figure 3).

The tunica media of precapillary arterioles is composed of smooth muscle cells wrapped circularly around the endothelial tube lining these vessels.[8,16,17] In contrast, the smooth muscle cells in larger arterioles and in small arteries are helically arranged with

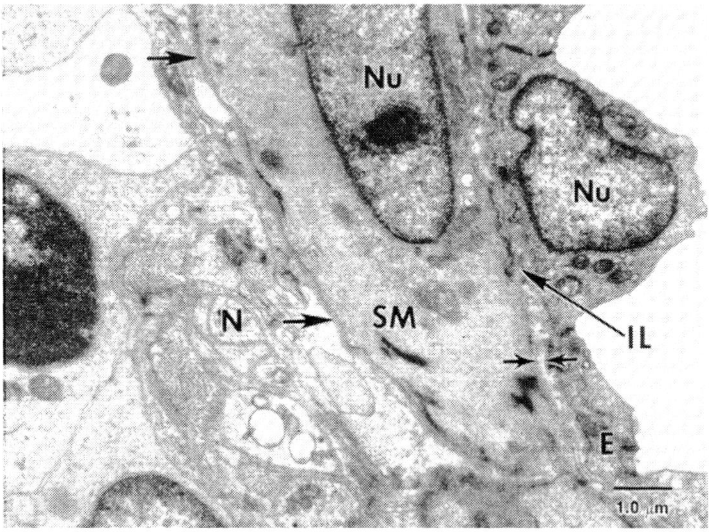

Figure 1-3 Arteriole illustrating close relationship between endothelium (E) and smooth muscle cells (SM) with intervening incomplete internal elastic lamella (IL) and basal laminae (arrow) of both the endothelial and smooth muscle cells. Note the lack of close approximation between the adjacent unmyelinated nerves (N) and the adjacent smooth muscle cells; Nuclei (Nu).

a pitch sometimes exceeding 45°.[8,16] The number of layers of smooth muscle cells decreases as the capillary bed is approached, becoming a single layer of continuous to discontinuous cells at the arteriolar-capillary junction. At this junction, the bore is often less than that of the capillary as well as less than the diameter of individual erythrocytes.[1,22] Thus, such vessels frequently produce a "bottleneck effect" which, coupled with their tapering bore, is responsible for the bulk of the "peripheral resistance" as evidenced by the large drop in systemic blood pressure that occurs along the course of these vessels.[19,23-28] Because precapillary arterioles supply numerous capillaries, variations in the internal arteriolar diameter can regulate simultaneously the flow of blood through a large segment of the capillary bed.

Vascular smooth muscle in the tunica media consists of discrete cells which are smaller than smooth muscle cells in viscera.[8,16,17,21] The cells are thin cylinders (3 to 5 µm × 30 to 60 µm) surrounded by a plasma membrane (sarcolemma) measuring about 80Å and have a cytoplasm that contains dense bodies and myofilaments that are randomly oriented. Thick (12 to 16 nm) myosin filaments are probably organized during contraction; they are difficult to observe in fixed material. The thin (5 to 7 nm) filaments containing actin and tropomyosin are intimately related to dense bodies attached to the plasmalemma. An elaborate array of 10 nm intermediate filaments containing desmin and vimentin also course through the cytoplasm. An ellipsoid nucleus is usually located superficially in the center of the cells and adjacent to it is a Golgi complex. In addition, the cytoplasm contains endoplasmic reticulum with ribosomes, mitochondria, and microtubules (20 to 40 nm), parallel to the long axis of the cell. A number of caveolae or sarcolemmal vesicles considerably increases the surface area of the cells.

In small arteries and arterioles where concentric layers of smooth muscle exist the cells are arranged circumferentially and separated by a thick envelope of glycoprotein in which are embedded collagen, reticular, and elastic fibers. Furthermore, at the periphery of the media are bands of elastic tissue, forming an internal and a less developed external elastic lamella, respectively (Figures 1–3). In the media there is abundant ground substance that contains chondroitin sulfate and the sole cell is the smooth muscle cell. This cell is responsible for the maintenance and production of the collagen and elastin fibers, as well as proteoglycans as it is virtually the only cell type present. A well-developed Golgi complex and rough endoplasmic reticulum reflect this synthetic capability.

Myo-myo and myo-endothelial contacts (direct contacts between the membranes of adjacent smooth muscle cells and between the membranes of smooth muscle cells and adjacent endothelial cells) are more numerous in precapillary arterioles than in larger vessels.[8,16,17,21] Such contacts contain gap junctions that provide a morphologic mechanism for impulse transmission and the rapid diffusion of pharmacodynamic substances, since normally a basal lamina tends to isolate individual muscle cells from each other and from the endothelium.[8,16] This may help explain the high sensitivity of these vessels to vasoactive substances.[29]

In some tissues and organs (e.g., skeletal and cardiac muscle, mesentery, kidney, exocrine pancreas) vascular smooth muscle cells frequently surround the orifices of capillaries that originate from precapillary arterioles. Such groups of cells have been termed "precapillary sphincters".[8,16,30] In contrast with the precapillary arterioles, the sphincteric action of these cells can serve to regulate flow to smaller portions of the capillary bed, i.e., blood flow into individual or small numbers of capillaries. The morphology of the smooth muscle cells of the sphincter is very similar to that of the media of precapillary arterioles and such cells have been considered to be extensions from the arteriolar tunica media.[8,16] Physiologically, however, the precapillary sphincters can respond independently of the musculature of adjacent arterioles[31] and may be more sensitive to vasoactive substances.[29] This may be a reflection of the morphology of the site since myo-endothelial membrane contacts are very numerous at the sites of precapillary sphincters.[8,16]

The connective tissue of the adventitia of small arteries and arterioles is limited and blends into that of the resident organ. The fibers are arranged in a direction both parallel and tangential in relation to the lumen of the vessel and are part of the complex of connective, elastic, and reticular fibers in the other tunics which add to the physical strength of a vessel as well as limiting the extent of its transverse and longitudinal expansions.

While all vessels, with the exception of capillaries, are innervated, the nerves are essentially limited to the adventitia (Figures 1–3).[8,16,17,21,32] Fibers from spinal and cranial nerves are found in the adventitia as a reticulated network. Unlike skeletal muscle, not all smooth muscle cells are innervated and the distance between the unmyelinated axons and the sarcolemma (Figure 3) is considerably greater than in the motor end plates of skeletal muscle. Three types of fibers can be distinguished; sensory, postganglionic sympathetic, and pre- and postganglionic parasympathetic fibers. The parasympathetic fibers have a more restricted distribution. Sensory fibers terminate in simple, free endings or in the form of complex convolutions (glomeruli).

The majority of arterioles have adrenergic innervation and in some sites also possess cholinergic innervation.[32,33] Other vasoactive peptides (Substance P, vasoactive intestinal peptide, etc.) also may be co-localized in these nerves in some sites. The distribution of sensory nerves to the microvascular wall is ill defined. In general, adrenergic innervation provides a degree of vascular tone in the arterioles while cholinergic innervation, when it exists, generally is dilatory. Some of the peptides are vasoconstrictive while others are vasodilatory. The amount of "resting" tone in these vessels varies from site to site in the body. This contributes to the variability in the responsiveness of vessels in different sites as do differences in the distribution and types of pharmacologic receptor sites and heterogeneity in vascular smooth muscle metabolism.[34-37]

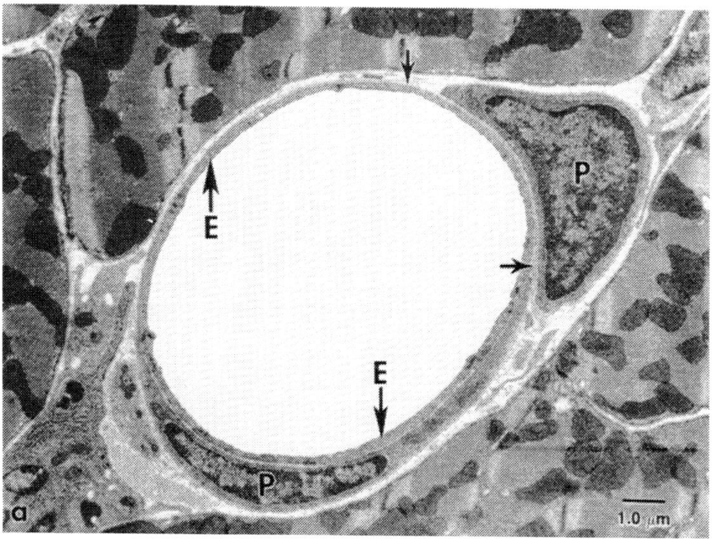

Figure 1-4 (**a**) Continuous capillary in cardiac muscle. Note continuous endothelium (E) and basal lamina (arrows). Pericytes (P) are enclosed in splits in the basal lamina. (**b**) Higher magnification of the endothelium (E) illustrating numerous cytoplasmic vesicles (arrows). Intercellular junction (J); basal lamina (BL); pericyte (P).

B. CAPILLARIES

The capillaries are cylindrical tubes, lined by endothelium, not surrounded by smooth muscle and with only a minimum of connective tissue investment (Figures 4–10).[16,17] In capillaries the endothelium is embraced, at irregular intervals, by a cell called a pericyte or Rouget cell (Figure 4). This is a multibranched cell containing numerous pinocytotic vesicles, a few dense bodies that are adjacent to the cell membrane, abundant rough endoplasmic reticulum, ribosomes, lysosomes, and a basal lamina that is common with the apposed endothelial cell. Because of the presence of occasional dense bodies, but especially by the presence of a basal lamina, these cells are considered to be a derivative of or related to smooth muscle cells as these characteristics are not present in fibroblasts. Controversy has existed for years as to whether or not these cells are contractile and play a role in regulating blood flow through capillaries and postcapillary (pericytic) venules. The presence of actin, myosin, and tropomyosin in pericytes further suggests that they have contractile capability.

Thus, the characteristic cell of capillaries is the endothelial cell. When these cells are examined with the light microscope they exhibit little detail. A prominent nucleus, usually oriented longitudinally, is observed, bulging into the lumen and when stained with silver nitrate the cell "borders" can be identified but their cytoplasm appears almost structureless and transparent.

Capillaries are the principal site of exchange between the blood and extravascular tissue due to the thinness of their walls and their lumens being approximately the diameter of a single erythrocyte.[16,17,21] The cytoplasm of endothelial cells consists of relatively few mitochondria adjacent to the nucleus, a sparse endoplasmic reticulum with ribonucleoprotein granules, a Golgi complex in proximity to the nucleus, microtubules, lysosomes, vesicles, and thick myosin and thin actin filaments as well as intermediate sized (9 to 11 nm) filaments containing vimentin.[38,39] Rod-shaped granules (0.1 μm × 3 μm) known as Weibel-Palade bodies also are found and are characteristic for most, but not all, endothelial

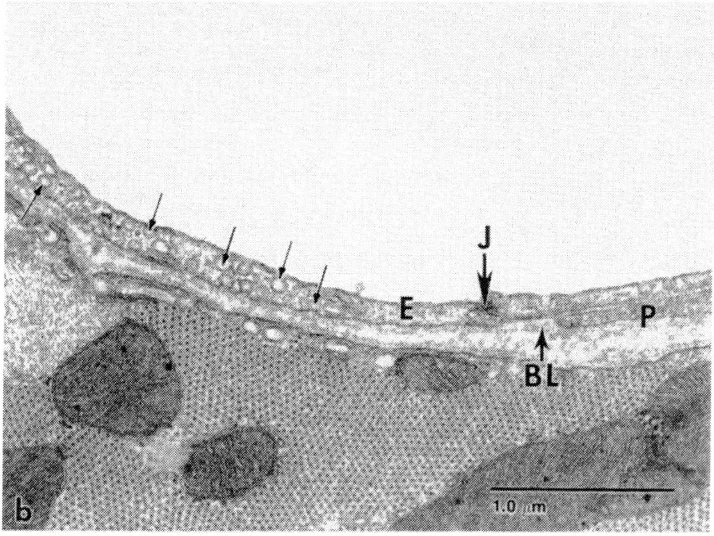

Figure 1-4 (Continued).

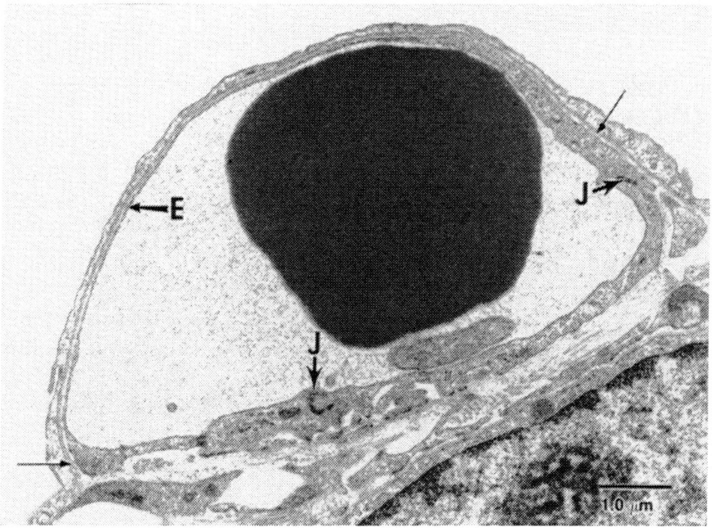

Figure 1-5 Continuous capillary in the lung. Note highly attenuated, but continuous, endothelium (E) and basal lamina (arrows); intercellular junctions (J).

cells. The greatest mass of cytoplasm is located adjacent to the nucleus. In other areas of the cell the cytoplasm may be very thin and in some vessels "perforated" (fenestrated). Finally, the entire cell is circumscribed by a trilaminar (unit) membrane about 90Å thick that appears as two dense bands separated by a clearer band, each having a thickness of about 30Å.

The junctions of endothelial cells (Figures 4 and 5), when viewed in profile by electron microscopy, reveal their complexity both in respect to their general configuration as well

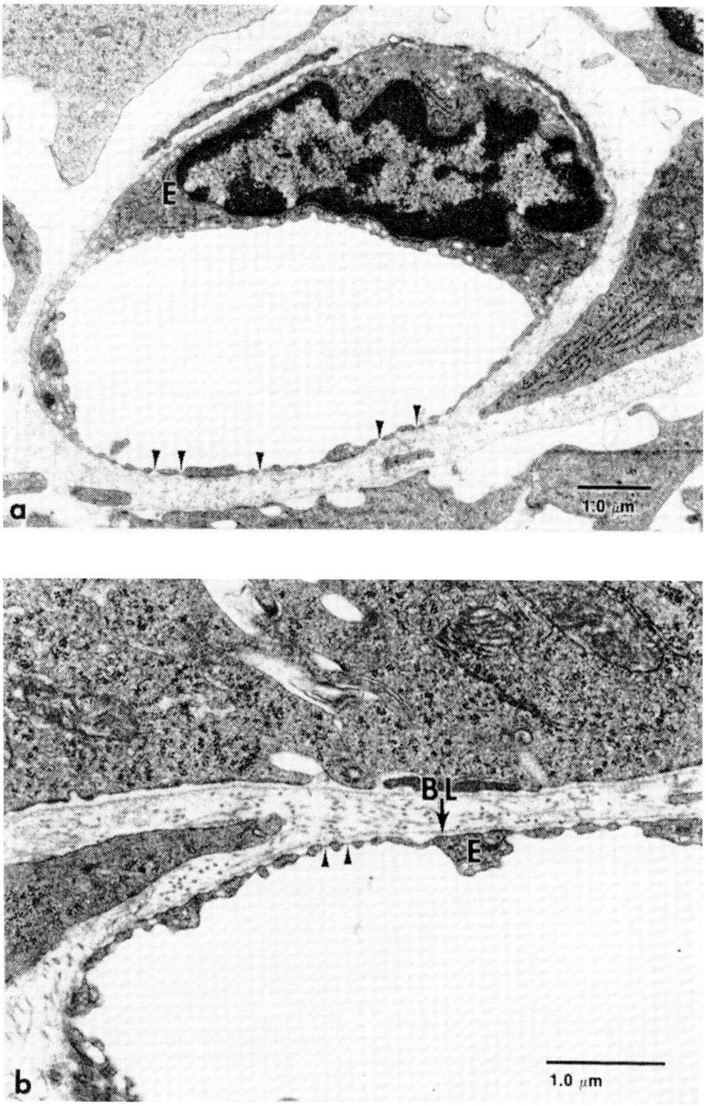

Figure 1-6 (**a**) Fenestrated capillary in an intestinal villus. (a) Note numerous fenestrae (arrows) bridged by diaphragms in the endothelium (E). (**b**) Higher magnification illustrating the closed fenestrae (arrows) overlying a continuous basal lamina (BL).

as the presence of localized modifications. The general shape of the junctions may be in the form of a mortis joint or a lap joint (Figure 5). Due to the complexity of these types of joints a relatively large area of each cell is involved, approximately 1 to 2 μm of overlap when viewed *en face*. It is this area which is rendered visible as a junction when endothelium is stained with silver nitrate and studied with the light microscope. This area contains the "intercellular cement" described by light microscopists, which is not intercellular since it consists primarily of the contiguous borders of endothelial cells where the actual intercellular "space" measures about 20 nm.

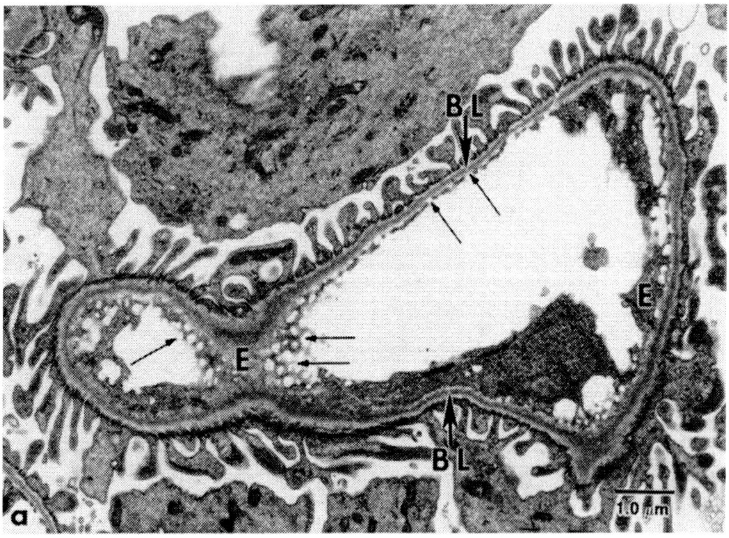

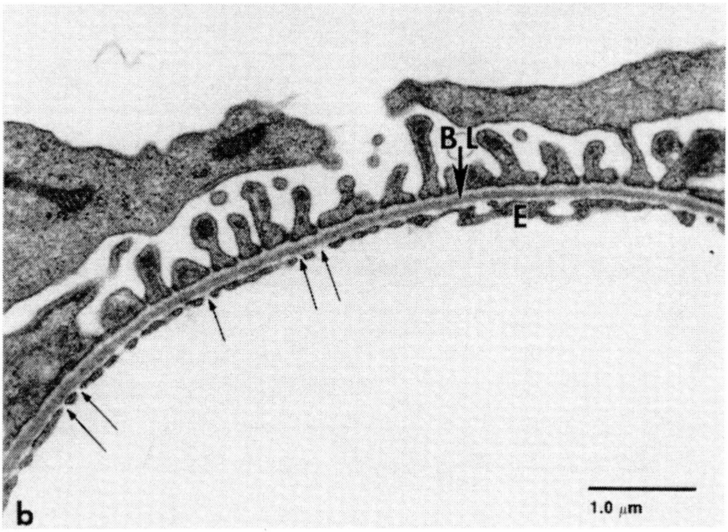

Figure 1-7 Fenestrated capillary in a renal glomerulus. (a) Note the numerous open fenestrate (arrows) usually lacking diaphragms through the endothelium (E), but covered on the abluminal surface by a thick basal lamina (BL). (b) Higher magnification of the fenestrae (arrows) and thick basal lamina (BL). (E) Endothelium.

Three types of junctions between endothelial cells have been described.[16,17,21,39] In one, the outer leaflets of the trilaminar unit membranes fuse along a portion of the joint to form a "tight junction", a *zonula occludens*. This *zonula occludens*, a band like fusion, is considered to encircle the cell. In another type of localized adherence the inner leaflet of the trilaminar unit membrane is thickened, a *zonula adherens*, while the two outer leaflets remain separated by an intercellular layer of about 20 nm. Finally, the unit membrane of

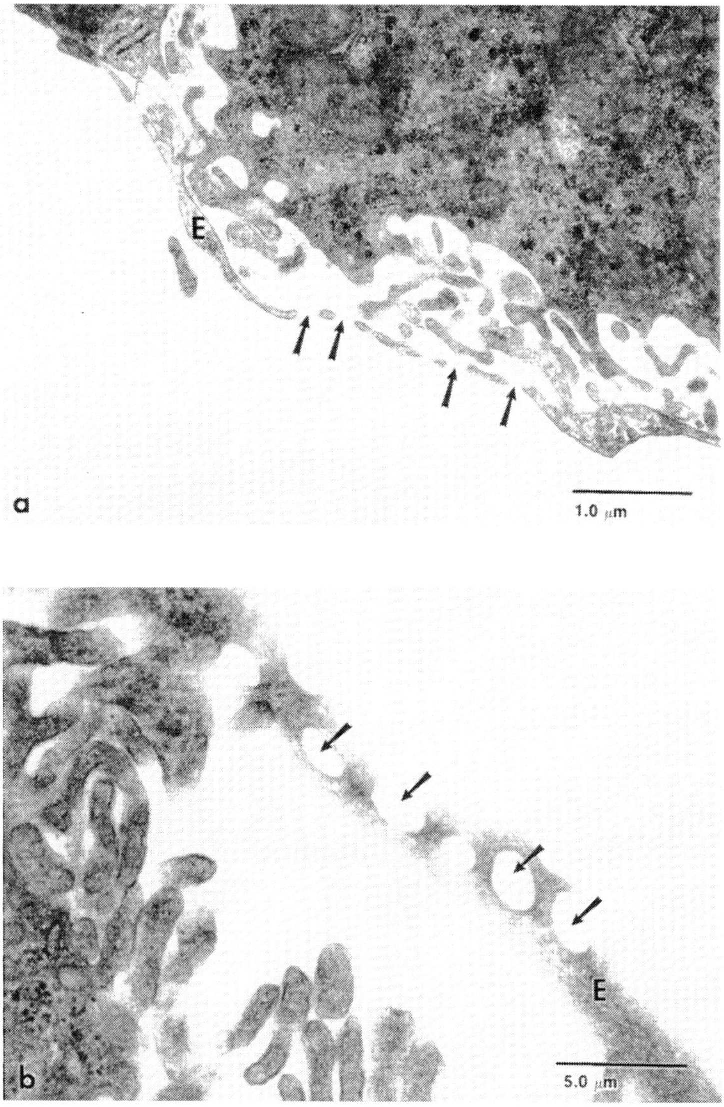

Figure 1-8 Sinusoid in the liver. (**a**) Note the attenuated endothelium (E) containing numerous open fenestrae (arrows) not covered by a basal lamina and, thus, providing for free exchange of large molecules between the blood and hepatocytes. (**b**) Tangential cut of open fenestrae (arrows) through the sinusoid endothelium (E).

each cell may remain unchanged and separated by a less electron dense substance or they may even be separated by gaps.

The intercellular junction is thought to represent the "small pore" (9 to 11 nm) postulated by physiological studies to be responsible for the transcapillary exchange of water and some other hydrophilic molecules less than 15Å in diameter and 10,000 in molecular weight.[40]

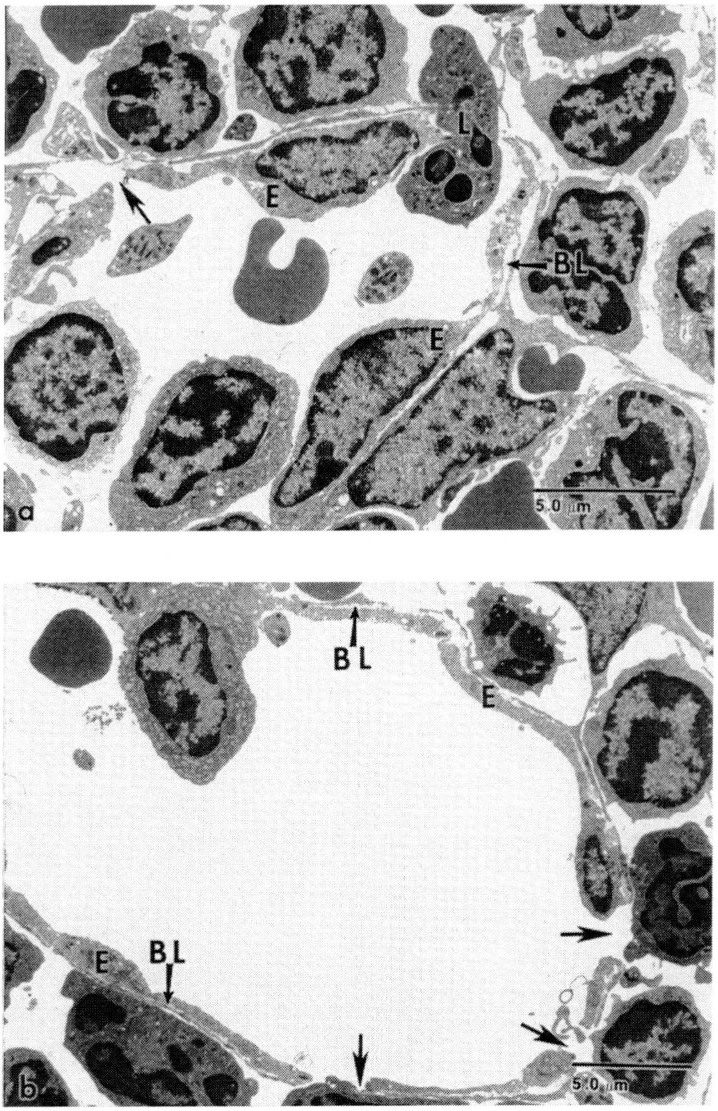

Figure 1-9 Discontinuous capillary (sinusoid) in the spleen (**a** and **b**). Note gaps (arrows) between adjacent endothelial cells (E) and the incomplete basal lamina (BL). In (**a**) note leukocyte (L) in transit between endothelial cells.

Transport of larger molecules from blood to tissue across the endothelial barrier is complex and is thought to be represented morphologically by several mechanisms termed transcytosis.[17,21,41] This includes transport in endocytotic vesicles shuttling between the lumenal and abluminal surfaces, through transient vesicle-derived channels extending through the cells, and through fenestrae. These, morphologically, are thought to represent the "large pore" (50 to 70 nm) proposed by physiologists.[40]

The interfacial relationship of endothelium differs at its luminal and basal surfaces. At the luminal surface an endocapillary layer has been described which is irregular in

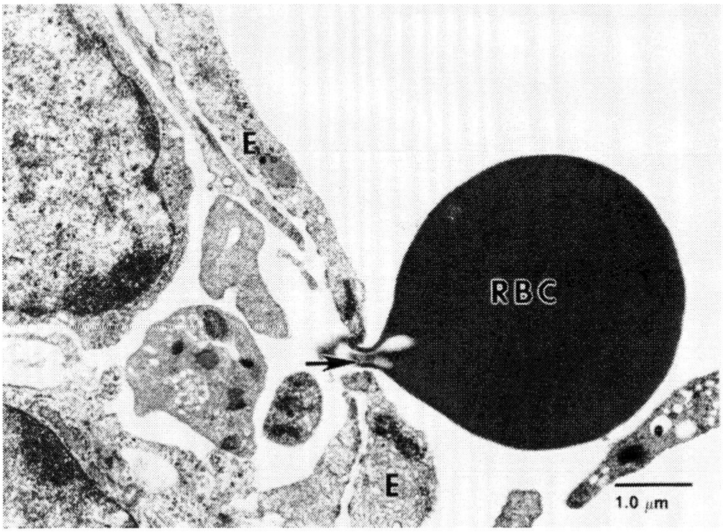

Figure 1-10 Erythrocyte (RBC) in transit through narrow intercellular gap (arrow) in splenic sinusoidal endothelium (E). Note lack of a basal lamina in this area.

contour and consists of plasma proteins sorbed to the outer leaflet of the unit membrane as well as exposed membrane associated glycoconjugates.[18,21,42] At the basal surface of endothelium of most capillaries there is a basal lamina. This lamina consists of a moderately electron dense band, 50- to 70-nm thick, that follows the contour of the bases of the endothelial cells and is separated from them by a less electron dense zone measuring approximately 40 nm consisting of an amorphous collagen matrix wherein thin filaments are embedded.

The ultrastructure of the endothelial lining of capillaries varies along sequential segments of the microvasculature, from tissue to tissue and between various organs.[16-18,21,43,44] Differences are found in the numbers of pinocytotic vesicles, intercellular junctions, and the numbers of fenestrae or pores in the endothelium. In addition, depending on the site, the thickness and continuity of the basal lamina may vary. All of these differences are thought to be related to the functional requirements of the tissue or organ being served by a particular capillary.[17-18,21,40,44]

This diversity of endothelial structure has been used to classify capillaries into several types — continuous, fenestrated, or discontinuous.[16,17] Examples of *continuous capillaries* include those of skeletal, smooth, and cardiac muscle (Figure 4), lung (Figure 5), and those in the central nervous system have endothelial cells which have a continuous basal lamina and whose cytoplasm contains invaginations and 50- to 70-nm vesicles (cavaeolae). In contrast, *fenestrated capillaries* in the renal glomeruli (Figure 7), endocrine glands, and gastrointestinal (Figure 6) system have a cytoplasm that is very thin and contain fenestrae (pores) that may or may not be covered with a diaphragm and a central knob. The basal lamina, in renal glomeruli (Figure 7) is quite thick and continuous, while in the sinusoids of the liver (Figure 8) it is incomplete or absent.

Sinusoids (Figures 8 through 10) are an example of a *discontinuous capillary* whose internal diameter generally is larger than that of an individual erythrocyte and whose walls have been modified for the passage of large molecules and/or blood cells as well as for phagocytosis. Such vessels are found in the spleen (Figures 9 and 10), bone marrow, and liver (Figure 8). The internal diameters of these vessels under normal conditions may vary so that a cylindrical appearance as seen in capillaries may not be exhibited. Discontinuities in the walls may take the form of fenestrae not bridged by diaphragms with little or no surrounding basal lamina (e.g., liver, Figure 8) or by gaps between adjacent endothelial cells (e.g., spleen, Figures 9 and 10).

To the above microscopic structural characteristics of endothelium it should be noted that these cells exhibit chemical differences as well. Differences in enzyme activity occur not only between arterioles, capillaries, and venules but also in respect to their location in the body. For example, acid phosphatase activity is found in the cytoplasm of endothelial cells containing vesicles, like those in the lung or skeletal muscle, but not in fenestrated capillaries like those in the renal glomerulus. In contrast, alkaline phosphatase activity occurs in capillaries and arterioles but not in venules.

Endothelial cells have been found in some internal organs to act as sphincters that regulate the flow of blood through individual capillaries or sinusoids.[30] Endothelial sphincters have been studied most extensively in the liver where they form the inlet and outlet sphincters of the sinusoids as well as forming sphincters in intersinusoidal sinusoids.[5] Like muscular "pre-capillary sphincters", endothelial sphincters open and close the lumen of the sinusoids, apparently in response to local metabolic requirements and are responsive to various vasoconstrictor and vasodilator substances. Similar cells have been seen in the sinusoids of the spleen and bone marrow, in the alveolar capillaries of the lung, and in the acinar and islet tissue of the pancreas.[30] They also may exist in other internal organs that have not yet been examined in detail by high resolution *in vivo* microscopic methods.[45]

Several lines of evidence suggest that endothelial cells are capable of active contraction and are not simply responding to changes in intracellular osmolarity by passively swelling. In addition to observation of the rapid response to vasoactive substances,[30] microfilaments and microtubules have been demonstrated by electron microscopy in the cytoplasm of these cells; the presence of these organelles suggests contractile activity.[8,16,17,21,46]

The fibrils generally are oriented parallel to the axis of the vessel. Thus, if contractile, they could cause the endothelial cell to bulge into the lumen as has been reported *in vivo*. More convincingly, however, is the demonstration of contractile protein in endothelium using immunofluorescent and histochemical methods.[38,39,47,48]

C. VENULES

Venules are efferent vessels that collect blood from the capillary bed (Figures 2 and 11). They begin as thin-walled pericytic venules (Figure 2), but as the diameters of venules increase, their walls acquire a discontinuous investment of vascular smooth muscle (Figure 11) which becomes progressively more continuous in larger vessels (muscular venules).[9,16,17,21,44] With the acquisition of smooth muscle, innervation also is acquired which is sparse when compared to arterioles.[33] It should be noted that a significant amount of transvasculature exchange occurs in the nonmuscular (pericytic) postcapillary venules; and, because of the less structured nature of their walls (Figure 2), venules are more fragile and subject to injury than are their accompanying arterioles.[49-51]

D. ARTERIOVENOUS ANASTOMOSES

Arteriovenous anastomoses (AVAs) usually have a diameter of less than 300 μm, are relatively short in length, provide direct communication between the arterial and venous system, and have been found in most tissues and organs.[52-54] Thus, AVAs provide a mechanism for shunting blood around the capillary network. Histologically, the tunica media of AVAs in some sites contains significant numbers of epithelioid cells which function like smooth muscle cells and serve to regulate the flow through the lumen. These cells function like smooth muscle cells but they contain fewer myofibrils, are larger than

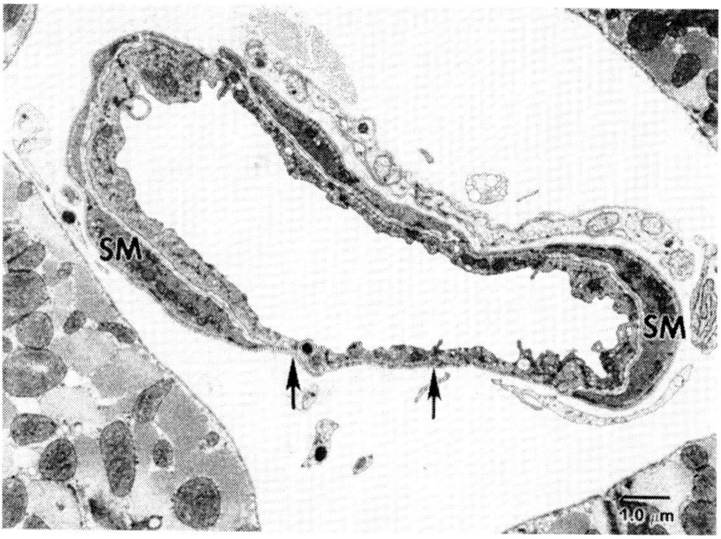

Figure 1-11 Venule in cardiac muscle which is in transition from pericytic to muscular type. Note incomplete layer of smooth muscle (SM) cells at the arrows.

smooth muscle cells as well as containing nuclei that stain lighter than those in smooth muscle. The transition from the arterial to the venous portion of these AVAs usually is marked by an abrupt loss of muscle cells and the appearance of a thin-walled vessel containing few if any smooth muscle cells. Another characteristic of arteriovenous anastomoses is that they contain many nerve fibers in their adventitia — more than in arterioles.

Blood flow through these shunts is intermittent and depends upon the functional requirements of the surrounding tissue. In contrast, some shunts are of capillary dimensions with scattered smooth muscle cells embracing the endothelium. In the mesentery they have been termed "thoroughfare" or "preferential" channels since blood is continuously flowing through these vessels while flow through the capillaries is intermittent.[7,10] However, these channels generally have not been found in other locations,[54] and in most sites, such as in the liver, blood flow through arterio-portal anastomoses is intermittent and appears to depend upon the functional activity of the hepatic parenchyma.[5]

IV. CHARACTERISTICS OF OPTIMAL BLOOD FLOW

Based on extensive studies in both man and experimental animals, blood flow through the microvasculature is characterized as optimal when the following criteria are met:[1,22] (1) erythrocytes, leukocytes, and platelets are distributed relatively homogeneously in the circulating blood; (2) the formed elements neither adhere to each other nor to the endothelium upon making random contact; (3) the velocity of flow in arterioles and venules is such that individual cells are not resolved optically and the flow appears streamlined; (4) when individual erythrocytes are seen, e.g., in capillaries, they exhibit a sharp outline and have no visible coating on their surface; and (5) the viscosity and composition of the blood is normal with respect to cellular composition and plasma constituents. As a result, the vascular walls are adequately nourished and their permeability is such that neither tissue edema nor hemoconcentration occurs. Failure of any of the above criteria to be met can lead to a suboptimal or pathologic microcirculation and resultant ischemia or hypoxia of cells, tissues, or organs.

REFERENCES

1. **Bloch, E. H.,** Principles of the microvascular system, *Invest. Opthalmol.*, 5, 250, 1966.
2. **Baez, S.,** Microvascular terminology, in *Microcirculation*, Vol. I, Kaley, G. and Altura, B. M., Eds., University Park Press, Baltimore, MD, 1977, 23.
3. **McCuskey, R. S.,** Microcirculation-basic considerations, in *Pathophysiology of Shock, Anoxia and Ischemia*, Cowley, R. A. and Trump, B. F., Eds., Williams & Wilkins, Baltimore, MD, 1982, 156.
4. **Bloch, E. H.,** The dynamic histology of organs *in situ*. II. The lung, liver and kidney, *Anat. Rec.*, 151, 498, 1965.
5. **McCuskey, R. S.,** A dynamic and static study of hepatic arterioles and hepatic sphincters, *Am. J. Anat.*, 119, 455, 1966.
6. **McCuskey, R. S.,** Hepatic microcirculation, in *Sinusoids in Human Liver: Health and Disease*, Bioulac-Sage, P. and Balabaud, C., Eds., Kupffer Cell Foundation, Leyden, 1988, 151.
7. **Chambers, R. and Zweifach, B. W.,** Topography and function of the mesenteric circulation, *Am. J. Anat.*, 75, 173, 1944.
8. **Rhodin, J. A. G.,** The ultrastructure of mammalian arterioles and precapillary sphincters, *J. Ultrastruct. Res.*, 18, 181, 1967.
9. **Rhodin, J. A. G.,** Ultrastructure of mammalian venous capillaries, venules and small collecting veins, *J. Ultrastruct. Res.*, 25, 452, 1968.
10. **Zweifach, B. W. and Metz, D. G.,** Selective distribution of blood through the terminal vascular bed of mesenteric structures and skeletal muscle, in *Vascular Patterns as Related to Function*, Fulton, G. P., Ed., Williams & Wilkins, Baltimore, MD, 1955, 282.
11. **McCuskey, R. S. and Chapman, T. M.,** Microscopy of the living pancreas *in situ*, *Am. J. Anat.*, 126, 395, 1969.
12. **Oestermeyer, C. F. and Bloch, E. H.,** *In vivo* microscopy of hamster renal allographs, *Microvasc. Res.*, 13, 153, 1977.
13. **Sobin, S. S. and Tremer, H. M.,** Three dimensional organization of microvascular beds as related to function, in *Microcirculation*, Vol. I, Kaley G. and Altura, B. M., Eds., University Park Press, Baltimore, MD, 1977, 43.
14. **Schmid-Schoenbein, G. W., Zweifach, B. W., and Kovalcheck, S.,** The application of stereological principles to morphometry of the microcirculation in different tissues, *Microvasc. Res.*, 14, 303, 1977.
15. **Johnson, P. C.,** Principles of peripheral circulatory control, in *Peripheral Circulation*, Johnson, P. C., Ed., John Wiley and Sons, New York, 1978, 111.
16. **Rhodin, J. A. G.,** Architecture of the vessel wall, in *Handbook of Physiology. The Cardiovascular System*, Vol. 2, Bohr, D. F., Sonnlyo, A., and Sparks, H., Eds., American Physiology Society, Washington, DC, 1980, 1.
17. **Simionescu, N. and Simionescu, M.,** The cardiovascular system, in *A Textbook of Histology*, 6th ed., Weiss, L., Ed., Urban and Schwarzenberg, Baltimore, MD, 1988, 23.
18. **Wagner, R. C.,** Ultrastructural studies of capillary endothelium: compartmental tracing, high voltage electron microscopy and cryofixation, in *Endothelial Cell Biology in Health and Disease*, Simionescu, N. and Simionescu, M., Plenum Press, New York, 1988, 23.
19. **Jeffords, J. G. and Knisely, M. H.,** Concerning the geometric shapes of arteries and arterioles. A contribution to the biophysics of health, disease and death, *Angiology*, 7, 105, 1956.
20. **Bloch, E. H.,** A quantitative study of the hemodynamics in the living microvascular system, *Am. J. Anat.*, 110, 125, 1962.

21. **Simionescu, M. and Simionescu, N.,** Ultrastructure of the microvascular wall: functional correlations, in *Handbook of Physiology, Vol. IV, The Cardiovascular System, The Microcirculation,* Renkin, E. M. and Michael, C. C., Eds., American Physiological Society, Washington, DC, 1984, 41.
22. **Bloch, E. H.,** Microscopic observations of the circulating blood in the bulbar conjunctiva in man in health and disease, *Ergeb. Anat. Entwicklungogeschicte*, 35, 1, 1956.
23. **Rappaport, M. G., Bloch, E. H., and Irwin, J. W.,** A manometer for measuring dynamic pressures in the microvascular system, *J. Appl. Physiol.*, 14, 651, 1959.
24. **Richardson, D. R. and Zweifach, B. W.,** Pressure relationships in macro-and microcirculation, *Microvasc. Res.*, 2, 474, 1970.
25. **Zweifach, B. W.,** Quantitative studies of microcirculatory structure and function. I. Analysis of pressure distribution in the terminal vascular bed in cat mesentery, *Circ. Res.*, 34, 843, 1974.
26. **Zweifach, B. W.,** Quantitative studies of microcirculatory structure and function. II. Direct measurement of capillary pressure in splanchnic mesenteric vessels, *Circ. Res.*, 34, 858, 1974.
27. **Gore, R. W. and Bohlen, H. G.,** Pressure regulation in the microcirculation, *Fed. Proc.*, 34, 2031, 1975.
28. **Bohlen, H. G. and Gore, R. W.,** Comparisons of pressures and diameters in the innervated and denervated microcirculation of rat intestine, *Microvasc. Res.*, 14, 251, 1977.
29. **Altura, B. M.,** Chemical and humoral regulation of blood flow through the precapillary sphincter, *Microvasc. Res.*, 3, 361, 1971.
30. **McCuskey, R. S.,** Sphincters in the microvascular system, *Microvasc. Res.*, 2, 428, 1971.
31. **Lutz, B. R. and Fulton, G. P.,** Smooth muscle and blood flow in small blood vessels, in *Factors Regulating Blood Flow*, Fulton, G. P. and Zweifach, B.W., Eds., American Physiology Society, Washington, DC, 1958, 13.
32. **Rosell, S.,** Nervous control of the microcirculation, in *Microcirculation*, Vol. 2, Kaley, G. and Altura, B. M., Eds., University Park Press, Baltimore, MD, 1978, 371.
33. **Burnstock, G.,** Innervation of vascular smooth muscle: histochemistry and electron microscopy, *Clin. Exp. Pharmacol. Physiol.*, 2 (Suppl. 2), 7, 1975.
34. **Vanhoutte, P. M.,** Heterogeneity in vascular smooth muscle, in *Microcirculation*, Vol. 2, Kaley, G. and Altura, B. M., Eds., University Park Press, Baltimore, MD, 1978, 181.
35. **Bevan, J. A.,** Some bases of differences in vascular response to sympathetic activity, *Circ. Res.*, 45, 161, 1979.
36. **Granger, D. N., Cook, B. H., and Taylor, A. E.,** Histochemistry of microvascular smooth muscle in the gastrointestinal tract, *Microvasc. Res.*, 12, 157, 1976.
37. **Cook, B. H., Granger, H. J., and Taylor, A. E.,** Metabolism of coronary arteries and arterioles. A histochemical study, *Microvasc. Res.*, 14, 145, 1977.
38. **Franke, W.W., Schmid, E., Osborn, M., and Weber, K.,** Intermediate-sized filaments of human endothelial cells, *J. Cell Biol.*, 81, 570, 1979.
39. **Franke, W. W., Cowin, P., Grund, C., Kuhn, C., and Kupprell, H. P.,** The endothelial junction: the plaque and its components, in *Endothelial Cell Biology in Health and Disease*, Simionescu, N. and Simionescu, M., Eds., Plenum Press, New York, 1988, 147.
40. **Renkin, E. M.,** Transport pathways and processes, in *Endothelial Cell Biology in Health and Disease*, Simionescu, N. and Simionescu, M., Eds., Plenum Press, New York, 1988, 51.
41. **Simionescu, M.,** Receptor-mediated transcytosis of plasma molecules by vascular endothelium, in *Endothelial Cell Biology in Health and Disease*, Simionescu, N. and Simionescu, M., Eds., Plenum Press, New York, 1988, 69.

42. **Luft, J. H.,** Fine structure of capillary and endocapillary layer as revealed by ruthenium red, *Fed. Proc.*, 25, 1773, 1966.
43. **Thorgeirsson, G. and Robertson, A. L.,** The vascular endothelium-pathobiologic significance, *Am. J. Pathol.*, 93, 803, 1978.
44. **Wolff, J. R.,** Ultrastructure of the terminal vascular bed as related to function, in *Microcirculation*, Vol. 1, Kaley G. and Altura, B. M., Eds., University Park Press, Baltimore, MD, 1977, 95.
45. **McCuskey, R. S.,** Microscopic methods for studying the microvasculature of internal organs, in *Physical Techniques in Biology and Medicine, Microvascular Technology*, Baker, C. H. and Nastuk, W. F., Eds., Academic Press, New York, 1986, 247.
46. **Majno, G., Shea, S. M., and Leventhal M.,** Endothelial contraction induced by histamine-type mediators. An electron microscopic study, *J. Cell Biol.*, 42, 647, 1969.
47. **Puchtler, H., Sweat, F., Terry, M. S., and Conner, H. M.,** Investigation of staining, polarization and fluorescence-microscopic properties of myoendothelial cells, *J. Microsc.*, 89, 95, 1968.
48. **Becker, C. G. and Nachman, R. L.,** Contractile proteins of endothelial cells, platelets and smooth muscle, *Am. J. Pathol.*, 71, 1, 1973.
49. **Majno, G., Gilmore, V., and Leventhal, M.,** On the mechanism of vascular leakage caused by histamine-type mediators, *Circ. Res.*, 21, 833, 1967.
50. **Simionescu, N., Simionescu, M., and Palade, G. E.,** Structural basis of permeability in sequential segments of the microvasculature. II. Pathways followed by microperoxidase across endothelium, *Microvasc. Res.*, 15, 17, 1978.
51. **Zweifach, B. W.,** Microvascular aspects of tissue injury, in *The Inflammatory Process*, Vol. 2, 2nd ed., Zweifach, B. W., Grant, L., and McCluskey, R. T., Eds., Academic Press, New York, 1973, 3.
52. **Clark, E. R.,** Arterio-venous anastomoses, *Physiol. Rev.*, 18, 229, 1938.
53. **Clara, M.,** *Die Arterio-venous Anastomosem*, Springer-Verlag, Wien, 1956.
54. **Weideman, M. P.,** Patterns of the arteriovenous pathways, in *Handbook of Physiology, Section 2: Circulation*, Vol. 2, Hamilton, W. F. and Dow, P., Eds., American Physiology Society, Washington, DC, 1963, 891.
55. **McCuskey, R. S. and McCuskey, P. A.,** *In vivo* and electron microscopic studies of the splenic microvasculature in mice, *Experientia,* 41, 179, 1985.

Chapter 2

Coronary Angiogenesis and Its Control

Harris J. Granger, James R. Hawker, Jr., Cynthia J. Meininger, David C. Zawieja, Linda E. Czisny, and Marina Ziche

CONTENTS

I. INTRODUCTION

The coronary vascular tree is designed to optimize nutrient delivery to the myocardium, as well as to ensure the efficient removal of metabolic waste-products produced by the beating parenchymal cells. The design parameters for coronary vascular architecture can best be appreciated by comparing resting skeletal muscle and left ventricular myocardium.[1] The oxygen consumption per unit mass of the latter is 30 to 60 times that of the former. Consequently, the rate of blood flow in left ventricular myocardium is 10- to 20-fold greater than in resting skeletal muscle. To ensure maximum extraction of the oxygen delivered to the microvascular level, the capillary density and exchange surface are 10 to 20 times greater in the heart. Because of the high vascularity of the myocardium, average blood-to-tissue diffusion distances are 1/3 to 1/4 the values in resting muscle.[2] In both tissues only a fraction of the entire capillary bed is perfused at any given moment. However, capillary recruitment is a more robust phenomenon in skeletal muscle, implying that a greater fraction of the myocardial capillaries are already perfused under normal conditions.

Rapidly acting, local vasoregulatory mechanisms allow adjustment of coronary blood flow and exchange parameters (i.e., capillary surface area and diffusion distance) in a matter of seconds to a few minutes when myocardial needs suddenly change.[3] These fast compensatory reactions rely on acute modulation of the state of contraction of smooth muscle cells located in the precapillary arterioles and upstream arteries.[4] Under certain conditions, acute vasomotor reactions are not adequate to ensure maintenance of balance between myocardial metabolic demand and coronary perfusion. Fortunately, nature has endowed the coronary vasculature with the ability to restructure over a period of time for the purpose of enhancing delivery of nutrients to the myocardium.[5] For example, the coronary microvasculature proliferates in response to long-term increases in cardiac work,[6-8] chronic reduction of ambient oxygen content,[9] and partial occlusion of the

0-8493-4547-2/94/$0.00+$.50

arterial supply.[10] The aim of this chapter is to explore the molecular and cellular mechanisms responsible for modulating the vascularity of the normal and dysfunctional heart.

II. VASCULAR DEVELOPMENT AND RESTRUCTURING

During embryonic growth, blood vessels first appear as simple tubes radiating from clusters of endothelial cells, a process known as vasculogenesis.[11] Throughout development, the vascular tree undergoes numerous stages of architectural refinement, including addition of smooth muscles cells or pericytes to produce resistance/capacitance vessels or exchange microvessels, respectively. From the embryonic stage to young adulthood, the formation of new vessels keeps pace with organ development and growth. In the adult, vascular restructuring takes on many forms depending upon the type of stimulus perceived by the blood vessels supplying the heart. For example, larger arteries can grow to a wider diameter after long periods of increased flow rate.[12] Occlusion of one coronary artery leads to enlargement of small collateral arterioles interconnecting two major perfusion pathways; after months of occlusion, the diameter of collateral vessels is measured in terms of millimeters, rather than micrometers.[13] Finally, new microvessels can form by budding from the pre-existing microvasculature.[14-17] Angiogenesis is the term used to specifically describe the latter phenomenon.

III. SITE OF ANGIOGENESIS

Angiogenesis occurs primarily in postcapillary or pericytic venules.[14-18] These microvessels are formed by the convergence of two or more capillaries. They are composed of a continuous layer of endothelium encircled over a fraction of their ablumenal surface by pericytes.[19] Pericytic venules are multifaceted elements of the microvasculature. These vessels have a higher permeability to water and proteins than upstream capillaries.[20] Postcapillary venules are extremely sensitive to inflammatory mediators; consequently, the fluid and protein leakage associated with inflammatory reactions is first observed in these special microvessels.[21-23] Extravasation of leukocytes[24] and tumor cells[25] is also a phenomenon restricted almost exclusively to pericytic venules.

In nonproliferating capillaries and pericytic venules, endothelial cells maintain a tubular morphology. This structure is stabilized by focal adhesions of the endothelial cell to the underlying basement membrane.[26] The molecular components of adhesion sites consist of receptor integrins associated with the endothelial cell surface and complementary ligands in the basement membrane such as collagen, fibronectin, vimentin, vitronectin, laminin, and fibrin.[27-30] Integrins are transmembrane glycoproteins composed of α and β subunits;[31] the extracellular domain serves as a receptor site for a specific basement membrane component, whereas the cytoplasmic domain interacts with the cytoskeleton of the endothelial cell. Thus, physical forces generated in the matrix can be transmitted to the cytoskeleton and vice versa. Inside the cell, the focal adhesion complex appears to be composed of actin bundles and other cytoskeletal proteins such as talin and α-actinin.[32] Several kinases, including src kinase and focal adhesion kinase,[33,34] are activated when specific integrins interact with their complementary basement membrane components. These kinases in turn can phosphorylate a number of substrates, including the contractile proteins of the cytoskeleton. Thus, integrins provide a unique means of physical communication between the extracellular matrix and the shape-determining framework of the cell.

At the periphery of the endothelial cell, cell/cell adhesion sites contribute to the integrity of the mature endothelial tube.[35,36] Depending on the type of exchange microvessel, these adhesion structures may consist of tight junctions, zonula adherans, or macula adherans.[37,38] Gap junctions, consisting of pore-like intercellular communicating proteins, are present in closely apposed endothelial cells.[39] These structures allow signals perceived by one cell to be passed on to adjacent cells by the free interchange of intracellular second messengers.[40,41] A special class of intercellular adhesion molecule known as cadherins serve as a calcium-dependent glue that binds adjacent endothelial cells to each other.[36,42,43] The cytoplasmic regions of cadherins interact with the actin, vinculin, and plakoglobin of the cytosol. Other interendothelial cell adhesion molecules, such as endoCAM,[35,44] are cell surface glycoproteins that do not require calcium to function as binding material.

Given the special role of pericytic venules in angiogenesis, we isolated and cultured endothelial cells from 15 μm postcapillary venules of the bovine heart.[45] To obtain these cells, we utilized an elegant bead-perfusion technique developed by Ryan and co-workers.[46] First, the isolated bovine heart is perfused with warm buffer to clear the circulation of trapped blood cells. Next, during retrograde perfusion through the coronary sinus or coronary vein, 15 μm polymer beads are introduced into cold buffer perfusate containing EDTA to loosen the vascular endothelium from its underlying basement membrane. The beads are allowed to lodge in venules of approximately the same size. In response to the presence of the bead in the lumen, the venular endothelial cells crawl off of their basement membrane and onto the bead. Thereafter, the venular cell/bead complexes are recovered from the coronary sinus during antegrade perfusion. These cells are endothelial in nature as evidenced by labeling with antibody to Factor VIII-related antigen and uptake of acetylated low-density lipoproteins. At confluency, they form a typical contact-inhibited monolayer with the usual cobblestone morphology. Throughout this chapter we shall refer to these coronary venular endothelial cells as CVEC.

IV. STAGES IN THE ANGIOGENESIS PROCESS[47]

Consider a source of angiogenic material located 50 μm from a 15 μm pericytic venule. A chemotactic gradient is established by simple diffusion, resulting in a lower concentration at the ablumenal surface of the venule and the highest concentration at the source. If the parent venule is to form daughter branches, an obvious requirement is movement of the endothelial cell toward the source of the chemoattractant. However, under normal conditions, the venular endothelial cell is confined by the basement membrane upon which it rests. Consequently, one of the first events in angiogenesis is secretion of endothelial-derived enzymes capable of dissolving the retaining matrix.[48] These enzymes include tissue plasminogen activator and collagenase.[49-51] The former leads to the appearance of the enzyme plasmin, which degrades a wide range of basement membrane constituents including fibronectin, laminin, and fibrin. The latter hydrolyzes collagen type IV found in the basal lamina, as well as interstitial collagen.

Upon destruction of the basement membrane, the endothelial cell is able to migrate into the interstitial space where motility is facilitated by continued secretion of proteolytic enzymes. As the cell advances toward the chemotactic source, the angiogenic agent induces cell division, thereby providing an adequate number of cells to form a new branch.[47] At this stage, the new cord-like endothelial cells are aligned in a linear configuration from the site of budding to the location of the angiogenic source. By a process of vacuolization or curling of the aligned cells, a lumen is formed and a tubular structure takes shape.[52] With budding occurring at two sites along the same venule, the two daughter tubes converge at the site of the angiogenic source and unite, thereby forming a primitive vascular loop capable of conducting blood flow. At this stage, the new microvessel is extremely permeable to fluid and plasma proteins.[53] With time, pericytes begin to appear and position themselves on the ablumenal surface of the endothelial tube. Upon contact of pericytes and endothelial cells, a fully differentiated, mature microvessel evolves.[54] The pericytes appear to be at least partially responsible for establishing the normal permeability phenotype characteristic of exchange vessels of the specific organ.[55]

A striking feature of the angiogenic process described above is that this complex sequence of events can be replicated *in vitro* by exposing cultured endothelial cells embedded in a basement membrane-like matrix or in a three-dimensional collagen gel to a single angiogenic factor such as basic fibroblast growth factor.[56-58] Thus, a single ligand interacting with its cell surface receptor is able to orchestrate secretion, motility, and tube formation in the proper spatial and temporal pattern such that a complex tubular network develops *in vitro*. This programmed recruitment of multiple cellular reactions by a single extracellular peptide promises to yield new insights into our understanding of intracellular signaling mechanisms.

V. ANGIOGENIC FACTORS

Table 1 lists the major angiogenic substances currently under investigation.[47,59] Since angiogenesis is a multistep process involving cell detachment from basement membrane and neighboring cells, secretion of proteolytic enzymes, cell migration, cell division, and tube formation, any agent that elicits one or more of these responses in endothelial cells could be considered an angiogenic factor. At the other extreme, the term could be restricted to substances that induce neovascularization *in vivo*. The difficulty here is that the biological response may be a reaction to a secondary stimulus that is made possible by the primary agent. Under *in vitro* conditions, some angiogenic factors stimulate cell division and are classified as mitogens; other agents are considered morphogens because they elicit tube formation. These considerations point to the problem of clearly defining what is an angiogenic factor. Substances such as histamine may cause a reduction in cell/cell and cell/matrix interactions in postcapillary venules but do not necessarily trigger angiogenesis. On the other hand, adenosine is known to cause endothelial cell chemotaxis[60,61] and proliferation,[60] as well as increased microvascular permeability;[62] however, the ability of adenosine to induce tube formation has not been demonstrated. Transforming growth factor β (TGFβ) stimulates tube formation *in vitro*,[62] but appears to inhibit endothelial cell proliferation.[63] Many cytokines appear to modulate angiogenic processes initiated by more competent growth factors.[65-67] Finally, peptides such as basic fibroblast growth factor (bFGF)[68-72] and vascular endothelial growth factor (VEGF)[73-76] appear to be able to activate all steps in the angiogenesis process under the appropriate conditions. Although bFGF activates proliferation of many cell types, VEGF appears to be specific for endothelial cells.

Table 2-1 **Chemical mediators of angiogenesis**

A.	Small molecules
	Adenosine
	Nicotinamide
	Nitric Oxide
B.	Peptides
	Angiogenin
	Fibroblast Growth Factors (acidic and basic FGF)
	Interferons (IFNγ)
	Interleukins (IL-6 and IL-8)
	Platelet-derived Endothelial Cell Growth Factor
	Transforming Growth Factors (TGFα and TGFβ)
	Tumor Necrosis Factors (TNFα)
	Vascular Endothelial Growth Factor

VI. BASIC SIGNALING MECHANISMS IN CORONARY VENULAR ENDOTHELIAL CELLS

In general, interaction of an extracellular ligand with its surface receptor triggers activation of guanosine triphosphate (GTP)-binding proteins (G-proteins), leading to modulation of membrane enzymes that catalyze the formation of intracellular second messengers. In turn, the second messengers act as a switch to turn on complementary protein kinases. These protein kinases catalyze the phosphorylation of functional proteins, leading to specific cellular reactions such as secretion, migration, or division. The adenylate cyclase,[77] phospholipase C,[78-80] nitric oxide (NO) synthase,[80-82] and guanylate cyclase[80,82] signaling cascades are present in CVEC and postcapillary venules of the porcine heart. Thus, protein kinases A, C, CaM, and G can be expected to participate in activation of CVEC by water-soluble ligands present in the extracellular fluid. Little is known about signal transduction in coronary venular pericytes.

Calcium, a common activator of intracellular processes,[83-85] interacts with the cytosolic Ca^{++}-binding protein calmodulin. The calcium/calmodulin complex (CaM) stimulates protein kinase CaM and NO synthase. Most surface receptors that interact with phospholipase C via a G-protein elicit the release of calcium from intracellular storage sites such as the endoplasmic reticulum.[86] Activation of phospholipase C leads to formation of two second messengers, inositol triphosphate (IP_3) and diacylglycerol (DAG).[87] DAG stimulates protein kinase C and inositol triphosphate opens a ligand-operated calcium channel in the endoplasmic reticulum, leading to a rapid transfer of calcium ion into the cytosol. In CVEC, bradykinin activates the phospholipase C signaling pathway, causing a typical transient in cytosolic calcium concentration.[78] The associated membrane hyperpolarization results from opening of a Ca^{++}-activated potassium channel. This hyperpolarization facilitates calcium entry into the CVEC by increasing the driving electrochemical gradient; this influx maintains a higher than normal calcium concentration in the new steady state, thereby sustaining cell activation. Calcium efflux out of the cell is accelerated by the rise in activity of the Ca^{++}-dependent calcium pumps in the plasma membrane and endoplasmic reticulum. A breakdown product of IP_3- or DAG-stimulated protein kinase C may further accelerate calcium extrusion. With increased extrusion from the cytosol, intracellular calcium concentration returns toward normal. In addition to the activation of protein kinases C and CaM, the phospholipase C signaling pathway may also recruit the NO synthase/guanylate cyclase signaling mechanism because NO synthase is stimulated by CaM and protein kinase C. In such a cascade,[80] the potential role of cyclic guanosine monophosphate (cyclic GMP) and the complementary protein kinase G must be considered.

VII. ROLE OF EXTRACELLULAR MATRIX COMPONENTS IN CELL SIGNALING

Not all extracellular signal molecules are soluble in nature. As described in a previous section, the extracellular matrix contains ligands, such as collagen and fibronectin, that are embedded in the solid-state phase. These ligands bind to specific integrin receptors located on the cell surface, and these solid-state interactions can modulate the characteristic response of an endothelial cell to a specific soluble growth factor. For example, CVEC grown on gelatin proliferate when exposed to angiogenic agents. By contrast, cell division does not occur when these same agents are presented to CVEC growing on Matrigel, a basement membrane-like matrix. This ability of extracellular matrix composition to modulate the basic nature of the cellular response to a given angiogenic factor points to the important role of the basement membrane in coordinating the various stages of angiogenesis described above. In addition, studies of CVEC responses on gelatin vs. Matrigel provide a paradigm for isolating signaling mechanisms responsible for mitogenesis versus morphogenesis, respectively.

VIII. ROLE OF ADENOSINE IN CORONARY ANGIOGENESIS

Adenosine, a breakdown product of intracellular adenosine triphosphate (ATP), is a powerful coronary vasodilator involved in moment-to-moment regulation of coronary blood flow.[2] In addition, adenosine stimulates angiogenesis in the chick chorioallantoic membrane[88,89] and embryo.[90] In CVEC seeded on gelatin, adenosine is chemotactic and mitogenic.[60] Adenosine signaling of CVEC proliferation[60] involves interaction of the ligand with a cell surface A_2 receptor and subsequent activation of adenylate cyclase via the stimulatory G-protein G_s. The short-lived increase in intracellular cyclic adenosine monophosphate (AMP) concentration presumably activates protein kinase A and leads to phosphorylation of proteins responsible for triggering cell division. Cholera toxin, a protein that facilitates G_s stimulation of adenylate cyclase, is itself mitogenic for CVEC and enhances the proliferative effects of adenosine. The central role of adenylate cyclase is further evidenced by the ability of inhibitors of the enzyme to block adenosine-induced CVEC proliferation.

CVEC exposed to oxygen tensions of approximately 10 mmHg proliferate faster than under normoxic conditions.[60] This mitogenic effect of *in vitro* hypoxia is mediated through adenosine since the response can be blocked with the adenosine receptor blocker 8-phenyltheophylline. In the intact heart, the myocardial cells are an important source of interstitial adenosine during hypoxia; this is an example of adenosine serving as a paracrine signal for coronary angiogenesis. However, given the ability of CVEC to release increased quantities of adenosine at low oxygen tensions, a part of the *in vivo* angiogenic response to chronic hypoxia may result from autocrine stimulation of A_2 receptors.

IX. ROLE OF BASIC FIBROBLAST GROWTH FACTOR IN CORONARY ANGIOGENESIS

Basic fibroblast growth factor is a peptide found in cardiac myocytes[91-93] and cells of the coronary vasculature.[94,95] The 18 kilodalton (kD) cationic peptide is also found in the basement membrane,[70,96] where it binds to anionic heparan sulfate and heparin.[97] FGF is elevated in myocytes[98] and endothelial cells[99] subjected to hypoxic stress. Moreover, *in vitro* studies of numerous types of endothelial cells demonstrate that bFGF is able to set in motion many of the cellular responses associated with angiogenesis, including secretion of proteolytic enzymes, migration, cell division, and tube formation.[100] Thus, the basic elements of a feedback control system for regulating coronary vascularity in accordance with myocardial metabolic demand appear to be in place in the heart.

The FGF receptor (FGFR) on CVEC is a 110 kD transmembrane protein; in ligand/receptor cross-linking studies of CVEC, a second band appears in the 240 kD range, suggesting that receptor dimerization may play a role in signaling of proliferation.[101-103] Each CVEC contains approximately 30,000 transmembrane receptors and more than 1,000,000 anionic binding sites in the basement membrane. The cytoplasmic domain of FGFR exhibits tyrosine kinase activity.[104] By contrast to second messenger-activated protein kinases which phosphorylate serine and threonine residues, FGFR transfers an active phosphate group to tyrosine residues of neighboring proteins. When FGF binds to its surface receptor, FGFR tyrosine kinase is activated, leading to autophosphorylation of the cytoplasmic domain and phosphorylation of other proteins. Thus, the multifunctional

FGFR serves as extracellular ligand sensor and intracellular phosphorylator of functional proteins. This signaling strategy differs markedly from the receptor/G-protein/membrane enzyme/second messenger/protein kinase cascade involving multiple proteins in the transduction pathway, as described above.

CVEC grown on gelatin proliferate rapidly in the presence of bFGF.[105] Half-maximal rates of cell division occur at 30 pM bFGF. We have not been able to obtain evidence for the involvement of the adenylate cyclase, phospholipase C, NO synthase, and guanylate cyclase signaling cascades in the early stages of bFGF-induced CVEC proliferation. Although other investigators have clearly demonstrated the ability of the FGFR tyrosine kinase to phosphorylate and activate phospholipase C,[106,107] mutant receptors that lack this ability retain their capacity to induce mitogenesis,[108-110] adding additional support to the view that phospholipase C is not required for bFGF-induced endothelial cell proliferation. How then does bFGF at the cell surface lead to activation of cell division? Analysis of the fate of radiolabeled bFGF in CVEC growing on gelatin reveals that the peptide is internalized and translocated to the nucleus.[105] During the first 2 to 4 h of exposure to external bFGF, more than 60% of the internalized peptide can be found in the nucleus of the cell. Nuclear bFGF activity plateaus at approximately 8 h, immediately before thymidine incorporation begins to rise. Blockade of bFGF internalization or nuclear translocation using tyrosine kinase inhibitors throttles FGF-induced CVEC proliferation.[111] In other cells, bFGF synthesized in the endoplasmic reticulum can translocate to the nucleus, suggesting an additional intracrine pathway for bFGF signaling,[112,113] in addition to the autocrine and paracrine routes of endothelial cell activation by the growth factor. In summary, internalization and nuclear translocation of extracellular bFGF made possible by activated receptor tyrosine kinase may play an important role in initiation of CVEC proliferation. However, phosphorylation of intracellular substrates other than phospholipase C by FGFR tyrosine kinase likely contributes to the signaling of cell division in CVEC.

On matrices derived from basement membrane (e.g. Matrigel) or in three-dimensional collagen gels, endothelial cells form tubular networks when exposed to bFGF.[57,58] Cell number remains constant during this morphogenetic process. For CVEC plated on Matrigel, bFGF-induced tube formation reaches a maximum at 18 to 24 h.[114] Tube formation in the presence of bFGF is throttled by inhibitors of protein kinase C, phospholipase C, and tyrosine kinase.[114] A critical role for protein kinase C is suggested by the fact that activators (e.g., phorbol esters) of this enzyme induce tube formation even in the absence of bFGF.[114,115] As discussed above, phospholipase C γ1 can be phosphorylated by the FGFR tyrosine kinase. This action of FGFR appears to occur in the presence of Matrigel but not on gelatin. Thus, the composition of the extracellular matrix appears to be a major determinant of whether mitogenesis or morphogenesis will be set in motion by bFGF. In summary, a signaling paradigm for CVEC tube formation on Matrigel could involve a FGFR tyrosine kinase/phospholipase C/protein kinase C signaling cascade.[114]

X. ROLE OF NITRIC OXIDE IN CORONARY ANGIOGENESIS

Continuous administration of a variety of coronary vasodilators leads to augmented myocardial vascularity.[116] This phenomenon is observed even under conditions of normal myocardial nutrient demand, thus leading to the possibility that shear rate or some other physical factor associated with increased coronary flow rate may activate angiogenic processes in postcapillary venules. In support of this concept, recent studies with isolated coronary venules and CVEC indicate that (1) venular permeability to albumin is shear-dependent[81] and (2) endothelial proliferation can be induced by stimulation of NO synthase or guanylate cyclase.[82] Since loosening of the venular endothelial cells from their basement membrane is one of the initial steps in angiogenesis, the observed increase in barrier conductance at higher shear rates is compatible with activation of the angiogenic cascade. The shear-dependent permeability increase is mediated by a NO synthase/guanylate cyclase cascade because inhibition of either enzyme prevents the change in albumin transport associated with higher luminal flow rates. CVEC exposed to sodium nitroprusside, an NO donor, exhibit an increased rate of cell division associated with an elevation of intracellular cyclic GMP concentration and, by inference, protein kinase G activity.[82]

The putative shear-dependent angiogenesis mechanism could act in synergy with adenosine and bFGF to maximize the stimulus for increased vascularity during chronic myocardial hyperfunction with attendant elevation of coronary blood flow. Under other conditions such as coronary hypoperfusion, the shear-sensitive pathway would play no role in eliciting coronary angiogenesis. The shear-dependent signaling cascade could also play a role in explaining microvascular rarefaction in chronic arterial hypertension. Elevated arterial pressure may result from defective NO signaling, leading to removal of a vasodilator influence and consequent arteriolar constriction. Throttling of NO formation could also lead to reduced vascularity if the shear-dependent mechanism plays a significant role in maintenance of normal vascularity.

XI. CORONARY ANGIOGENESIS AS A MULTICELLULAR PROCESS

Much of the preceding discussion emphasized the role of endothelial cells and cardiac myocytes in coronary angiogenesis. However, in the intact heart, postcapillary venules are subjected to chemical stimuli originating from mural pericytes, nearby mast cells, interstitial fibroblasts, and macrophages. Thus, a given stress leading to angiogenesis is likely to involve cross-talk between several cell types. Consequently, although one angiogenic factor may initiate the overall process, induced expression and release of secondary mediators may play a pivotal role in affecting the final outcome.

As emphasized in a previous section, the functions of pericytes are poorly understood. Some pericyte processes penetrate the endothelial cell basement membrane and actually make physical contact with the plasma membrane of the underlying endothelium. This intimate interaction of pericyte and endothelial cell apparently is required to maintain the differentiated state of the microvascular tube. TGFβ, a potent endothelial morphogen, is released by both cell types in a latent, inactive form.[54] With physical contact between pericytes and endothelial cells, the latent form of TGFβ is converted to the active form.[54] The cytoplasmic extensions of the spider-shaped pericyte are most numerous near interendothelial junctions,[55] implying that pericytes may also be poised to modulate the physical contacts between adjacent endothelial cells. Thus, pericytes appear to have the potential for influencing the early (e.g., detachment of endothelial cells from basement membrane) and late (e.g., morphogenesis) stages of microvessel formation.

Mast cells are usually found lined up along the external surface of the entire microvascular tree.[117] These cells release histamine, heparin, and heparanase when activated and thereby stimulate surrounding endothelial cells.[118,119] Histamine aids in the detachment process and heparin acts as an endothelial cell chemoattractant and facilitates the interaction of FGF to its surface receptor.[97,120] Heparanase degrades the basement membrane of endothelial cells and releases extracellular bFGF from its heparan sulfate binding sites,[121] thereby making more of the growth factor available for binding the surface receptor. Mast cell density in myocardium is increased in several conditions known to provoke coronary angiogenesis.[122] Adenosine may also play a role in mast cell/endothelial cell interactions because it is a positive modulator of mast degranulation.[123] To date few studies have focused on mast cell/pericyte interactions; consequently, the impact of mast cells on pericyte functions is unclear.

Fibroblasts may also play a key role in *in vivo* coronary angiogenesis. These interstitial cells are well situated to monitor the internal environment of the myocardium. For example, the known relationship between myocardial hypoxia and coronary neovascularization could, in part, reflect increased production of TGFβ by hypoxic fibroblasts.[124] As the manufacturer of the interstitial matrix through which endothelial cells must migrate and upon which endothelial tubes must form, fibroblasts could modulate the composition of collagen, glycosaminoglycans, and proteoglycans in an optimal temporal pattern to accommodate the new vascular structures. This type of interaction would require the release of chemical messages from endothelial cells to modify fibroblast behavior, and presentation of signals by fibroblasts or associated matrix to alter endothelial functions.

Finally, activated macrophages secrete substances that induce angiogenesis. Macrophages exposed to low oxygen tension release substances that elicit neovascularization.[125] Numerous cytokines secreted by macrophages, including the tumor necrosis factors,[65] interleukins,[66] and interferons,[67] may play an important role in coronary angiogenesis, but very few studies have focused on this question.

XII. CLINICAL IMPLICATIONS

Coronary angiogenesis is an important homeostatic response to inadequate nutrient delivery in myocardium under stress conditions commonly found in clinical disorders of the heart. For example, analysis of ischemic myocardium demonstrates elevated thymidine incorporation in postcapillary venular endothelium of the border zone within a few hours after onset of the stress.[126] In this region, the myocardium is hyperfunctional as it takes over the load normally carried by neighboring muscle fibers. To meet the increased metabolic demand over an extended period of time, new capillaries and venules must be produced. A similar situation occurs in hyperthyroidism[6] and chronic alveolar hypoxia associated with high altitude,[9] as well as in left ventricular hypertrophy secondary to elevated arterial afterload.[7,8] In contrast, excessive angiogenesis is life-threatening in conditions such as cardiac hemangiomas, angiosarcomas, and hemangiopericytomas.[127-129] These cardiac tumors result from uncontrolled proliferation of microvascular endothelial cells, leading to formation of a cavernous ventricular wall and abnormal cardiac mechanics and excitation. The molecular controls of angiogenesis in all of the aforementioned clinical conditions remain to be elucidated. Yet, it is clear that the ability to manipulate coronary angiogenesis in a clinical setting could be an important new tool in combating the detrimental impact of heart disease.[10,13,130-132] As we gain more insight into the intercellular and intracellular signaling mechanisms responsible for governing endothelial cell functions in the various stages of angiogenesis, our ability to design therapeutic strategies for a significant number of cardiac disorders will improve.

REFERENCES

1. **Folkow, B. and Neil, E.,** *Circulation*, University Press, London, 1971.
2. **Tomanek, R. J.,** Anatomical principles of the coronary circulation, *Coronary Circulation. Basic Mechanisms and Clinical Relevance*, Springer Verlag, Tokyo, 1990.
3. **Berne, R. M., Knabb, R. M., Ely, S. W., and Rubio, R.,** Adenosine in the local regulation of blood flow: a brief overview, *Fed. Proc.*, 42, 3136, 1983.
4. **Granger, H. J., Goodman, A. H., and Granger, D. N.,** Role of resistance and exchange vessels in local microvascular control of skeletal muscle oxygenation, *Circ. Res.*, 38, 379, 1976.

5. **Schaper, W.**, *The Collateral Circulation of the Heart*, Elsevier, New York, 1971.
6. **Chilian, W. M., Wangler, R. D., Peters, K. G., Tomanek, R. J., and Marcus, M. L.**, Thyroxine-induced left ventricular hypertrophy in the rat. Anatomical and physiological evidence for angiogenesis, *Circ. Res.*, 57, 591, 1985.
7. **Mall, G., Zimmer, G., Baden, S., and Mattfeldt, T.**, Capillary neoformation in the rat heart-stereological studies on papillary muscles in hypertrophy and physiologic growth, *Basic Res. Cardiol.*, 85, 531, 1990.
8. **Tomanek, R. J., Schalk, K. A., Marcus, M. L., and Harrison, D. G.**, Coronary angiogenesis during long-term hypertension and left ventricular hypertrophy in dogs, *Circ. Res.*, 65, 352, 1989.
9. **Kayar, S. R. and Banchero, N.**, Myocardial capillarity in acclimation to hypoxia, *Pflügers Arch.*, 404, 319, 1985.
10. **Schaper, W.**, Angiogenesis in the adult heart, *Basic Res. Cardiol.*, 86 (Suppl. 2), 51, 1991.
11. **Risau, W., Sariola, H., Zerwes, H. G., Sasse, J., Ekblom, P., Kemler, R., and Doetschman, T.**, Vasculogenesis and angiogenesis in embryonic-stem-cell-derived embryoid bodies, *Development*, 102, 471, 1988.
12. **Kamiya, A., Ando, J., Shibata, M., and Masuda, H.**, Roles of fluid shear stress in physiological regulation of vascular structure and function, *Biorheology*, 25, 271, 1988.
13. **Schaper, W., Sharma, H. S., Quinkler, W., Markert, T., Wunsch, M., and Schaper, J.**, Molecular biologic concepts of coronary anastomoses, *J. Am. Coll. Cardiol.*, 15, 513, 1990.
14. **Clark, E. R. and Clark, E. L.**, Microscopic observations on the growth of blood capillaries in the living mammal, *Am. J. Anat.*, 64, 251, 1939.
15. **Myrhage, R. and Hudlicka, O.**, Capillary growth in chronically stimulated adult skeletal muscle as studied by intravital microscopy and histological methods in rabbits and rats. *Microvasc. Res.*, 17, 73, 1978.
16. **Phillips, G. D., Whitehead, R. A., and Knighton, D. R.**, Initiation and pattern of angiogenesis in wound healing in the rat, *Am. J. Anat.*, 192, 257, 1991.
17. **Folkman, J.**, Angiogenesis: initiation and control, *Ann. N.Y. Acad. Sci.*, 401, 212, 1982.
18. **Diaz-Flores, L., Gutierrez, R., and Varela, H.**, Behavior of postcapillary venule pericytes during postnatal angiogenesis, *J. Morphol.*, 213, 33, 1992.
19. **Wagner, R. C. and Hossler, F. E.**, SEM of capillary pericytes prepared by ultrasonic microdissection: evidence for the existence of a pericapillary syncytium, *Anat. Rec.*, 234, 249, 1992.
20. **Simionescu, N., Simionescu, M., and Palade, G. E.**, Open junctions in the endothelium of the postcapillary venules of the diaphragm, *J. Cell. Biol.*, 79, 27, 1978.
21. **Yuan, Y., Chilian, W. M., Granger, H. J., and Zawieja, D. C.**, Permeability to albumin in isolated coronary venules, *Am. J. Physiol.*, 265, H543, 1993.
22. **Majno, G., Shea, S. M., and Leventhal, M.**, Endothelial contraction induced by histamine-type mediators, *J. Cell. Biol.*, 42, 647, 1969.
23. **Arfors, K. E., Rutili, G., and Svensjo, E.**, Microvascular transport of macromolecules in normal and inflammatory conditions, *Acta Physiol. Scand.*, 463 (Suppl.), 93, 1979.
24. **Lewis, R. E. and Granger, H. J.**, Diapedesis and the permeability of venous microvessels to protein macromolecules: the impact of leukotriene B_4 (LTB_4), *Microvasc. Res.*, 35, 27, 1988.
25. **Ward, K. A., Jain, R. K., and Zhou, Q.**, Cancer cell interactions with the microvasculature, *FASEB J.*, 3, A543, 1989.

26. **Basson, C. T., Knowles, W. J., Bell, L., Albelda, S. M., Castronovo, V., Liotta, L. A., and Madri, J. A.,** Spatiotemporal segregation of endothelial cell integrin and nonintegrin extracellular matrix-binding proteins during adhesion events, *J. Cell. Biol.*, 110, 789, 1990.
27. **Hayashi, K., Madri, J. A., and Yurchenco, P. D.,** Endothelial cells interact with the core protein of basement membrane perlecan through beta 1 and beta 3 integrins: an adhesion modulated by glycosaminoglycan, *J. Cell. Biol.*, 119, 945, 1992.
28. **Massia, S. P. and Hubbell, J. A.,** Vascular endothelial cell adhesion and spreading promoted by the peptide REDV of the IIICS region of plasma fibronectin is mediated by integrin alpha 4 beta 1, *J. Biol. Chem.*, 267, 14019, 1992.
29. **Cheng, Y. F. and Kramer, R. H.,** Human microvascular endothelial cells express integrin-related complexes that mediate adhesion to the extracellular matrix, *J. Cell. Physiol.*, 139, 275, 1989.
30. **Dejana, E.,** Endothelial cell adhesive receptors, *J. Cardiovasc. Pharmacol.*, 21 (Suppl. 1), S18, 1993.
31. **Tarone, G., Stefanuto, G., Mascarello, P., Defilippi, P., Altruda, F., and Silengo, L.,** Expression of receptors for extracellular matrix proteins in human endothelial cells, *J. Lipid. Mediat.*, 2 (Suppl.), S45, 1990.
32. **Gates, R. E., Hanks, S. K., and King, L. E., Jr.,** Focal-adhesion components are enriched in ventral membranes isolated from transformed keratinocytes in culture, *Biochem. J.*, 289, 221, 1993.
33. **Kornberg, L., Earp, H. S., Parsons, J. T., Schaller, M., and Juliano, R. L.,** Cell adhesion or integrin clustering increases phosphorylation of a focal adhesion-associated tyrosine kinase, *J. Biol. Chem.*, 267, 23439, 1992.
34. **Guan, J. L. and Shalloway, D.,** Regulation of focal adhesion-associated protein tyrosine kinase by both cellular adhesion and oncogenic transformation, *Nature*, 358, 690, 1992.
35. **Albelda, S. M., Muller, W. A., Buck, C. A., and Newman, P. J.,** Molecular and cellular properties of PECAM-1 (endoCAM/CD31): a novel vascular cell-cell adhesion molecule, *J. Cell Biol.*, 114, 1059, 1991.
36. **Liaw, C. W., Cannon, C., Power, M. D., Kiboneka, P. K., and Rubin, L. L.,** Identification and cloning of two species of cadherins in bovine endothelial cells, *EMBO J.*, 9, 2701, 1990.
37. **Muller, W. A., Ratti, C. M., McDonnell, S. L., and Cohn, Z. A.,** A human endothelial cell-restricted, externally disposed plasmalemmal protein enriched in intercellular junctions, *J. Exp. Med.*, 170, 399, 1989.
38. **Lampugnani, M. G., Resnati, M., Raiteri, M., Pigott, R., Pisacane, A., Houen, G., Ruco, L. P., and Dejana, E.,** A novel endothelial-specific membrane protein is a marker of cell-cell contacts, *J. Cell. Biol.*, 118, 1511, 1992.
39. **Pepper, M. S., Montesano, R., el Aoumari, A., Gros, D., Orci, L., and Meda, P.,** Coupling and connexin 43 expression in microvascular and large vessel endothelial cells, *Am. J. Physiol.*, 262, C1246, 1992.
40. **Bruzzone, R., Haefliger, J. A., Gimlich, R. L., and Paul, D. L.,** Connexin40, a component of gap junctions in vascular endothelium, is restricted in its ability to interact with other connexins, *Mol. Biol. Cell*, 4, 7, 1993.
41. **Schulze, C. and Firth, J. A.,** Junctions between pericytes and the endothelium in rat myocardial capillaries: a morphometric and immunogold study, *Cell Tissue Res.*, 271, 145, 1993.
42. **Bavisotto, L. M., Schwartz, S. M., and Heimark, R. L.,** Modulation of Ca2(+)-dependent intercellular adhesion in bovine aortic and human umbilical vein endothelial cells by heparin-binding growth factors, *J. Cell. Physiol.*, 143, 39, 1990.

43. **Salomon, D., Ayalon, O., Patel-King, R., Hynes, R. O., and Geiger, B.,** Extrajunctional distribution of N-cadherin in cultured human endothelial cells, *J. Cell. Sci.*, 102, 7, 1992.
44. **Albelda, S. M., Oliver, P. D., Romer, L. H., and Buck, C. A.,** EndoCAM: a novel endothelial cell-cell adhesion molecule, *J. Cell. Biol.*, 110, 122, 1990.
45. **Schelling, M. E., Meininger, C. J., Hawker, J. R., and Granger, H. J.,** Venular endothelial cells from bovine heart, *Am. J. Physiol.*, 254, H1211, 1988.
46. **Ryan, U. S., White, L. A., Lopez, M., and Ryan, J. W.,** Use of microcarriers to isolate and culture pulmonary microvascular endothelium, *Tissue Cell*, 14, 597, 1982.
47. **Folkman, J. and Brem, H.,** Angiogenesis and inflammation, in *Inflammation: Basic Principles and Clinical Correlates*, Gallin, J. I., Goldstein, I. M., and Snyderman, R., Eds., Raven Press, New York, 1992, 821.
48. **Mignatti, P. and Rifkin, D. B.,** Biology and biochemistry of proteinases in tumor invasion, *Physiol. Rev.*, 73, 161, 1993.
49. **Gross, J. L., Moscatelli, D., and Rifkin, D. B.,** Increased capillary endothelial cell protease activity in response to angiogenic stimuli in vitro, *Proc. Natl. Acad. Sci. U.S.A.*, 80, 2623, 1983.
50. **Unemori, E. N., Ferrara, N., Bauer, E. A., and Amento, E. P.,** Vascular endothelial growth factor induces interstitial collagenase expression in human endothelial cells, *J. Cell. Physiol.*, 153, 557, 1992.
51. **Pepper, M. S., Sappino, A. P., Montesano, R., Orci, L., and Vassalli, J. D.,** Plasminogen activator inhibitor-1 is induced in migrating endothelial cells, *J. Cell. Physiol.*, 153, 129, 1992.
52. **Merwin, J. R., Anderson, J. M., Kocher, O., Van Itallie, C. M., and Madri, J. A.,** Transforming growth factor beta 1 modulates extracellular matrix organization and cell-cell junctional complex formation during in vitro angiogenesis, *J. Cell. Physiol.*, 142, 117, 1990.
53. **Mayerhofer, A. and Bartke, A.,** Developing testicular microvasculature in the golden hamster, Mesocricetus auratus: a model for angiogenesis under physiological conditions, *Acta Anat. (Basel)*, 139, 78, 1990.
54. **Orlidge, A. and D'Amore, P. A.,** Inhibition of capillary endothelial cell growth by pericytes and smooth muscle cells, *J. Cell. Biol.*, 105, 1455, 1987.
55. **Sims, D. E.,** Recent advances in pericyte biology — implications for health and disease, *Can. J. Cardiol.*, 7, 431, 1991.
56. **Folkman, J. and Haudenschild, C.,** Angiogenesis in vitro, *Nature*, 288, 551, 1980.
57. **Madri, J. A., Pratt, B. M., and Tucker, A. M.,** Phenotypic modulation of endothelial cells by transforming growth factor-beta depends upon the composition and organization of the extracellular matrix, *J. Cell. Biol.*, 106, 1375, 1988.
58. **Montesano, R., Vassalli, J. D., Baird, A., Guillemin, R., and Orci, L.,** Basic fibroblast growth factor induces angiogenesis in vitro, *Proc. Natl. Acad. Sci. U.S.A.*, 83, 7297, 1986.
59. **Klagsbrun, M. and D'Amore, P. A.,** Regulators of angiogenesis, *Annu. Rev. Physiol.*, 53, 217, 1991.
60. **Meininger, C. J., Schelling, M. E., and Granger, H. J.,** Adenosine and hypoxia stimulate proliferation and migration of endothelial cells, *Am. J. Physiol.*, 255, H554, 1988.
61. **Teuscher, E. and Weidlich, V.,** Adenosine nucleotides, adenosine and adenine as angiogenesis factors, *Biomed. Biochim. Acta*, 44, 493, 1985.
62. **Vinores, S. A., Sen, H., and Campochiaro, P. A.,** An adenosine agonist and prostaglandin E1 cause breakdown of the blood-retinal barrier by opening tight junctions between vascular endothelial cells, *Invest. Ophthalmol. Vis. Sci.*, 33, 1870, 1992.

63. **Pepper, M. S., Vassalli, J. D., Orci, L., and Montesano, R.,** Biphasic effect of transforming growth factor-beta 1 on in vitro angiogenesis, *Exp. Cell. Res.*, 204, 356, 1993.
64. **Madri, J. A., Pratt, B. M., and Tucker, A. M.,** Phenotypic modulation of endothelial cells by transforming growth factor-beta depends upon the composition and organization of the extracellular matrix, *J. Cell. Biol.*, 106, 1375, 1988.
65. **Leibovich, S. J., Polverini, P. J., Shepard, H. M., Wiseman, D. M., Shively, V., and Nuseir, N.,** Macrophage-induced angiogenesis is mediated by tumour necrosis factor-alpha, *Nature*, 329, 630, 1987.
66. **Koch, A. E., Polverini, P. J., Kunkel, S. L., Harlow, L. A., DiPietro, L. A., Elner, V. M., Elner, S. G., and Strieter, R. M.,** Interleukin-8 as a macrophage-derived mediator of angiogenesis, *Science*, 258, 1798, 1992.
67. **Maheshwari, R. K., Srikantan, V., Bhartiya, D., Kleinman, H. K., and Grant, D. S.,** Differential effects of interferon gamma and alpha on in vitro model of angiogenesis, *J. Cell. Physiol.*, 46, 164, 1991.
68. **Burgess, W. H. and Maciag, T.,** The heparin-binding (fibroblast) growth factor family of proteins, *Annu. Rev. Biochem.*, 58, 575, 1989.
69. **Gospodarowicz, D., Massoglia, S., Cheng, J., and Fujii, D. K.,** Effect of fibroblast growth factor and lipoproteins on the proliferation of endothelial cells derived from bovine adrenal cortex, brain cortex, and corpus luteum capillaries, *J. Cell Physiol.*, 127, 121, 1986.
70. **Moscatelli, D.**, Metabolism of receptor-bound and matrix-bound basic fibroblast growth factor by bovine capillary endothelial cells, *J. Cell. Biol.*, 107, 753, 1988.
71. **Gospodarowicz, D.,** Humoral control of cell proliferation: the role of fibroblast growth factor in regeneration, angiogenesis, wound healing, and neoplastic growth, *Prog. Clin. Biol. Res.*, 9, 1, 1976.
72. **Gaudric, A., N'guyen, T., Moenner, M., Glacet-Bernard, A., and Barritault, D.,** Quantification of angiogenesis due to basic fibroblast growth factor in a modified rabbit corneal model, *Ophthalmic Res.*, 24, 181, 1992.
73. **Pepper, M. S., Ferrara, N., Orci, L., and Montesano, R.,** Potent synergism between vascular endothelial growth factor and basic fibroblast growth factor in the induction of angiogenesis in vitro, *Biochem. Biophys. Res. Commun.*, 189, 824, 1992.
74. **Breier, G., Albrecht, U., Sterrer, S., and Risau, W.,** Expression of vascular endothelial growth factor during embryonic angiogenesis and endothelial cell differentiation, *Development*, 114, 521, 1992.
75. **Berse, B., Brown, L. F., Van de Water, L., Dvorak, H. F., and Senger, D. R.,** Vascular permeability factor (vascular endothelial growth factor) gene is expressed differentially in normal tissues, macrophages, and tumors, *Mol. Biol. Cell*, 3, 211, 1992.
76. **Ferrara, N., Houck, K. A., Jakeman, L. B., Winer, J., and Leung, D. W.,** The vascular endothelial growth factor family of polypeptides, *J. Cell. Biochem.*, 47, 211, 1991.
77. **Meininger, C. J. and Granger, H. J.,** Mechanisms leading to adenosine-stimulated proliferation of microvascular endothelial cells, *Am. J. Physiol.*, 258, H198, 1990.
78. **Ziche, M., Zawieja, D., Hester, K., and Granger, H.,** Calcium entry, mobilization and extrusion in postcapillary venular endothelium, *Am. J. Physiol.*, 265, H569, 1993.
79. **Yuan, Y., Granger, H. J., Zawieja, D. C., and Chilian, W. M.,** Flow modulates coronary venular permeability by a nitric oxide-related mechanism, *Am. J. Physiol.*, 263, H641, 1992.
80. **Yuan, Y., Granger, H. J., Zawieja, D. C., DeFily, D. V., and Chilian, W. M.,** Histamine increases venular permeability via a phospholipase C-NO synthase-guanylate cyclase cascade, *Am. J. Physiol.*, 265, H1734, 1993.

81. **Wu, G. and Meininger, C. J.,** The regulation of L-arginine synthesis from L-citrulline by L-glutamine in endothelial cells, *Am. J. Physiol.,* 265, H1965, 1993.
82. **Ziche, M., Morbidelli, L., Masini, E., Granger, H., Geppetti, P., and Ledda, F.,** Nitric oxide promotes DNA synthesis and cyclic GMP formation in endothelial cells from postcapillary venules, *Biochem. Biophys. Res. Comm.,* 192, 1198, 1993.
83. **Putney, J. W.,** The capacitative model for receptor-activated calcium entry, *Adv. Pharmacol.,* 22, 251, 1991.
84. **Berridge, M. J. and Galione, A.,** Cytosolic calcium oscillators, *FASEB J.,* 2, 3074, 1988.
85. **Colden-Stanfield, M., Schilling, W. P., Ritchie, A. K., Eskin, S. G., Navarro, L. T., and Kunze, D. L.,** Bradykinin-induced increases in cytosolic calcium and ionic currents in cultured bovine aortic endothelial cells, *Circ. Res.,* 61, 632, 1987.
86. **Bundgaard, M.,** The three-dimensional organization of smooth endoplasmic reticulum in capillary endothelia: its possible role in regulation of free cytosolic calcium, *J. Struct. Biol.,* 107, 76, 1991.
87. **Berridge, M. J.,** Inositol trisphosphate and diacylglycerol as second messengers, *Biochem. J.,* 220, 345, 1984.
88. **Dusseau, J. W., Hutchins, P. M., and Malbasa, D. S.,** Stimulation of angiogenesis by adenosine on the chick chorioallantoic membrane, *Circ. Res.,* 59, 163, 1986.
89. **Dusseau, J. W. and Hutchins, P. M.,** Hypoxia-induced angiogenesis in chick chorioallantoic membranes: a role for adenosine, *Respir. Physiol.,* 71, 33, 1988.
90. **Adair, T. H., Montani, J. P., Strick, D. M., and Guyton, A. C.,** Vascular development in chick embryos: a possible role for adenosine, *Am. J. Physiol.,* 256, H240, 1989.
91. **Kardami, E. and Fandrich, R. R.,** Basic fibroblast growth factor in atria and ventricles of the vertebrate heart, *J. Cell. Biol.,* 109, 1865, 1989.
92. **Speir, E., Tanner, V., Gonzalez, A. M., Farris, J., Baird, A., and Casscells, W.,** Acidic and basic fibroblast growth factors in adult rat heart myocytes. Localization, regulation in culture, and effects on DNA synthesis, *Circ. Res.,* 71, 251, 1992.
93. **Consigli, S. A. and Joseph-Silverstein, J.,** Immunolocalization of basic fibroblast growth factor during chicken cardiac development, *J. Cell. Physiol.,* 146, 379, 1991.
94. **Nilsson, J., Herzfeld, I., Grip, L., Aberg, B., and Ryden, L.,** Immunohistochemical analysis of a human coronary artery exposed to excimer laser angioplasty in vivo: evidence for release of fibroblast growth factor at the site of injury, *Am. Heart J.,* 125, 908, 1993.
95. **Spirito, P., Fu, Y. M., Yu, Z. X., Epstein, S. E., and Casscells, W.,** Immunohistochemical localization of basic and acidic fibroblast growth factors in the developing rat heart, *Circulation,* 84, 322, 1991.
96. **Folkman, J., Klagsbrun, M., Sasse, J., Wadzinski, M., Ingber, D., and Vlodavsky, I.,** A heparin-binding angiogenic protein — basic fibroblast growth factor — is stored within basement membrane, *Am. J. Pathol.,* 130, 393, 1988.
97. **Yayon, A., Klagsbrun, M., Esko, J. D., Leder, P., and Ornitz, D. M.,** Cell surface, heparin-like molecules are required for binding of basic fibroblast growth factor to its high affinity receptor, *Cell,* 64, 841, 1991.
98. **Morrow, N. G., Kraus, W. E., Moore, J. W., Williams, R. S., and Swain, J. L.,** Increased expression of fibroblast growth factors in a rabbit skeletal muscle model of exercise conditioning, *J. Clin. Invest.,* 85, 1816, 1990.
99. **Hawker, J. R., Meininger, C. J., and Granger, H. J.,** Unpublished observations.
100. **Ingber, D. E. and Folkman, J.,** Mechanochemical switching between growth and differentiation during fibroblast growth factor-stimulated angiogenesis in vitro: role of extracellular matrix, *J. Cell. Biol.,* 109, 317, 1989.

101. **Schelling, M. E., Hawker, J., and Granger, H. J.,** High and low affinity binding of a and b FGF to their receptor on coronary venular endothelial cells, *FASEB J.*, 3, A1317, 1989.
102. **Schelling, M. E., Hawker, J. R., and Granger, H. J.,** Characterization of the endothelial cell growth factor (acidic fibroblast growth factor) receptor of coronary venular endothelial cells, *J. Cell. Biochem.*, 12A (Suppl.), 113, 1988.
103. **Hawker, J. R., Jr.,** Mechanisms by which Fibroblast Growth Factors Stimulate DNA Synthesis in Coronary Venular Endothelial Cells, dissertation, Texas A&M University, College Station, TX, 1992.
104. **Coughlin, S. R., Barr, P. J., Cousens, L. S., Fretto, L. J., and Williams, L. T.,** Acidic and basic fibroblast growth factors stimulate tyrosine kinase activity in vivo, *J. Biol. Chem.*, 263, 988, 1988.
105. **Hawker, J. R. and Granger, H. J.,** Internalized basic fibroblast growth factor translocates to nuclei of venular endothelial cells before initiation of DNA synthesis, *Am. J. Physiol.*, 262, H1525, 1992.
106. **Mohammadi, M., Honegger, A. M., Rotin, D., Fischer, R., Bellot, F., Li, W., Dionne, C. A., Jaye, M., Rubinstein, M., and Schlessinger, J.,** A tyrosine-phosphorylated carboxy-terminal peptide of the fibroblast growth factor receptor (Flg) is a binding site for the SH2 domain of phospholipase C-gamma 1, *Mol. Cell. Biol.*, 11, 5068, 1991.
107. **Burgess, W. H., Dionne, C. A., Kaplow, J., Mudd, R., Friesel, R., Zilberstein, A., Schlessinger, J., and Jaye, M.,** Characterization and cDNA cloning of phospholipase C-gamma, a major substrate for heparin-binding growth factor 1 (acidic fibroblast growth factor)-activated tyrosine kinase, *Mol. Cell. Biol.*, 10, 4770, 1990.
108. **Mohammadi, M., Dionne, C. A., Li, W., Li, N., Spivak, T., Honegger, A. M., Jaye, M., and Schlessinger, J.,** Point mutation in FGF receptor eliminates phosphatidylinositol hydrolysis without affecting mitogenesis, *Nature*, 358, 681, 1992.
109. **Peters, K. G., Marie, J., Wilson, E., Ives, H. E., Escobedo, J., Del Rosario, M., Mirda, D., and Williams, L. T.,** Point mutation of an FGF receptor abolishes phosphatidylinositol turnover and Ca^{2+} flux but not mitogenesis, *Nature*, 358, 678, 1992.
110. **Magnaldo, I., L'Allemain, G., Chambard, J. C., Moenner, M., Barritault, D., and Pouyssegur, J.,** The mitogenic pathway of fibroblast growth factor is not mediated through polyphosphoinositide hydrolysis and protein kinase C activation in hamster fibroblasts, *J. Biol. Chem.*, 261, 16916, 1986.
111. **Hawker, J. R., Jr. and Granger, H. J.,** Tyrosine kinase inhibitors impair fibroblast growth factor signaling in coronary endothelial cells, *Am. J. Physiol.*, 266, H107, 1994.
112. **Dell'Era, P., Presta, M., and Ragnotti, G.,** Nuclear localization of endogenous basic fibroblast growth factor in cultured endothelial cells, *Exp. Cell Res.*, 192, 505, 1991.
113. **Logan, A.,** Intracrine regulation at the nucleus — a further mechanism of growth factor activity?, *J. Endocrinol.*, 125, 339, 1990.
114. **Czisny, L. E., Hawker, J. R., Zawieja, D. C., and Granger, H. J.,** Tube formation by coronary venular endothelial cells seeded on matrigel is mediated by a FGF receptor/phosphlipase C/protein kinase C signaling cascade, *FASEB J.*, 7, A125, 1993.
115. **Montesano, R. and Orci, L.,** Tumor-promoting phorbol esters induce angiogenesis in vitro, *Cell*, 42, 469, 1985.
116. **Hudlicka, O., Brown, M., and Egginton, S.,** Angiogenesis in skeletal and cardiac muscle, *Physiol. Rev.*, 72, 369, 1992.
117. **Rakusan, K., Sarkar, K., Turek, Z., and Wicker, P.,** Mast cells in the rat heart during normal growth and in cardiac hypertrophy, *Circ. Res.*, 66, 511, 1990.

118. **Marks, R. M., Roche, W. R., Czerniecki, M., Penny, R., and Nelson, D. S.,** Mast cell granules cause proliferation of human microvascular endothelial cells, *Lab. Invest.*, 55, 289, 1986.
119. **Meininger, C. J., Sherwood, S. J., Hawker, J. R., and Granger, H. J.,** Mast cells release basic fibroblast growth factor (bFGF) from endothelial cells and matrix, *FASEB J.*, 4, A487, 1990.
120. **Schelling, M. E., Hawker, J. R., and Granger, H. J.,** Heparin potentiation of the binding of endothelial cell growth factor to its receptor on coronary venular endothelial cells, *FASEB J.*, 2, A1878, 1988.
121. **Bashkin, P., Razin, E., Eldor, A., and Vlodavsky, I.,** Degranulating mast cells secrete an endoglycosidase that degrades heparan sulfate in subendothelial extracellular matrix, *Blood*, 75, 2204, 1990.
122. **Olivetti, G., Lagrasta, C., Ricci, R., Sonnenblick, E. H., Capasso, J. M., and Anversa, P.,** Long-term pressure-induced cardiac hypertrophy: capillary and mast cell proliferation, *Am. J. Physiol.*, 257, H1766, 1989.
123. **Peachell, P. T., Columbo, M., Kagey-Sobotka, A., Lichtenstein, L. M., and Marone, G.,** Adenosine potentiates mediator release from human lung mast cells, *Am. Rev. Respir. Dis.*, 138, 1143, 1988.
124. **Falanga, V., Qian, S. W., Danielpour, D., Katz, M. H., Roberts, A. B., and Sporn, M. B.,** Hypoxia upregulates the synthesis of TGF-beta 1 by human dermal fibroblasts, *J. Invest. Dermatol.*, 97, 634, 1991.
125. **Knighton, D. R., Hunt, T. K., Scheuenstuhl, H., Halliday, B. J., Werb, Z., and Banda, M. J.,** Oxygen tension regulates the expression of angiogenesis factor by macrophages, *Science*, 221, 1283, 1983.
126. **Casscells, W., Kimura, H., Sanchez, J. A., Yu, Z. X., and Ferrans, V. J.,** Immunohistochemical study of fibronectin in experimental myocardial infarction, *Am. J. Pathol.*, 37, 801, 1990.
127. **Sulayman, R. and Cassels, D. E.,** Myocardial coronary hemangiomatous tumors in children, *Chest*, 68, 113, 1975.
128. **Soberman, M. S., Plauth, W. H., Winn, K. J., Forest, G. C., Hatcher, C. R., Jr., and Sink, J. D.,** Hemangioma of the right ventricle causing outflow tract obstruction, *J. Thorac. Cardiovasc. Surg.*, 96, 307, 1988.
129. **Yang, H. Y., Wasielewski, J. F., Lee, W., Lee, E., and Paik, Y. K.,** Angiosarcoma of the heart: ultrastructural study, *Cancer*, 47, 72, 1981.
130. **Fujita, M., Yamanishi, K., Hirai, T., Ohno, A., Miwa, K., and Sasayama, S.,** Comparative effect of heparin treatment with and without strenuous exercise on treadmill capacity in patients with stable effort angina, *Am. Heart J.*, 122, 453, 1991.
131. **Unger, E. F., Sheffield, C. D., and Epstein, S. E.,** Creation of anastomoses between an extracardiac artery and the coronary circulation. Proof that myocardial angiogenesis occurs and can provide nutritional blood flow to the myocardium, *Circulation*, 82, 1449, 1990.
132. **Yanagisawa-Miwa, A., Uchida, Y., Nakamura, F., Tomaru, T., Kido, H., Kamijo, T., Sugimoto, T., Kaji, K., Utsuyama, M., and Kurashima, C.,** Salvage of infarcted myocardium by angiogenic action of basic fibroblast growth factor, *Science*, 257, 1401, 1992.

Chapter 3

Neoplasia

Roberto F. Nicosia and Giuseppe G. Pietra

CONTENTS

I. INTRODUCTION

Tumors of the microcirculation are among the most common and heterogeneous neoplasms of man. They include a spectrum of conditions ranging from benign vascular proliferations to highly malignant spindle cell sarcomas. Between these two extremes there are lesions with a variable clinical course growing rapidly or regressing spontaneously, possibly under the influence of autocrine and paracrine factors, or the host's hormonal status. While the mechanisms that modulate endothelial proliferation in tumors

0-8493-4547-2/94/$0.00+$.50

of nonvascular origin have been extensively investigated, those operating in vascular neoplasms have received little attention. For years, our knowledge of tumors of the vasoformative tissue was based primarily on clinical-pathological observations and on experimental models of chemical carcinogenesis. Now, advances in cell and molecular biology provide the opportunity to apply new concepts on angiogenic mechanisms to the study of microvascular neoplasms. In this chapter, we review tumor angiogenesis and its mechanisms, describe the pathology of the most common vascular tumors, and discuss how experimental work on angiogenesis is contributing to our current understanding of the biology of microvascular tumors.

II. ANGIOGENESIS IN TUMORS OF NONVASCULAR ORIGIN

A. SYMBIOTIC RELATIONSHIP BETWEEN NONVASCULAR TUMOR CELLS AND MICROVESSELS

Angiogenesis and tumor growth are mutually dependent processes supported by the symbiotic relationship between tumor cells and vascular endothelium. Adult vascular endothelial cells, which are under normal conditions a quiescent population of cells, proliferate in response to tumor angiogenic stimulation forming new blood vessels.[1] The acquisition of angiogenic activity during tumor progression precedes the transition from *in situ* to invasive carcinoma.[2] It can be demonstrated before transformation and tumorigenesis in cell lines at high risk of becoming neoplastic,[3] in hyperplastic lesions of the breast,[4] and in proliferative lesions of the endocrine pancreas.[5]

The fraction of endothelial cells synthesizing DNA (labeling index) in tumors of nonvascular origin, dramatically increases from baseline values of less than 0.1% to values of 20 to 30% or more.[1,6] The endothelial labeling index is highest at the periphery of the tumor, where there is active vascular proliferation, and lowest in the tumor center.[6] The newly formed blood vessels are continuously stimulated by tumor angiogenic factors which promote their growth and prevent their regression.[7] At the same time, the growth and spread of tumor cells is dependent on the newly formed microvessels which supply oxygen and nutrients, dispose of metabolic waste products, and provide a trellis-like three-dimensional substrate for tumor cell attachment, migration, and proliferation.[8,9]

B. BLOOD VESSEL MORPHOLOGY IN TUMORS OF NONVASCULAR ORIGIN

The vasculature of tumors is characterized by a variety of structural alterations. *In vivo* studies have shown continuous vascular remodeling with incorporation or obliteration by the tumor of preexisting blood vessels and formation of new ones.[10] Some authors have emphasized differences between the vasculature of benign and malignant tumors. For example, the vasculature of colonic adenomas in rats resembles the normal colonic vasculature, whereas that of colonic adenocarcinomas is chaotic and disorganized.[11] One possible explanation for this difference is that the vasculature of benign tumors expands as a result of orderly endothelial cell proliferation and intercalation within preexisting microvessels, which become longer. Conversely, malignant tumors induce continuous vascular sprouting with formation of new vascular networks, whose disorganized architecture reflects the chaotic growth of the tumor.[12,13]

Tumor blood vessels are characteristically dilated and tortuous (Figure 1). The dilated, coiled, bulbous appearance of some tumor blood vessels is believed to be the result of a shape change in preexisting vessels, which precedes the sprouting of new vessels. The change in cylindrical geometry is probably due to the proliferative expansion of the endothelial surface area in blood vessels whose ends are fixed due to their connection to neighboring vessels.[14] This results in uniform dilatation, tortuosity, or buckling with formation of varicose structures. In a detailed review of the histology of the tumor

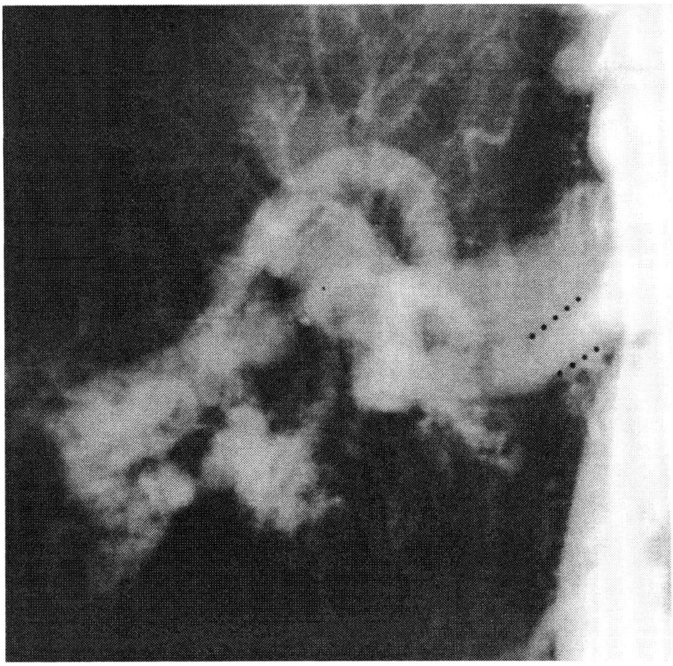

Figure 3-1 Venous phase of a renal artery angiogram showing tortuous and dilated blood vessels in a richly vascularized renal cell carcinoma. *(Courtesy of Dr. W. Miller, Jr.)*

microvasculature, Warren described abnormal microvessels including sinusoids, arteriovenous anastomoses, and a variety of wide-bore, thin-walled microchannels (giant capillaries) prone to neoplastic intravasation.[10]

Ultrastructurally, endothelial cells of tumor microvessels are characteristically plump and activated. The endothelial cytoplasm is abundant and contains an increased number of cytoplasmic organelles. Capillary sprouts show marked irregularities of their surfaces with heaping up of the endothelial plasma membrane and formation of microvilli or saccular outgrowths.[15] The basement membrane is absent or attenuated around developing sprouts. When present, the capillary basement membrane may be thickened and multilayered. Pericytes are either absent or dissociated from the endothelium.[11,16]

C. STEPS IN THE ANGIOGENIC PROCESS

Angiogenesis is characterized by an orderly sequence of growth and morphogenetic events which can be summarized as follows:[17]

(1) Engorgement and dilatation of venules or capillaries with activation of endothelial cells.
(2) Focal dissolution of the basement membrane followed by migration of endothelial cells from the parent vessel into the interstitium and formation of immature sprouts (Figure 2).
(3) Proliferation of endothelial cells behind the migrating endothelium of the sprout.
(4) Continuous remodeling of the extracellular matrix (ECM) with digestion of the matrix around the invasive tip of the endothelial sprout and deposition of a new ECM. Because

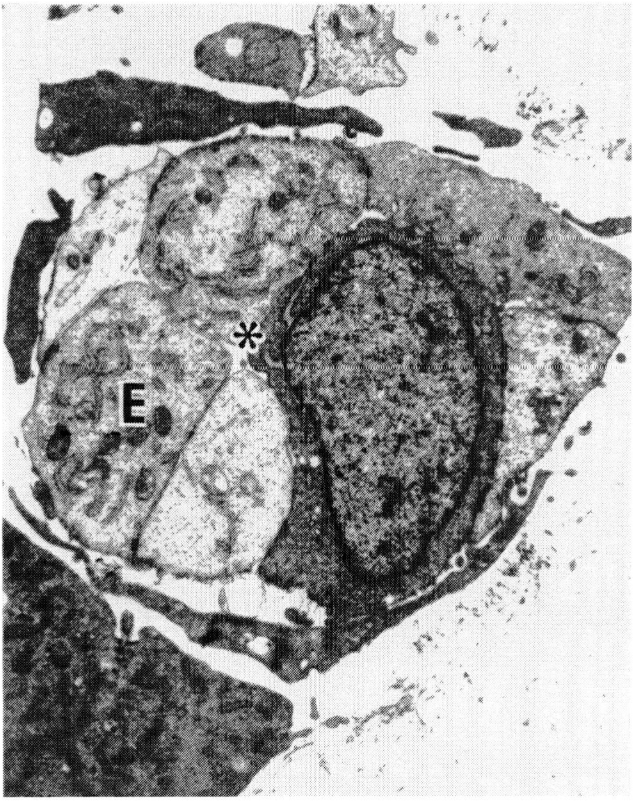

Figure 3-2 Electron micrograph of newly formed microvessel in human granulation tissue. Notice the plump, activated endothelium (E) and the small lumen (asterisk). (× 8,200)

of this continuous remodeling, particularly in regions of active penetration of the ECM by endothelial cells, the basement membrane of immature sprouts is typically faint and discontinuous.

(5) Canalization of solid sprouts and formation of anastomoses. Blind-end endothelial sprouts contain plasma and occasional blood cells which are exposed to the pulsatile force of the heart beat but are unable to circulate due to the lack of blood flow. Formation of loops from the fusion of adjacent sprouts is immediately followed by the establishment of blood flow. Because of the leakiness of the immature sprouts, red blood cells and fibrinogen may extravasate.[18]

(6) Appearance of pericytes coinciding with the maturation of the newly formed microvessels.

(7) Continuous remodeling of the newly formed vasculature.

D. MECHANISMS OF TUMOR ANGIOGENESIS

The formation of new blood vessels is the result of a complex process of interaction between soluble angiogenic regulators, insoluble ECM molecules, and ECM-degrading endothelial enzymes. Soluble regulators of angiogenesis affect endothelial cell migration, proliferation, and ECM digestion. Solid phase regulators (ECM molecules) modulate the

Table 3-1 **Soluble polypeptide regulators of angiogenesis**

Molecule	Molecular Weight (kDa)	Secretion	Endothelial Migration	Endothelial Proliferation
bFGF	18–25	No	+	+
aFGF (ECGF)	17	No	+	+
VEGF (VPF)	45	Yes	+	+
PD-ECGF	45	No	+	+
TGF-alpha	5.5	Yes	+	+
Angiogenin	14.1	Yes	0	0
Angiotropin	4.5	Yes	+	0
TGF-beta	25	Yes	–	–
TNF-alpha	17	Yes	+	–

For abbreviations of growth factors see text. Symbols indicate stimulation (+), no effect (0), or inhibition (–).
(Modified from Klagsburn, M. and D'Amore, P. A., *Annu. Rev. Physiol.*, 53, 217, 1991.)

migratory and proliferative response of endothelial cells to soluble growth factors and play a major role in the morphogenesis of capillary tubes.

1. Soluble Regulators of Tumor Angiogenesis

Angiogenic factors, which are better defined as soluble regulators of angiogenesis because of their diverse mechanisms of action, are for the most part polypeptides that have been isolated from tumors of vascular and nonvascular origin or from normal sources such as the central nervous system, the retina, the pituitary gland, the corpus luteum, and the placenta (Table 1). For a more detailed list of original references on polypeptide regulators of angiogenesis, the reader is referred to comprehensive reviews on the subject.[19,20] Here we give a brief summary of the most salient features of these factors.

a. Fibroblast Growth Factors

Fibroblast growth factors (FGF) are heparin-binding polypeptides capable of stimulating endothelial migration and proliferation, production of ECM degrading enzymes, and angiogenesis both *in vivo* and *in vitro*.[21] Basic FGF (bFGF, cationic molecule with pI of 9.6) and acidic FGF (aFGF, anionic molecule with pI of 5) are the best known members of this family of mitogenic polypeptides, which also includes the products of oncogenes hst (gastric adenocarcinoma), int-2, K-FGF (Kaposi's sarcoma), and FGF-5.[16] bFGF is widely distributed and produced by different cell types including endothelial and smooth muscle cells. aFGF, also known as endothelial cell growth factor (ECGF) is found primarily in the central nervous system, but it can be demonstrated also in endothelial and smooth muscle cells.[22] bFGF and aFGF are intracellular protein with no secretory signal peptide and a virtually unknown mechanism of secretion. One possibility is that they are released after cell injury. In contrast, oncogene-associated FGFs have signal peptides and are probably secreted through conventional pathways.[23] FGFs are mitogenic not only for endothelial but also for other mesenchymal cells.

b. Vascular Endothelial Growth Factor

Vascular endothelial growth factor (VEGF), a dimeric polypeptide initially isolated from cells of the pituitary gland, is expressed in a variety of normal and tumor cells.[24] In contrast to FGF, VEGF has a signal peptide and is secreted. VEGF stimulates specifically endothelial cells and angiogenesis without apparently affecting other cell types. VEGF belongs to the same polypeptide family as vascular permeability factor (VPF), a molecule isolated from tumors, which causes an increase in vascular permeability and angiogenesis.[25] Both VEGF and VPF bind to heparin and have 21 to 24% homology with platelet-derived growth factor (PDGF).

c. Platelet-Derived Endothelial Cell Growth Factor

Platelet-derived endothelial cell growth factor (PD-ECGF), not to be confused with PDGF, is a single-chain specific endothelial mitogen isolated from platelets but present also in fibroblasts and tumor cells.[26] It appears to be the major angiogenic factor in platelets. Like FGF, PD-ECGF has no signal peptide and is sequestered intracellularly. It does not bind to heparin.

d. Transforming Growth Factor Alpha

Transforming growth factor alpha (TGF-alpha) is a small single-chain polypeptide secreted by normal cells such as macrophages and by a variety of tumor cells. TGF-alpha is more angiogenic than epidermal growth factor (EGF), which is 40% homologous to TGF-alpha.[27]

e. Transforming Growth Factor Beta

Transforming growth factor beta (TGF-beta) includes at least five homologous, homodimeric polypeptides (TGF-beta 1, 2, 3, 4, 5). It is secreted as an inactive molecule which can be activated by proteases (plasmin) or acid treatment.[28] Its effect on angiogenesis is complex and incompletely understood. The active form of TGF beta is angiogenic *in vivo*, it inhibits endothelial proliferation in two-dimensional culture, and promotes the reorganization of preexisting endothelial cells with formation of capillary tubes in three-dimensional collagen cultures.[28,29] Its effect on capillary morphogenesis in three-dimensional culture may be mediated by the ECM, which is known to modulate capillary tube formation. Thus, TGF-beta stimulates deposition of ECM and inhibits its degradation. The angiogenic effect of TGF-beta *in vivo* is probably indirect. TGF-beta is chemotactic for monocytes, which in turn release angiogenic factors capable of stimulating endothelial migration and proliferation.[30]

f. Tumor Necrosis Factor-Alpha

Tumor necrosis factor-alpha (TNF-alpha), also known as cachectin for its ability to induce cachexia, is a macrophage-derived polypeptide which plays an important role in inflammatory and immune-mediated processes. TNF-alpha is also produced by some tumor cells. Endothelial effects of TNF-alpha include the induction of class I major histocompatibility antigens, procoagulant activity, interleukin 1, and leukocyte adhesiveness. In addition, TNF-alpha stimulates angiogenesis *in vivo* and endothelial migration and capillary tube formation *in vitro*. Like TGF-beta, TNF-alpha inhibits endothelial proliferation in two-dimensional culture.[31]

g. Angiogenin

Angiogenin, a single-chain polypeptide, originally isolated from an adenocarcinoma cell line, is 68% homologous to pancreatic ribonuclease. In spite of its angiogenic activity *in vivo*, angiogenin does not stimulate endothelial migration or proliferation *in vitro*. It is also found in plasma, lymphocytes, and in the liver.[32]

Besides FGF, VEGF, PD-ECGF, TGFalpha and beta, TNFalpha, and angiogenin, other molecules are likely to contribute to the redundant mechanisms of tumor angiogenesis, which are schematically summarized in Figure 3. Among them, *angiotropin*, a copper-containing polyribonucleo-polypeptide produced by activated monocytes, has been proposed as a mediator of inflammatory angiogenesis.[33] Angiotropin promotes angiogenesis *in vivo*; *in vitro* it promotes endothelial migration and formation of capillary tubes without inducing endothelial proliferation.

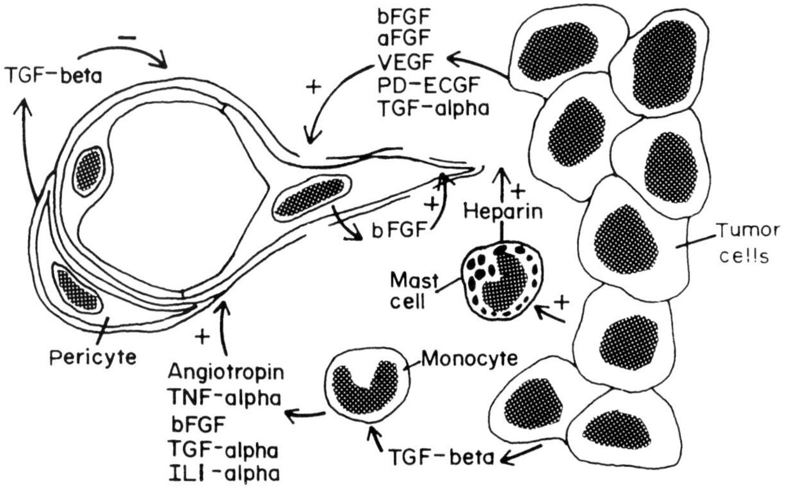

Figure 3-3 Schematic drawing showing putative autocrine and paracrine pathways of activation (+) and inhibition (–) of angiogenesis involving tumor cells, endothelial cells, and accessory cells (pericyte, mast cell, monocyte).

Ceruloplasmin or copper-carrying fragments of ceruloplasmin have been shown to be angiogenic *in vivo.*[34] The role played by copper and ceruloplasmin in angiogenesis is incompletely understood. The growth of brain tumors and their vascular supply is inhibited in copper-depleted animals.[35]

Small molecules such as *endothelial cell stimulating angiogenesis factor, prostaglandins E1* and *E2, and nicotinamide* have been shown to induce angiogenesis *in vivo.*[36]

Heparin, a highly sulfated glycosaminoglycan, potentiates the effect of FGF *in vivo* and probably plays a physiologic role as an angiogenesis co-factor. Heparin is present in the cytoplasmic granules of mast cells and it is found as heparan sulfate proteoglycan on the surface of endothelial cells and in vascular basement membranes. It was the discovery of heparin-affinity chromatography that allowed the purification of potent angiogenic factors from tumors.[37] Heparin binds FGF and may act physiologically as a low affinity receptor for this molecule, which is more soluble and stable when bound to heparin. FGF bound to heparin or to heparan sulfate may undergo conformational changes that would allow the FGF to better interact with its high affinity receptor on the cell surface. The angiogenic activity of heparin may be related to its sulfate groups and does not require the anticoagulant moiety of the molecule.[38] However, the role of heparin in angiogenesis is incompletely understood: it potentiates the angiogenic effect of growth factors but it can also enhance the anti-angiogenic effect of hydrocortisone and other angiostatic steroids.[39]

2. Solid-Phase Regulators of Angiogenesis: Extracellular Matrix Molecules

Quiescent microvessels are enveloped by a sheath of basement membrane and are surrounded by interstitial collagen. Constituents of the microvascular basement membrane include the collagens types IV and V, the heparan sulfate proteoglycan and the glycoproteins laminin, and fibronectin. The interstitial space around the microvascular basement membrane contains the fibrillar collagens type I and III. The microvascular ECM is focally digested during the early stages of angiogenesis and subsequently undergoes complex maturational changes.[40] These changes are likely to play an important role in regulating endothelial migration, proliferation, and organization during angiogenesis.

Capillaries acquire their tubular shape through complex mechano-chemical interactions with the ECM.[41] Rapid formation of capillary tubes can be obtained by culturing endothelial cells on collagen gels[42] or on basement membrane substrates.[43,44] Moreover, angiogenesis can be inhibited both *in vivo* and *in vitro* with inhibitors of collagen metabolism.[45,46]

Angiogenesis can also be inhibited *in vitro* with GRGDS (Gly-Arg-Gly-Asp-Ser), a pentapeptide containing the amino acid sequence RGD (Figure 4) which is present in the cell binding domain of several ECM molecules.[47] RGD-containing peptides interfere with the attachment of endothelial cells to substrates by competing with ECM molecules for their receptors. The RGD effect supports the notion that angiogenesis is an anchorage-dependent process requiring adhesive interactions between endothelial cells and the ECM.

The ECM interacts with growth factors modulating their vasoproliferative effect. For instance, the basement membrane has been shown to store bFGF bound to heparan sulfate molecules. Injury or the secretion of heparan sulfate degrading enzymes from tumor cells may release bFGF, which would then stimulate angiogenesis by interacting with its high affinity receptor on the endothelial cell surface.[48] Moreover, the response of endothelial cells to soluble growth factors can be modulated by modifying, with different concentrations of ECM molecules, the adhesiveness of the substrate on which the cells are cultured.[41] Angiogenesis can be also promoted by fibrin, which accumulates in the provisional ECM of wounds or tumors around leaky microvessels in areas of extravascular activation of coagulation.[49,50] Furthermore, enzymatic degradation of the ECM may play an important role in the angiogenic process. Fragments of ECM molecules such as hyaluronic acid and fibrin have been shown to stimulate angiogenesis and/or endothelial migration.[51,52]

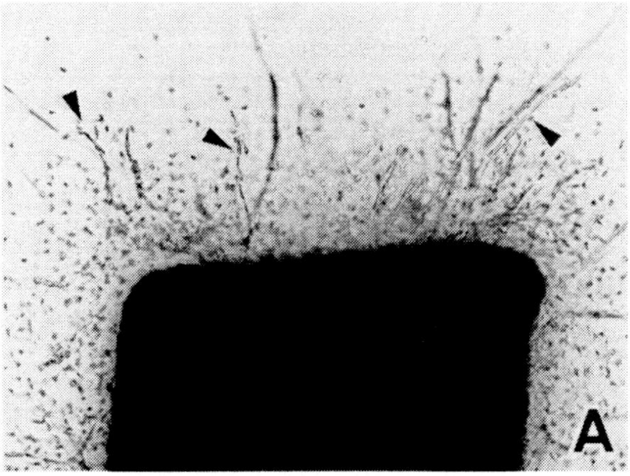

Figure 3-4 Effect of RGD-containing peptide in the serum-free rat aorta model of angiogenesis. Angiogenesis in collagen gel culture is markedly inhibited by the pentapeptide GRGDS (B). In contrast, there are many newly formed microvessels (arrowheads) in the absence of GRGDS (A) and in the presence of GRGES, a control peptide lacking the RGD sequence (C). ×35 *(From Nicosia, R. F. and Bonanno, E., Am. J. Pathol., 138, 829, 1991, with permission.)*

III. THE PATHOLOGY OF VASCULAR TUMORS

Most vascular neoplasms arise in the microcirculation. They are classified as benign or malignant on the basis of morphologic and biologic criteria, such as the degree to which they resemble well-organized microvascular channels, the intensity of proliferative activity, the degree of nuclear pleomorphism of the endothelial cells, and the tendency of the tumor cells to spread locally or systemically. Thus, benign tumors are nonmetastasizing lesions, characterized by their great resemblance to normal microvasculature. Malignant tumors, on the contrary, deviate markedly from the normal; they grow as solid cords of cells containing poorly developed vascular spaces and metastasize at distant sites. Between these two extremes there are tumors of an intermediate malignant grade which are usually locally invasive and form poorly developed vascular channels. Because of their marked heterogeneity in location and degree of differentiation, vascular tumors have an extremely variable clinical behavior.[57]

A. BENIGN VASCULAR TUMORS

1. Hemangioma and Hemangiomatosis

Hemangiomas are localized benign vascular neoplasms. They can be congenital or acquired. When they involve large segments of the body, such as an entire extremity, they are defined as hemangiomatosis.

Hemangiomas are the most common tumors in infancy and childhood and one of the most common benign soft tissue tumors in adults. They are further subdivided into capillary, cavernous, and venous, depending on the dimensions of the vascular spaces formed by the tumor and the thickness of the vascular wall, but admixtures of different types are common.

a. Capillary Hemangiomas

Capillary hemangiomas are vascular tumors composed of small blood vessels resembling capillaries (Figure 6). They occur usually in the skin or subcutaneous tissue and represent by far the largest single group of benign vascular tumors. Congenital lesions are seen most commonly on the head and neck. These tumors usually regress spontaneously by fibrosis during the first decade of life. Depending on their clinical presentation they are further subdivided into juvenile or strawberry hemangioma, acquired tufted hemangioma, and senile hemangioma or cherry hemangioma.

Juvenile angiomas, also known as strawberry hemangiomas because of their elevated reddish appearance, are extremely common. They are usually single but may be multiple and may occur in any part of the body with preferential involvement of the head and neck. They become manifest within a few weeks after birth, rapidly increase in size in about 5 to 6 months and slowly regress over a period of several years leaving a small area of pigmentation. The microscopic appearance reflects the macroscopic evolution. Early lesions are characterized by plump endothelial cells lining small blood vessels, whereas older lesions are composed of vascular spaces lined by flat endothelial cells and separated by a variable amount of connective tissue.

Acquired tufted hemangiomas differ from the juvenile hemangioma only in their clinical presentation. The tumors develop in adult or elderly individuals in the form of slowly growing erythematous skin plaques. Histopathologically they are composed of a mixture of mature and immature capillaries growing in the dermis.

Senile hemangiomas or cherry hemangiomas are red papular lesions measuring few millimeters in diameter, usually distributed over the trunk and extremities. Although they are called senile, they may occur in adolescent life.

b. Cavernous Hemangiomas

Cavernous hemangiomas are composed of large, irregular blood-filled cystic spaces lined by flattened endothelial cells (Figure 7), frequently located in the skin of the face, neck,

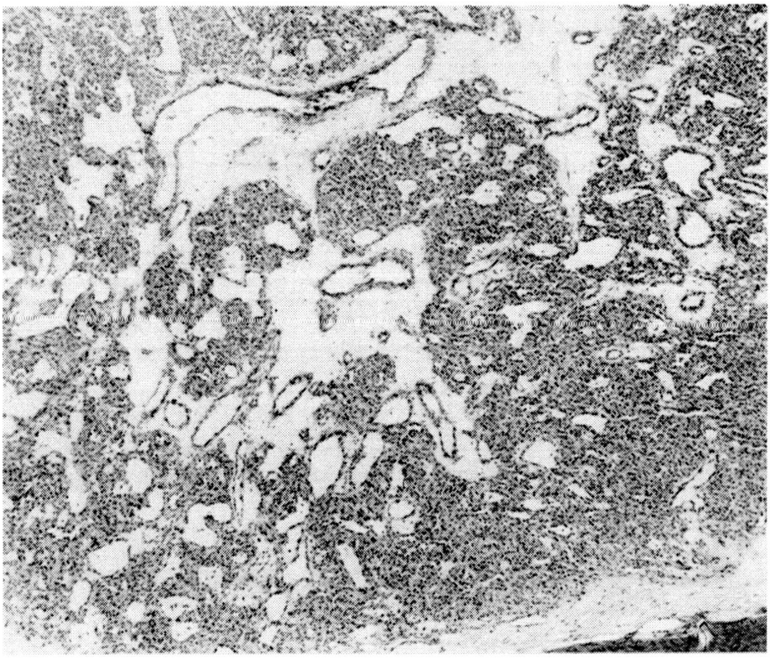

Figure 3-6 Capillary hemangioma of the skin showing a multitude of well differentiated capillaries. Hematoxylin-eosin stain, (HE, ×55).

thorax. They are most common in childhood and may be congenital. Because of their large size and frequent location in deep organs cavernous hemangiomas can compress and destroy adjacent structures requiring surgical treatment.

Cavernous hemangiomas may be associated with multiple enchondromas (Maffucci's syndrome) or with consumption coagulopathy as a result of intralesional thrombosis (Kasabach-Merrit syndrome).

c. Hemangiomatosis

Hemangiomatosis as indicated earlier is a rare condition in which large segments of the body are involved by proliferating blood vessels. Hemangiomatosis probably begins early in intrauterine life when the limb buds form, grow proportionally with the fetus, and at birth affect large areas of the trunk or extremities. Not unexpectedly, hemangiomatosis presents itself during childhood or infancy as swelling, induration, or discoloration of the affected areas. In some individuals it may be associated with hypertrophy of the affected limb. Although most common in the extremities, any site can be affected, including lungs, liver, and other viscera.

The microscopic appearance is not distinctive consisting in a proliferation of small blood vessels of different shapes and sizes that infiltrate the affected tissue. Mortality is high when the lesions are multiple and compress vital structures, or when consumption coagulopathy develops as a result of sequestration of platelets in the abnormal vessels. Pulmonary hypertension may occur when the lungs are involved.

2. Pyogenic Granuloma

Pyogenic granuloma is a polypoid vascular lesion of the skin and mucosal surfaces which is regarded by some as a form of exaggerated granulation tissue, by others as a benign neoplasm. The nonneoplastic nature is suggested by the fact that the lesion often develops after trauma, grows rapidly, and regresses spontaneously. However, the proponents of a

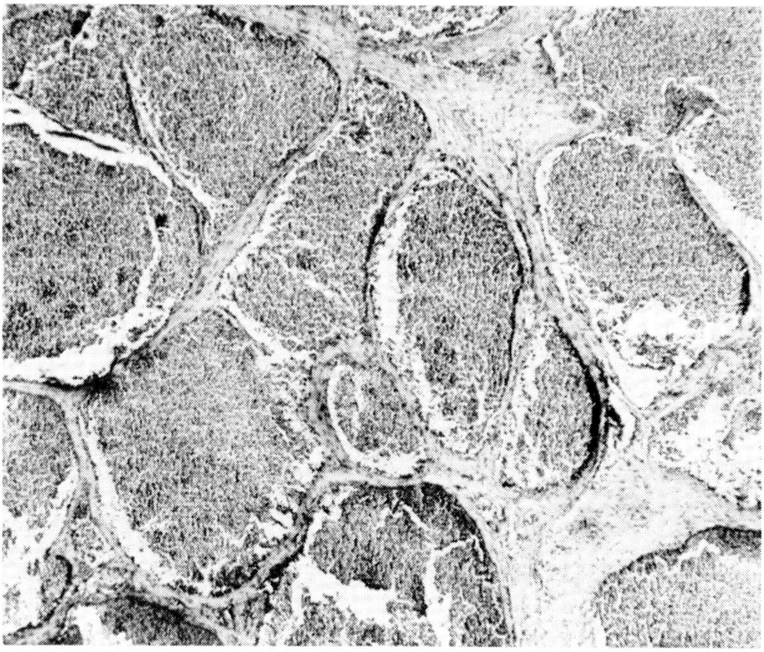

Figure 3-7 Cavernous hemangioma of the liver composed of markedly dilated endothelial-lined vascular channels. (HE, ×35)

neoplastic etiology emphasize the fact that some pyogenic granulomas may recur after surgical excision and form numerous small noncontiguous satellite nodules. Multiple pyogenic granulomas of the skin and oral mucosa have been described in elderly individuals with visceral malignancies, suggesting systemic release of angiogenic factors by nonvascular tumors.[58] Microscopically, pyogenic granuloma is composed of numerous capillaries and venules separated by edematous connective tissue containing acute and chronic inflammatory cells (Figure 8).

Granuloma gravidarum is a pyogenic granuloma occurring in the gingival mucosa of pregnant women. The role of the host's endocrine status on the growth of these lesions is suggested by their spontaneous regression following parturition and their recurrence in subsequent pregnancies.

3. Glomus Tumor

Glomus tumors are rare vascular lesions that occur in both sexes but more frequently in women. They are believed to arise from the glomus body, a specialized form of arteriovenous anastomosis involved in the thermal regulation. These structures have abundant nerve fibers, and are particularly abundant in the dermis of the subungueal regions, the digits and palms. Glomus tumors are blue-red, usually single nodules located in the deep dermis of the upper or lower extremities, most often in the subungueal region. The most common symptom is intense pain triggered by changes in temperature or tactile stimulation. Microscopically, the tumor repeats in varying degrees the structure of the glomus body with a mixture of proliferating blood vessels and glomus cells. Familial occurrence has been reported.[57]

4. Histiocytoid Hemangioma

Histiocytoid or epithelioid hemangiomas are unusual but distinct vascular tumors characterized by a poorly circumscribed proliferation of plump endothelial cells associated

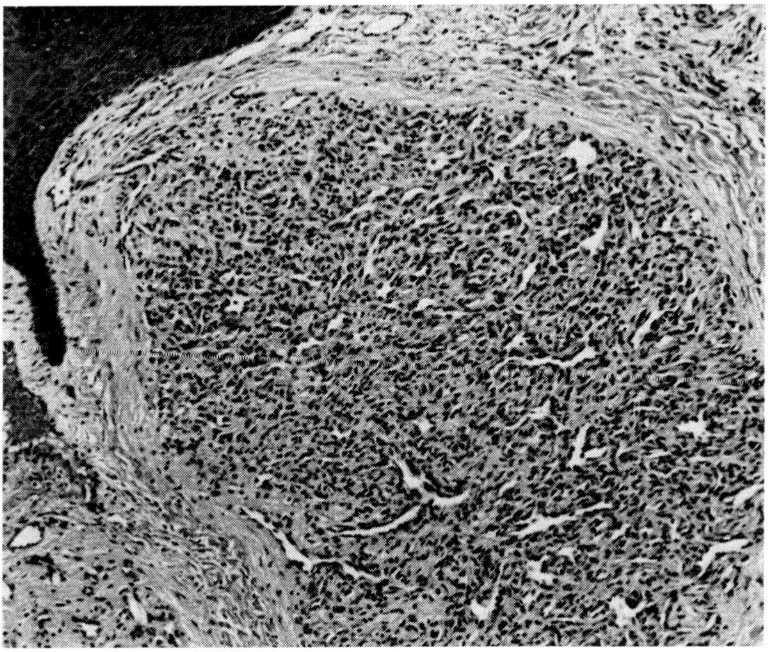

Figure 3-8 Pyogenic granuloma. The tumor is composed of a circumscribed lobulated proliferation of capillaries separated by a matrix containing inflammatory cells. (HE, ×60)

with variable admixture of inflammatory cells. Depending on the histologic features, they have been designated angiolymphoid hyperplasia with eosinophilia, histiocytoid hemangioma, and Kimura's disease.[59] Histiocytotid hemangiomas occur during early to mid-adult life, more often in women, in the form of single or multiple small, dull red, pruritic dermal plaques, usually in the head and neck regions, which may recur or regress spontaneously. Kimura's disease differs from typical histiocytoid hemangioma by its male preponderance, earlier age of development and greater eosinophilia. The characteristic histopathologic feature is that of solid sprouts of plump endothelial cells with large vesicular nuclei and prominent nucleoli. The solid sprouts undergo intracellular vacuolization and eventually form vascular lumens. The vessels are surrounded by a mixture of inflammatory cells including eosinophils. It is not clear whether the inflammation is a primary event triggering vascular proliferation through the release of angiogenic factors or a secondary response of the host's immune system to the vascular proliferation.[57]

B. VASCULAR TUMORS OF BORDERLINE MALIGNANT POTENTIAL

1. Hemangioendothelioma

Hemangioendotheliomas are vascular tumors with the biologic potential of low-grade malignant neoplasms and great morphologic variability. They range from benign hemangiomas with active mitotic activity to tumors composed of ill-demarcated masses of malignant endothelial cells. Since these neoplasms are cured by complete local excision, it is important to differentiate them from the more aggressive angiosarcomas. Three major types of hemangioendotheliomas have been identified: epithelioid hemangioendothelioma, spindle cell hemangioendothelioma, and malignant endovascular papillary hemangioendothelioma (Dabska tumor).[57] Only the epithelioid hemangioendothelioma will be discussed here.

Epithelioid hemangioendothelioma is an angiocentric vascular tumor which affects both sexes equally and occurs at any age but rarely in childhood. The tumor is characterized by solid cords or strands of plump epithelial-like endothelial cells with poorly defined vascular channels. Because of their epithelial-like appearance, in the past these tumors have been confused with peculiar variants of carcinomas. However, with careful microscopic examination, the vascular nature of the tumor and the presence of intracellular spaces containing red blood cells can be detected. Further confirmation of the endothelial nature is provided by the immunohistochemical demonstration of Factor VIII-related antigen (FVIII-RA) and binding of Ulex europaeus lectin. Usually, cellular atypia and mitotic activity are not prominent, but in about one fourth of cases atypical cellular features, necrosis, and mitoses are present.

Tumors with these features have been recognized in a large number of sites. Those occurring in the soft tissue of the head and neck often arise from the wall of a vein. Those occurring in the liver have been associated with the use of oral contraceptives.[60] In the lungs they have been confused with a peculiar variant of bronchioloalveolar carcinoma growing intravascularly and designated intravascular bronchioloalveolar tumor or IVBAT.[61]

The clinical behavior of epithelioid hemangioendothelioma is variable. Most tumors are cured by complete surgical resection but may recur if incompletely excised and about 30% metastasize to regional lymph-nodes, liver, lungs, and bone.

2. Hemangiopericytoma

Stout and Murray[62] have proposed the term hemangiopericytoma to designate a vascularized spindle cell neoplasm which they thought was derived from the pericyte. The pericytic origin of these tumors is a controversial issue since there are no specific cellular features or markers that allow the identification of these cells in a neoplasm. Thus, the recognition of this entity rests only on architectural patterns which are shared by other highly vascularized neoplasms, namely, the presence of tightly packed, basement membrane bound, round to oval cells surrounding thin-walled arborizing vascular channels.

C. MALIGNANT VASCULAR TUMORS

1. Angiosarcoma

Angiosarcomas are relatively rare malignant neoplasms derived from vascular endothelium. Theoretically, malignant tumors arising from vascular endothelium (hemangiosarcomas) should be separated from those of lymphatic endothelial derivation (lymphangiosarcomas). In practice, this distinction is not possible on histological or immunohistochemical grounds because malignant endothelial cells may not express FVIII-RA or other markers specific for nonneoplastic vascular endothelial cells.

Angiosarcomas may exhibit a spectrum of morphologic variants ranging from well differentiated to highly undifferentiated tumors. For these reasons a variety of terms has been used to designate tumors with different degrees of differentiation, i.e., hemangioendothelioma, hemangioblastoma, hemangiosarcoma. Use of these ambiguous terms should be discouraged.[57]

Angiosarcomas comprise less than 1% of all soft tissue sarcomas and may occur in any location. The skin and superficial soft tissue of elderly individuals are most frequently involved whereas the endothelium of large blood vessels rarely becomes neoplastic. The presentation and clinical behavior varies with the location. In general the tumor grows locally, invading vital structures and rapidly spreading to distant sites.

The tumors are characterized microscopically by the presence of irregular, freely anastomosing vascular channels lined by large flat cells with hyperchromatic nuclei (Figure 9). The degree of nuclear pleomorphism and mitotic activity varies with the

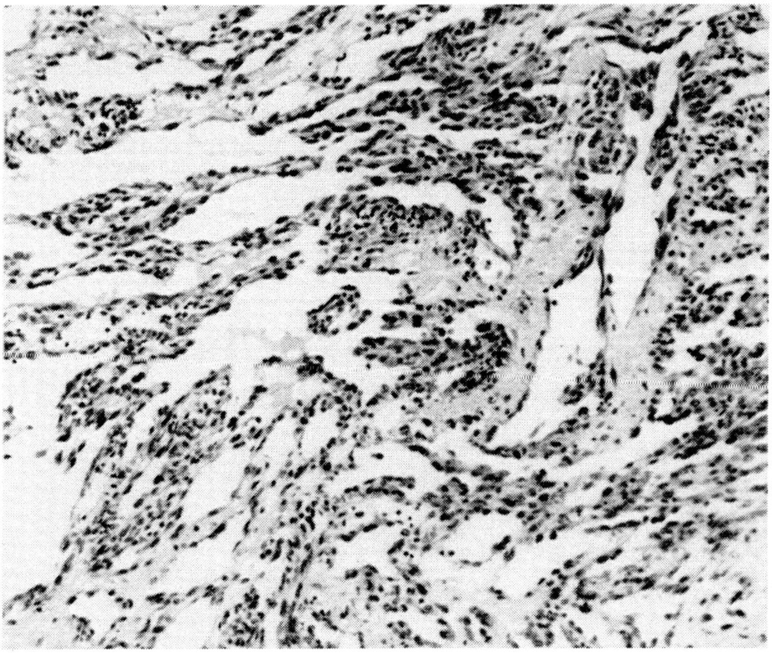

Figure 3-9 Angiosarcoma of the liver in a patient exposed to vinyl chloride. Notice the highly irregular, freely anastomosing vascular channels lined by atypical and hyperchromatic endothelial cells. (HE, ×55)

degree of de-differentiation of the tumor cells. Immunohistochemical and electron microscopic techniques contribute little to the diagnosis of poorly differentiated tumors since demonstration of FVIII-RA is highly variable, binding of Ulex europeaus lectin is nonspecific and typical ultrastructural features, i.e., junctional complexes, basal lamina, cytoplasmic vesicles, and Weibel-Palade bodies may be absent.

Of interest is the relatively frequent occurrence of angiosarcomas or lymphangiosarcomas in extremities afflicted with chronic lymphatic obstruction, as in women who have undergone radical mastectomy for breast carcinoma. Obstruction of lymphatic drainage has been found to often cause a reactive vascular proliferation within regional lymph nodes, called nodal angiomatosis. Development of angiosarcomas in extremities afflicted with chronic lymphatic obstruction has been explained by the combination of reactive vascular proliferation stimulated by local growth factors and loss of immunosurveillance of unstable mutant populations of endothelial cells in limbs with obstructed lymph flow.

Angiosarcomas have been reported following radiation injury from Thorotrast previously used as an intravascular contrast medium[63] or following therapeutic irradiation of benign or malignant lesions.[64] Radiation-induced angiosarcomas have an average latent period of 12 years but the latent period may be longer depending on the dose and modalities of administration.

Among carcinogenic agents in the environment or in the work place, of particular importance is vinyl chloride, used in the production of synthetic rubber. Several cases of hepatic angiosarcomas have been reported in workers employed in the rubber industry.[65] Sporadic cases of angiosarcomas of the liver have been reported in vineyard workers apparently from exposure to arsenic oxide-containing pesticides.[66]

D. KAPOSI'S SARCOMA AND ITS IMITATORS

1. Kaposi's Sarcoma

Kaposi's sarcoma has gained wide publicity in recent years because of its frequent occurrence in homosexual males with acquired immunodeficiency syndrome (AIDS). The tumor was originally recognized in 1872[67] by the Hungarian dermatologist Kaposi who described the presence of a peculiar skin sarcoma in a group of elderly Jewish males. Subsequently, the tumor was recognized in all races but more frequently in older men of eastern European or Mediterranean descent. Currently, four clinical forms of Kaposi's sarcoma are recognized:

a. The Cutaneous European Form

The cutaneous European form, originally described by Kaposi, consisting of multiple red-brown skin plaques or nodules, most commonly located in the skin of the lower extremities. The tumor nodules increase slowly in size and number and usually remain localized to the skin and subcutaneous tissue. They have an erratic course with remissions and recurrences but rarely cause death by spreading to the viscera. This form of the disease is rare in the U.S., accounting for only 0.02% of all malignant tumors. Its peak incidence occurs in the sixth-seventh decade.

b. The African Form

The African form occurs in younger men in equatorial Africa in the same regions where there is a high prevalence of malaria and of Burkitt's lymphoma. In these regions its incidence is high, representing 10% of all malignant tumors. The clinical presentation is similar to the classic European form but in children it has the tendency to spread to cervical, inguinal, and hilar lymph nodes and has a rapidly fatal course.

c. Transplantation-Associated Form

Transplantation-associated form is found in about 4% of renal transplant recipients receiving immunosuppressive therapy. However, the majority of these individuals are also of Jewish or Mediterranean descent.

The disease develops months to a few years after the transplant and is either localized to the skin or systemic. The extent and severity of the disease is correlated to the loss of cellular immunity and the lesions often regress when immuno-suppressive treatment is stopped.

d. AIDS-Associated Form

Homosexual males with AIDS develop cutaneous and visceral Kaposi's sarcoma. In contrast to the classic form of Kaposi, the skin lesions of AIDS patients have no predilection for the lower extremities but occur frequently on the face, nose, and ear lobes. Involvement of the oral mucosa, gastrointestinal wall, lungs, and lymph nodes is common.

In the early phases of the AIDS epidemic the incidence of Kaposi's sarcoma among male homosexuals was nearly 40%; in more recent years the incidence has decreased for unexplained reasons. About a third of the patients with the African and the AIDS-associated forms develop malignant lymphomas.

Regardless of the clinical presentation, all types of Kaposi's sarcoma have a similar microscopic appearance. In the early stages the tumor is characterized by a proliferation of irregular, jagged, thin-walled, vascular spaces lined by endothelial cells (Figure 10). The intervening connective tissue contains sheets of periendothelial cells, extravasated red blood cells, hemosiderin, lymphocytes, and plasma cells. The more advanced nodular lesions consist of strands or nests of plump and spindle shaped cells separated by slit-like spaces (Figure 11) and extravasated red blood cells. Lymphocytes, plasma cells, and dilated thin-walled vessels are present at the periphery of the nodules.

Immunohistochemical studies have yielded equivocal results leading to the suggestion by some that the tumor arises from lymphatic endothelium.[68] Electron microscopic

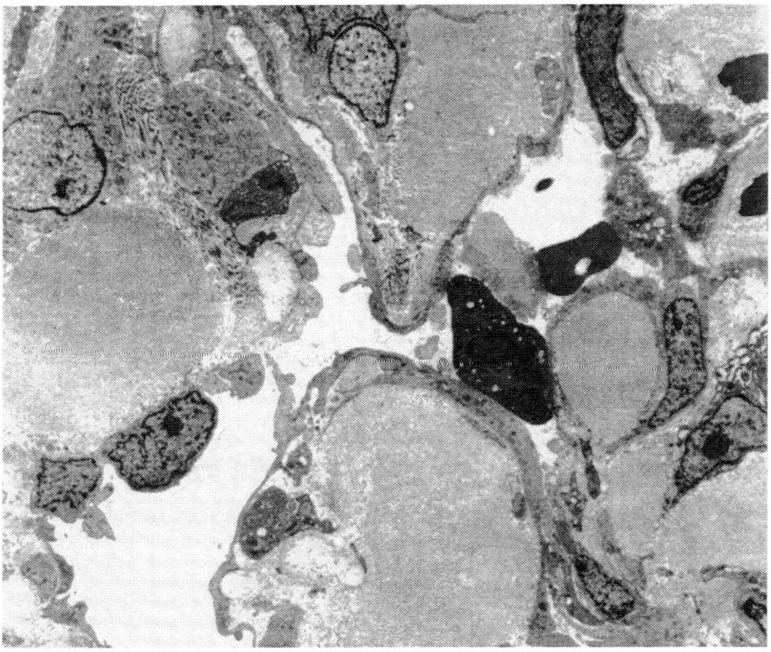

Figure 3-10 Electron micrograph of early lesion of cutaneous Kaposi's sarcoma showing an irregular vascular space lined by endothelial cells that have dissected the collagen bundles of the dermis. (×21,000)

studies of early lesions have lent support to the origin of Kaposi's sarcoma from endothelium (Figures 10 and 12) but have not convincingly resolved the issue of its derivation from vascular or lymphatic vessels.

2. Bacillary Angiomatosis

This angioproliferative lesion has been recently described in men seropositive for human immunodeficiency virus 1 (HIV-1).[69] The tumor was originally designated *epithelioid angiomatosis* because it was composed both of proliferating small blood vessels lined by plump endothelial cells and of cuboidal cells expressing endothelial and histiocytic markers, namely, FVIII-RA and alpha-1 anti-chymotripsin. More recently, the lesion has been reclassified as *bacillary angiomatosis* because of the frequent association of the proliferating vessels with bacilli that can be visualized with the Warthin-Starry silver stain. The microorganisms have been shown to share antigenic characteristics with the bacteria causing cat-scratch disease.[70]

The clinical behavior of this vascular proliferation is variable. Usually there are multiple purplish nodules over the skin of the trunk, face, neck, and extremities. In other cases widespread visceral involvement may be present and it may be associated with disseminated intravascular coagulation, or compression of vital organs. Spontaneous regression of the lesions has been reported.

Bacillary angiomatosis has been confused with Kaposi's sarcoma but it is now apparent that HIV seropositive individuals with or without AIDS develop a variety of vascular lesions ranging from telangiectases to Kaposi's sarcoma. It is likely that these vascular proliferations are pathogenetically related to the local or systemic release of angiogenic factors by endothelial or accessory cells infected either with the HIV-1 virus[71]

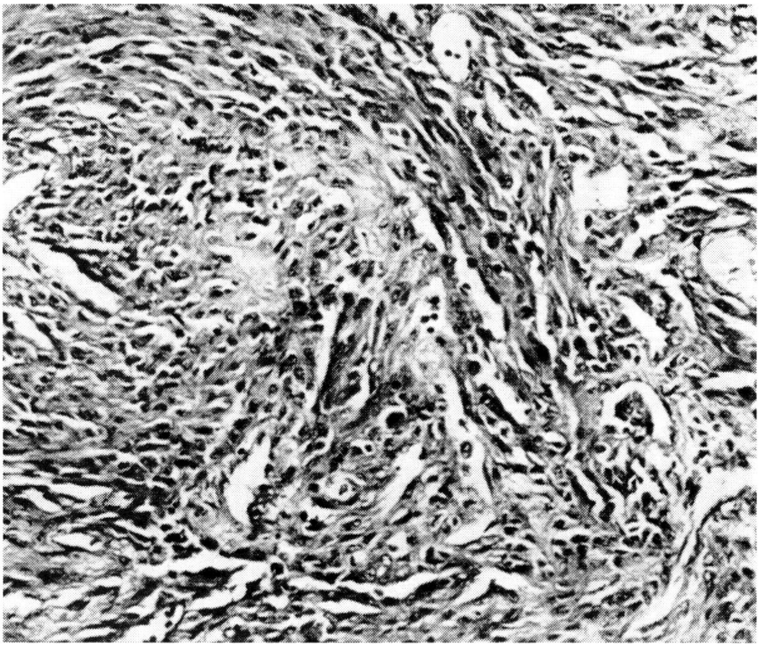

Figure 3-11 Kaposi's sarcoma metastatic to lung. The tumor is composed of interlacing bundles of malignant spindle cells and slit-like vascular spaces containing occasional red blood cells. (HE, ×300)

or with other microorganisms as a result of the depressed immune response caused by the HIV infection.

3. Vascular Neoplasia Mimicking Kaposi's Sarcoma

Several cases of vascular neoplasia with histologic features closely resembling Kaposi's sarcoma have been recently reported in immunocompetent HIV-negative individuals with either benign angiofollicular hyperplasia (Castleman's Disease)[72] or malignant lymphoma.[73] The striking microscopic feature of these lesions is the close association between proliferating vessels lined by spindle-shaped endothelial cells and lymphoid cells. In two of the reported cases the vascular lesions behaved aggressively and the patients died with widespread metastases.[72] This association between microvascular proliferation and lymphoid hyperplasia or neoplasia may be mediated by angiogenic factors released by lymphoid cells. Alternatively, neoplastic microvascular endothelial cells might stimulate the growth and differentiation of lymphocytes.

IV. CONTRIBUTION OF ANGIOGENIC MODELS TO THE UNDERSTANDING OF VASCULAR TUMOR BIOLOGY

In recent years, the transfer of genetic information into embryos or cells and the development of *in vivo* and *in vitro* models of angiogenesis have provided new insights into the pathogenesis of vascular tumors.

Transgenic and chimeric mice expressing the polyoma virus mT oncogene developed multiple cavernous hemangiomas.[74] Montesano et al. observed that mT-expressing endothelioma cells formed cystic structures in fibrin gel culture resembling the dilated

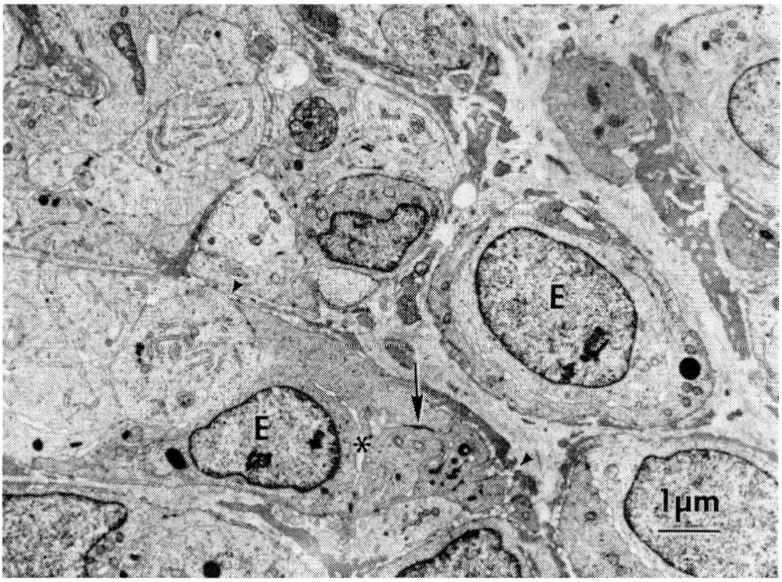

Figure 3-12 Electron micrograph of Kaposi's sarcoma. The tumor is composed of vascular spaces lined by plump endothelial cells (E) rich in cell organelles. The vessels have slit-like lumina (asterisk) and incomplete basal lamina (arrowheads). The endothelial cells show well-developed junctional complexes (arrow). (×14,000)

vascular spaces of the hemangiomas *in vivo*.[75] They also found that neutralization of the endothelioma cells' excess proteolytic activity with serine protease inhibitors corrected the tendency of these cells to form cysts and instead allowed formation of small endothelial tubes that resembled normal capillaries. Formation of cysts by mT-expressing endothelial cells was attributed to excessive production of U-PA and a decreased production of plasminogen activator inhibitors, which resulted in excessive fibrinolysis.

Physical models of morphogenesis predict that the shape of a biological structure is the result of a balance of stimulatory and inhibitory stimuli.[14,76] Pattern-generating systems such as developing microvessels can theoretically be explained if there is a short range stimulatory effect balanced by a wider range inhibitory effect. According to this model, activation at the tip of a growing microvascular sprout should be balanced by a diffuse lateral inhibitory effect of enzymatic activity along the trailing part of the sprout. The observations by Montesano et al.[75] with the polyoma virus mT-induced hemangioma are in favor of this hypothesis and suggest that an uncontrolled degradation of the ECM during angiogenesis may result in the formation of vascular cysts rather than small capillary tubes. A similar mechanism may be responsible for the naturally occurring cavernous hemangiomas, the telangiectases, and for the giant capillaries observed in tumors of nonvascular origin.

Experimental studies on Kaposi's sarcoma are providing new clues concerning the autocrine and paracrine mechanisms that regulate the growth of vascular tumors. Transgenic mice carrying the HIV-1 tat gene developed Kaposi's sarcoma-like lesions.[77,78] Surprisingly, the tat gene was expressed in the skin of the animals but not in the Kaposi's sarcoma cells. *In vitro* studies showed that the tat protein stimulated growth of Kaposi's sarcoma cells suggesting that the proliferation of spindle cells in Kaposi's sarcoma might be mediated by virally encoded growth factor-like proteins. Moreover, Kaposi's sarcoma cells could amplify the proliferative response to the HIV-1 tat protein by stimulating their own growth and the growth of normal cells (endothelial, smooth muscle, and fibroblasts) with a variety of growth factors and cytokines. Recently, Kaposi's sarcoma-like lesions have been produced by injecting nude mice with SV-40 T-antigen-transformed endothelial cells.[79] A subpopulation of tumor cells in these lesions did not contain SV 40 T antigen supporting the hypothesis that Kaposi's sarcoma may form as a result of stimulation and recruitment of host endothelial cells by growth factors secreted by endothelial or other cells altered by viral infection.

The mechanism of growth stimulation by the HIV-encoded tat protein is virtually unknown. A possible clue comes from the observation that the tat protein contains an RGD sequence and binds to cells in an RGD-dependent manner.[80] If the RGD sequence is important for the function of the tat protein, RGD-containing peptides could be designed to competitively inhibit the binding of tat to Kaposi's sarcoma cells and abolish its growth-promoting effects.[81]

The study of Kaposi's sarcoma is also disclosing possible mechanisms through which endothelial cells may undergo uncontrolled growth. The isolation from Kaposi's sarcoma of a gene coding for an FGF-like growth factor with signal peptide sequence (K-FGF) suggests that unregulated proliferation of blood vessels in some tumors may be mediated by FGF-like growth factors, which by carrying a signal peptide are freely secreted through conventional pathways. This is in contrast with aFGF and bFGF, whose release into the extracellular space may be more tightly controlled due to the lack of a signal peptide. Similar mechanisms may also operate in tumors of nonvascular origin that express FGF-like growth factors with signal peptide sequences.[23]

A novel approach to the study of vasoformative tumors comes from bacillary angiomatosis, a benign Kaposi's sarcoma-like vascular lesion associated with bacterial infection and characterized by marked vascular proliferation. Because of their association with newly formed microvessels, bacteria found in these lesions have been proposed as possible sources of angiogenic factors. A factor that stimulates endothelial proliferation and t-PA production *in vitro* and angiogenesis *in vivo* has been isolated from *Bartonella bacilliformis*, a motile intracellular bacterium that causes Verruga peruana, a south american vasoproliferative dermal eruption that resembles bacillary angiomatosis.[82]

V. CONCLUSIONS AND FUTURE DIRECTIONS

In this chapter we have examined tumor angiogenesis and vascular tumors, in an attempt to apply current hypotheses on angiogenic mechanisms to the pathogenesis of vasoproliferative neoplasias. Recently developed experimental models of vascular tumors represent a new area of research for the endothelial biologist interested in how growth, maturation, and regression of blood vessels are altered by neoplastic transformation. Tumors such as hemangiomas, which have the ability to independently grow but also to spontaneously regress, are offering a new opportunity to investigate the molecular mechanisms that turn angiogenesis on and off. New questions are being raised by the study of angiogenesis in vascular tumors.

The observation that unregulated degradation of the ECM is responsible for the formation of cystically dilated vessels in experimental hemangiomas suggests that during physiologic angiogenesis this process is tightly controlled and localized, possibly at the advancing tip of the endothelial sprout. But, how do microvessels accomplish the task of localized degradation of the ECM required for sprouting? Do microvessel-derived bFGF and TGFbeta, which have opposite effects on endothelial cell migration, proliferation, and enzymatic activity, cooperate through intracrine, autocrine, or paracrine mechanisms to ensure an adequate temporal and spatial modulation of activatory and inhibitory stimuli? What turns angiogenesis off during wound healing or in hemangiomas? Can experimental hemangiomas be used to study the mechanisms of vascular regression? Are hemangiomas the result of a local dysfunction of the autocrine and paracrine mechanisms that normally regulate microvascular quiescence and proliferation? Which growth factors are responsible for the uncontrolled angiogenesis in vascular tumors? Is the release of FGF from injured microvascular cells responsible for the formation of pyogenic granulomas after traumas? Does the expression of freely secreted FGF in Kaposi's sarcoma or in tumors of nonvascular origin correlate with the transition from a preneoplastic to a neoplastic state and with tumor progression? What is the role of accessory cells such as mast cells, monocytes, and pericytes in the growth and regression of vascular tumors? Can angiogenesis in hemangiomas or Kaposi's sarcoma be suppressed by inhibiting the attachment of endothelial cells to the ECM with RGD peptide analogues? The recent report that pulmonary angiomatosis can be treated with alpha-interferon, an inhibitor of angiogenesis[83] suggests that vascular tumors may be fertile ground for the clinical application of drugs designed to specifically interfere with basic mechanisms of the angiogenic process.

ACKNOWLEDGMENT

This work was supported in part by Grants HL-43392 and HL-32482 from the NHLB1.

REFERENCES

1. **Folkman, J. and Cotran, R.,** Relation of vascular proliferation to tumor growth, *Int. Rev. Exp. Pathol.,* 16, 207, 1976.
2. **Weidner, N., Semple, J. P., Welch, W. R., and Folkman, J.,** Tumor angiogenesis and metastasis: correlation in invasive breast carcinoma, *N. Engl. J. Med.,* 324, 1, 1991.
3. **Ziche, M. and Gullino, P. M.,** Angiogenesis and neoplastic progression *in vitro*, *JNCI*, 69, 483, 1982.
4. **Brem, S. S., Jensen, H. M., and Gullino, P. M.,** Angiogenesis as a marker of preneoplastic lesions of the human breast, *Cancer*, 41, 239, 1978.
5. **Folkman, J., Watson, K., Ingber, D., and Hanahan, D.,** Induction of angiogenesis during the transition from hyperplasia to neoplasia, *Nature*, 339, 58, 1989.
6. **Brien, S. E., Zagzag, D., and Brem, S.,** Rapid in situ cellular kinetics of intracerebral tumor angiogenesis using a monoclonal antibody to bromodeoxyuridine, *Neurosurgery*, 25, 715, 1989.
7. **Ausprunk, D. H., Falterman, K., and Folkman, J.,** The sequence of events in the regression of corneal capillaries, *Lab. Invest.,* 38, 284, 1978.
8. **Folkman, J.,** What is the evidence that tumors are angiogenesis-dependent?, *JNCI*, 82, 4, 1990.
9. **Nicosia, R. F., Tchao, R., and Leighton, J.,** Angiogenesis-dependent tumor spread in reinforced fibrin clot culture, *Cancer Res.*, 43, 2159, 1983.
10. **Warren, B. A.,** The vascular morphology of tumors, in *Tumor Blood Circulation: Angiogenesis, Vascular Morphology and Blood Flow of Experimental and Human Tumors*, Peterson, H. I., Ed., CRC Press, Boca Raton, FL, 1979, chap. 1.
11. **Wang, W. and Campiche, M.,** Microvasculature of human colorectal epithelial tumors, *Virchows Arch. Pathol. Anat.*, 397, 131, 1982.
12. **Egawa, J., Ishioka, K., and Ogata, T.,** Vascular structure of experimental tumours, *Acta Radiol. Oncol.,* 18, 367, 1978.
13. **Skinner, S. A., Tutton, P. J., and O'Brien, P. E.,** Microvascular architecture of experimental colon tumors in the rat, *Cancer Res.,* 50, 2411, 1990.
14. **Waxman, A. M.,** Blood vessel growth as a problem in morphogenesis: a physical theory, *Microvasc. Res.,* 22, 32, 1981.

15. **Cavallo, T., Sade, R., Folkman, J., and Cotran, R.,** Ultrastructural autoradiographic studies of the early vasoproliferative response in tumor angiogenesis, *Am. J. Pathol.,* 70, 345, 1973.
16. **D'Amore, P. and Thompson, R. W.,** Mechanisms of angiogenesis, *Ann. Rev. Physiol.,* 49, 453, 1987.
17. **Furcht, L. T.,** Critical factors controlling angiogenesis: cell products, cell matrix, and growth factors, *Lab. Invest.,* 55, 505, 1986.
18. **Schoefl, G. I.,** Studies on inflammation. III. Growing capillaries: their structure and permeability, *Virchows Arch. Pathol. Anat.,* 337, 97, 1963.
19. **Klagsburn, M. and D'Amore, P. A.,** Regulators of angiogenesis, *Annu. Rev. Physiol.,* 53, 217, 1991.
20. **Blood, C. H. and Zetter, B. R.,** Tumor interactions with the vasculature: angiogenesis and tumor metastasis, *Biochim. Biophys. Acta,* 1032, 89, 1990.
21. **Montesano, R., Vassalli, J. D., Baird, A., Guillemin, R., and Orci, L.,** Basic fibroblast growth factor induces angiogenesis *in vitro*, *Proc. Natl. Acad. Sci. U.S.A.,* 83, 7297, 1986.
22. **Speir, E., Sasse, J., Shrivastav, S., and Casscells, W.,** Culture-induced increase in acidic and basic fibroblast growth factor activities and their association with the nuclei of vascular endothelial and smooth muscle cells, *J. Cell. Physiol.,* 147, 362, 1991.
23. **Rogelj, S., Weinberg, R. A., Fanning, P., and Klagsburn, M.,** Characterization of tumors produced by signal peptide-basic fibroblast growth factor-transformed cells, *J. Cell. Biochem.,* 39, 13, 1989.
24. **Ferrara, N. and Henzel, W. J.,** Pituitary follicular cells secrete a novel heparin-binding growth factor specific for vascular endothelial cells, *Biochem. Biophys. Res. Commun.,* 161, 851, 1989.
25. **Connolly, D. T., Heuvelman, D. M., Nelson, R., Olander, J. V., Eppley, B. L., et al.,** Tumor vascular permeability factor stimulates endothelial cell growth and angiogenesis, *J. Clin. Invest.,* 84, 1478, 1989.
26. **Usuki, K., Heldin, N. E., Miyazono, K., Ishikawa, F., Takaku, F., et al.,** Production of platelet-derived endothelial cell growth factor by normal and transformed human cells in culture, *Proc. Natl. Acad. Sci. U.S.A.,* 86, 7427, 1989.
27. **Schreiber, A. B., Winkler, M. E., and Dernick, R.,** Transforming growth factor-alpha: a more potent angiogenic mediator than epidermal growth factor, *Science,* 232, 1250, 1986.
28. **Sporn, M. B. and Roberts, A. B.,** Peptide growth factors are multifunctional, *Nature,* 332, 217, 1988.
29. **Madri, J. A., Pratt, B. M., and Tucker, A. M.,** Phenotypic modulation of endothelial cells by TGF-beta depends upon the composition and organization of the extracellular matrix, *J. Cell Biol.,* 106, 1375, 1988.
30. **Wahl, S. M., Hunt, D. A., Wakefield, I. M., McCartney-Francis, N., Wahl, I. M., et al.,** Transforming growth factor beta induces monocyte chemotaxis and growth factor production, *Proc. Natl. Acad. Sci. U.S.A.,* 84, 5788, 1987.
31. **Leibovich, S. J., Polverini, P. J., Shepard, H. M., Wiseman, D. M., Shively, V., and Nuseir, N.,** Macrophage-induced angiogenesis is mediated by tumor necrosis factor-alpha, *Nature,* 329, 630, 1987.
32. **Fett, J. W., Strydom, D. J., Lobb, R. F., Alderman, E. M., Bethune, J. L., et al.,** Isolation and characterization of angiogenin an angiogenic protein from human carcinoma cells, *Biochemistry,* 24, 5480, 1985.
33. **Hockel, M., Jung, W., Vaupel, P., Rabes, H., Khaledpour, C., and Wissler, J. H.,** Purified monocyte-derived angiogenic sustance (angiotropin) induces controlled angiogenesis associated with regulated tissue proliferation in rabbit skin, *J. Clin. Invest.,* 82, 1075, 1988.

34. **Raju, K. S., Alessandri, G., Ziche, M., and Gullino, P. M.,** Ceruloplasmin, copper ions and angiogenesis, *JNCI*, 69, 1183, 1982.
35. **Brem, S., Zagzag, D., Tsanaclis, A. M. C., Gately, S., Elkouby, M. P., and Brien, S. E.,** Inhibition of angiogenesis and tumor growth in the brain. Suppression of endothelial cell turnover by penicillamine and the depletion of copper, an angiogenic factor, *Am. J. Pathol.,* 137, 1121, 1990.
36. **Odedra, R. and Weiss, J. B.,** Low molecular weight angiogenic factors, *Pharmacol. Ther.,* 49, 111, 1991.
37. **Shing, Y., Folkman, J., Sullivan, R., Butterfield, C., Murray, J., and Klagsburn, M.,** Heparin affinity: purification of a tumor capillary endothelial cell growth factor, *Science,* 223, 543, 1984.
38. **Yayon, A., Klagsburn, M., Esko, J. D., Leder, P., and Ornitz, D. M.,** Cell surface, heparin-like molecules are required for binding of basic fibroblast growth factor to its high affinity receptor, *Cell*, 64, 841, 1991.
39. **Folkman, J.,** Regulation of angiogenesis: a new function of heparin, *Biochem. Pharmacol.,* 34, 905, 1985.
40. **Nicosia, R. F. and Madri, J. A.,** The microvascular extracellular matrix: developmental changes during angiogenesis in the aortic ring-plasma clot model, *Am. J. Pathol.,* 128, 78, 1987.
41. **Ingber, D. E. and Folkman, J.,** How does extracellular matrix control capillary morphogenesis?, *Cell*, 58, 803, 1989.
42. **Montesano, R., Orci, L., and Vassalli, P.,** *In vitro* rapid organization of endothelial cells into capillary-like networks is promoted by collagen matrices, *J. Cell Biol.,* 97, 1648, 1983.
43. **Madri, J. A. and Williams, S. K.,** Capillary endothelial cell cultures: phenotypic modulation by matrix components, *J. Cell Biol.,* 97, 153, 1983.
44. **Kubota, Y., Kleinman, H. K., Martin, G. R., and Lawley, T. J.,** Role of laminin and basement membrane in the morphological differentiation of human endothelial cells into capillary-like structures, *J. Cell Biol.,* 107, 1589, 1988.
45. **Ingber, D. E. and Folkman, J.,** Inhibition of angiogenesis through modulation of collagen metabolism, *Lab. Invest.,* 59, 44, 1988.
46. **Nicosia, R. F., Belser, P., Bonanno, E., and Diven, J.,** Regulation of angiogenesis *in vitro* by collagen metabolism, *In Vitro Cell. Dev. Biol.,* 27A, 961, 1991.
47. **Nicosia, R. F. and Bonanno, E.,** Inhibition of angiogenesis *in vitro* by Arg-Gly-Asp-containing synthetic peptide, *Am. J. Pathol.,* 138, 829, 1991.
48. **Vlodavsky, I., Fuks, Z., Rivka, I. M., Bashkin, P., Levi, E., Korner, G., Bar-Shavit, R., and Klagsburn, M.,** Extracellular matrix-resident basic fibroblast growth factor: implication for the control of angiogenesis, *J. Cell. Biochem.,* 45, 167, 1991.
49. **Dvorak, H. F.,** Tumors: wounds that do not heal, *N. Engl. J. Med.,* 315, 1650, 1986.
50. **Nicosia, R. F. and Ottinetti, A.,** Growth of microvessels in serum-free matrix culture of rat aorta: a quantitative assay of angiogenesis *in vitro*, *Lab. Invest.*, 63, 115, 1990.
51. **Thompson, W. D., Campbell, R., and Evans, T.,** Fibrin degradation and angiogenesis: quantitative analysis of the angiogenic response in the chick chorioallantoic membrane, *J. Pathol.,* 145, 27, 1985.
52. **West, D. C., Hampson, I., Arnold, F., and Kumar, S.,** Angiogenesis induced by degradation products of hyaluronic acid, *Science*, 228, 1324, 1985.
53. **Moscatelli, D. and Rifkin, D. B.,** Membrane and matrix localization of proteinases: a common theme in tumor cell invasion and angiogenesis, *Biochim. Biophys. Acta*, 948, 67, 1988.
54. **BenEzra, D., Hemo, I., and Maftzir, G.,** *In vivo* angiogenic activity of interleukins, *Arch. Ophtalmol.,* 108, 573, 1990.

55. **Lutty, G. A., Liu, S. A., and Prendergast, R. A.,** Angiogenic lymphokines of activated T-cell origin., *Inv. Ophtal. Visual Sci.*, 24, 1595, 1983.
56. **Sato, N., Sawasaki, Y., Senoo, A., Fuse, Y., Hirano, Y., and Goto, T.,** Development of capillary networks from rat microvascular endothelial fragments *in vitro*: the role of myofibroblastic cells, *Microvasc. Res.*, 33, 194, 1987.
57. **Enzinger, F. M. and Weiss, S. W.,** *Soft Tissue Tumors,* C. V. Mosby, St. Louis, MO, 1988.
58. **Nappi, O. and Wick, N. R.,** Disseminated lobular capillary hemangioma (pyogenic granuloma): a clinico-pathologic study of two cases, *Am. J. Dermatopathol.,* 8, 379, 1986.
59. **Rosai, J., Gold, J., and Landy, R.,** The histiocytoid hemangioma: a unifying concept embracing several previously described entities of skin, soft tissue, large vessels, bone and heart, *Human Pathol.,* 10, 707, 1979.
60. **Dean, P. J., Haggitt, R. C., and O'Hara, C. J.,** Malignant epithelioid hemangioendothelioma of the liver in young women. Relationship to oral contraceptive use, *Am. J. Surg. Pathol.,* 10, 695, 1985.
61. **Dail, D. H., Liebow, A. A., and Gmelich, J. T.,** Intravascular, bronchiolar and alveolar tumors of the lung (IVBAT). An analysis of twenty cases of a peculiar sclerosing endothelial tumor, *Cancer,* 51, 451, 1983.
62. **Stout, A. P. and Murray, M. R.,** Hemangiopericytoma, a vascular tumor featuring Zimmermann's pericytes, *Ann. Surg.,* 116, 26, 1942.
63. **Ito, Y., Kojiro, M., Nakashima, T., and Nori, T.,** Pathomorphologic characteristics of 102 cases of Thorotrast-related hepatocellular carcinoma, cholangiocarcinoma, and hepatic angiosarcoma, *Cancer*, 62, 1153, 1988.
64. **Nanus, D. M., Kelsen, D., and Clark, D. G. C.,** Radiation-induced angiosarcoma, *Cancer*, 60, 777, 1987.
65. **Thomas, L. B. and Popper, H.,** Pathology of angiosarcoma of the liver among vinyl chloride-polyvinyl chloride workers, *Ann. N.Y. Acad. Sci.,* 246, 268, 1975.
66. **Pimentel, J. C. and Menezes, A. P.,** Liver disease in vineyard sprayers, *Gastroenterology*, 72, 275, 1977.
67. **Kaposi, M.,** Idiopatisches multiples Pigmentsarkom der Haut, *Arch. Dermatol. Syphil.,* 4, 265, 1872.
68. **Dorfman, R. F.,** Kaposi's sarcoma revisited, *Human Pathol.,* 15, 1013, 1984.
69. **Cockerell, C. J., Whitlow, M. A., Webster, G. F., and Friedman-Kien, A. E.,** Epithelioid angiomatosis: a distinct vascular disorder in patients with the acquired immunodeficiency syndrome or AIDS-related complex, *Lancet,* Sept 19(2), 654, 1987.
70. **Koehler, J. E., Le Boit, P. E., Egbert, B. M., and Berger, T. G.,** Cutaneous vascular lesions and disseminated cat-scratch disease in patients with the acquired immunodeficiency syndrome (AIDS) and AIDS-related complex, *Ann. Int. Med.,* 109, 449, 1988.
71. **Roth, W. K.,** HIV-associated Kaposi's sarcoma: new developments in epidemiology and molecular pathology, *J. Cancer Res. Clin. Oncol.,* 117, 186, 1991.
72. **Gerald, W., Kostianovsky, M., and Rosai, J.,** Development of vascular neoplasia in Castleman's disease, *Am. J. Surg. Pathol.,* 14, 603, 1990.
73. **Zerri, L., Guigon, V., Lepidi, H., Horschowski, N., Lejeune, C., and Hassoun, J.,** Lymphadenopathic tumor exhibiting intermingled features of Kaposi's sarcoma, malignant lymphoma and angiofollicular hyperplasia, *Arch. Pathol. Lab. Med.,* 115, 1162, 1991.
74. **Bautch, V. L., Toda, S., Hassell, J. A., and Hanahan, D.,** Endothelial cell tumors develop in transgenic mice carrying the polyoma virus middle-T oncogene, *Cell*, 51, 529, 1987.

75. **Montesano, R., Pepper, M. S., Mohle-Steinlein, U., Risau, W., Wagner, E. F., and Orci, L.,** Increased proteolytic activity is responsible for the aberrant morphogenetic behavior of endothelial cells expressing the middle T oncogene, *Cell*, 62, 435, 1990.
76. **Gierer, A. and Meinhardt, H.,** Biological pattern formation involving lateral inhibition, *Lect. Math. Life Sci.*, 7, 163, 1974.
77. **Vogel, J., Hinrichs, S. H., Reynolds, R. K., Luciw, P. A., and Jay, G.,** The HIV tat gene induces dermal lesions resembling Kaposi's sarcoma in transgenic mice, *Nature*, 335, 606, 1988.
78. **Ensoli, B., Barillari, G., and Gallo, R. C.,** Pathogenesis of AIDS-associated Kaposi's sarcoma, *Hematol./Oncol. Clin. N. Am.*, 5(2), 281, 1991.
79. **O'Connell, K., Landman, G., Farmer, E., and Edidin, M.,** Endothelial cells transformed by SV 40 T antigen cause Kaposi's sarcomalike tumors in nude mice, *Am. J. Pathol.*, 139, 743, 1991.
80. **Brake, D. A., Debouck, C., and Biesecker, G.,** Identification of an Arg-Gly-Asp (RGD) cell adhesion site in human immunodeficiency virus type I transactivation protein, tat, *J. Cell Biol.*, 111, 1275, 1990.
81. **Ruoslathi, E.,** Integrins, *J. Clin. Invest.*, 87, 1, 1991.
82. **Garcia, F. U., Wojta, J., Broadley, K. N., Davidson, J. M., and Hoover, R.,** *Bartonella bacilliformis* stimulates endothelial cells *in vitro* and is angiogenic *in vivo*, *Am. J. Pathol.*, 136, 1125, 1990.
83. **White, C. W.,** Treatment of hemangiomatosis with recombinant interferon alfa, *Sem. Hematol.*, 27(3) (Suppl. 4), 15, 1990.

Chapter 4

Hypertension

Russell L. Prewitt, Donna H. Wang, and Michael A. Hill

CONTENTS

I. IMPORTANCE OF THE MICROCIRCULATION IN HYPERTENSION

A. CONTRIBUTION TO VASCULAR RESISTANCE

1. Definitions and Nomenclature

Although essential hypertension and several forms of experimental hypertension are most likely of renal origin,[1] elevated total peripheral resistance becomes the hallmark of established hypertension. A major portion of vascular resistance resides in the microcirculation and it is of interest to determine the extent and mechanism whereby these vessels contribute to elevations in peripheral vascular resistance.

0-8493-4547-2/94/$0.00+$.50

The resistance vessels, the arterioles and small arteries, are the site of blood flow control due to the possession of a large fraction of the adjustable vascular resistance. For comparisons between hypertensive and normotensive subjects, it is essential to classify the arterioles according to their position in the network. This varies with the different organs, but it is fairly well established for skeletal muscle, a tissue widely studied in hypertensive animals.[2,3] The feeding arteries to muscles of rats are often near 100 μm in diameter and are designated first-order arterioles, or 1As. Branches from the 1A, designated second-order or 2As, form an arcading network. Transversely branching arterioles which form terminal arborizations are designated third-order or 3As. Fourth-order branches (4As) from the 3As give rise to capillaries or sometimes fifth-order branches.

2. Pressure Profiles

The series distribution of resistance through an organ can be determined by the drop in pressure across each subsequent branch. There are significant differences in the pressure profiles between various organs and even between different skeletal muscles, precluding classification of resistance vessels on the basis of vessel size alone. The cerebral[4] and coronary[5] circulations have large pressure drops above the level of the microcirculation, while cat skeletal muscle has approximately a 10% pressure drop in vessels larger than 115 μm.[6-8] Although early studies[9] of pressure profiles in spontaneously hypertensive rat (SHR) and Kyoto Wistar rat (WKY) cremaster muscle indicated a nearly 60% drop in pressure above the 1A, recent studies[10,11] have demonstrated that the pressures were decreased because of the loss of the distal feeding artery when the cremaster was prepared according to the method of Baez.[12] As shown in Figure 1, there is less than a 40% pressure drop above the 1A when both feeders are intact, and an even smaller drop in the arteries leading to the rat gracilis muscle.[11]

A widely quoted set of pressure data are those of Davis et al.[13] shown in Figure 2. There are no points in this data set between 249 and 94 μm. When a straight line is used to connect the two points as in the dashed line of Figure 2, it suggests that significant

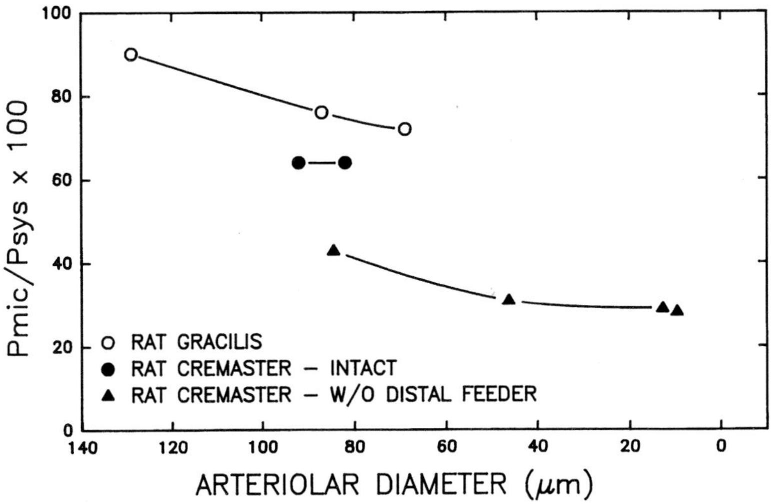

Figure 4-1 Microvascular pressures as a percent of systemic arterial pressure in rat gracilis muscle,[11] cremaster muscle with intact distal feeding artery (cremasteric artery branching from the deferential artery),[11] and cremaster muscle after ligation of the cremasteric artery.[9]

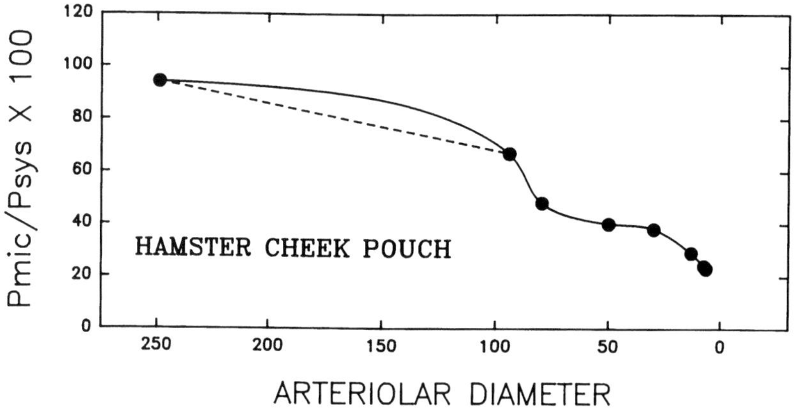

Figure 4-2 Microvascular pressure profile as a percent of systemic arterial pressure in the hamster cheek pouch[13] with curved and straight lines fitted between the 249 μm external maxillary artery and the 94 μm inferior saccular artery.

amounts of vascular resistance reside in arteries larger than 150 μm. If a curved line, more typical of pressure profiles is used, however, little pressure drop occurs above the 150 μm level.

Vessels from the rat mesentery are widely used as representative of resistance arteries in hypertensive studies. Pressure profiles in this bed indicate that the first order arterioles, with an average internal diameter of 35 μm in the SHR and 31 μm in the controls, had pressures only 12 mmHg below systemic values in the SHR and 13 mmHg below systemic in the controls.[14] There was however, a 66 mmHg pressure drop from the 1A to the 2A in these 16- to 20-week-old SHR, suggesting that these are very important resistance vessels in the hypertensive animal. Again these data indicate little vascular resistance above the arteriolar level.

A study by Borders and Granger[15] in the rat cremaster muscle demonstrated that the power dissipation per unit length in large arterioles is greater than in small arterioles. They mentioned but did not calculate, however, that the total power dissipation of a branch type is equal to the average power dissipation multiplied by the number of vessels in that average. Recent measurements on the cremaster muscle[16] show that there are just over 400 3As and nearly 4000 4As in the cremaster muscle. If these numbers are taken into consideration, the total power dissipated in the small arterioles is greater and the data are consistent with the micropressure measurements. In addition, the data of Borders and Granger[15] were obtained on the cremaster with the distal feeder ligated, so the resistance of the remaining feeding arteriole is overestimated. It should be kept in mind that all of the known data on pressure profiles have been obtained from exteriorized preparations in anesthetized animals and the profile might be quite different in the conscious state. If sympathetic tone were inhibited by anesthesia, the resultant dilation would shift the pressure profile to the right, favoring the microvessels. In any case, the arterioles contain a significant portion of vascular resistance, and convincing evidence that small arteries contribute to vascular resistance are available only for the coronary and cerebral circulations.

B. GRADIENTS IN CONTROL MECHANISMS

In addition to its importance as a site of vascular resistance in hypertension, the arteriolar bed is where activities of control mechanisms to adjust vascular resistance are concentrated in an increasing gradient toward the smaller vessels. These gradients are seen in responses to activity of the sympathetic nervous system, metabolic autoregulation, and myogenic responses to changes in intravascular pressure.

1. Sympathetic Nerve Stimulation

The small arterioles of the rat cremaster respond more rapidly and with greater constriction than larger arterioles to stimulation of the lumbar sympathetic chain,[17] posterior hypothalamic stimulation,[17] or direct application of norepinephrine.[18] A similar gradient favoring the small arterioles occurs in the rat mesentery.[19] Sympathetic nerve stimulation at 1 to 2 Hz to the lateral gastrocnemius of the cat increased resistance preferentially in arterioles smaller than 25 μm.[20] When increased to 8 to 16 Hz the vessels larger than 25 μm constricted strongly and their resistance increased 7.8-fold compared to a still slightly greater 10.9 fold increase in the small arterioles. In skeletal muscle, the rapid vasoconstriction of the 4As to norepinephrine or sympathetic nerve stimulation quickly fades, most probably because these same vessels are also the most sensitive to metabolic factors such as a fall in tissue PO_2.[21]

2. Metabolic Autoregulatory Responses

Vasodilation associated with metabolic activity also shows an increasing gradient in the smaller arterioles. Electrical stimulation of the rat spinotrapezius[22] or cat skeletal muscle[23] induces preferential vasodilation of the smaller arterioles. Arterioles above 25 μm in diameter dilate when the intensity of exercise is increased to near maximal levels.[23]

3. Myogenic Responses

Vascular adjustments to increased or decreased intravascular pressure are concentrated in the smaller arterioles. Myogenic responses in the rat cremaster were confined to 3A and smaller arterioles,[24] but the response of the 1A and 2As may have been inhibited by the loss of the distal feeder in this preparation. In the cat gastrocnemius, however, the myogenic response is greatest in arterioles smaller than 25 μm.[25] Reactive hyperemia, which is predominantly myogenic for short occlusions and combined myogenic-metabolic for longer occlusions, is also mediated primarily by small arterioles.[26,27]

A major exception to the increasing gradient in the microcirculation is the release of endothelial-derived nitric oxide, whose basal release appears to be greater in large arterioles and small arteries.[28,29] As such, this would be a mechanism to allow these vessels to respond appropriately to changes in blood flow initiated by the smaller arterioles. The increased shear rate may activate an endothelial potassium channel as the initiating event in release of nitric oxide.[30,31]

II. MECHANISMS OF INCREASED VASCULAR RESISTANCE

A. FUNCTIONAL

Vascular hindrance to the flow of blood is due to a combination of the structure of the blood vessels and the level of vascular tone superimposed on this structure. In both normotension and hypertension, resting vascular tone in the microcirculation accounts for up to 40% of vascular resistance.[32] During development of renal hypertension, however, vascular tone is at first greatly enhanced, followed by a return toward control levels as the structural increases in resistance take place. This is best seen in the 1K1C and 2K1C models of experimental hypertension where these alterations take place within 8 weeks.[33,34] Immediately upon stenosis of the renal artery, pressure rises and arteriolar narrowing takes place.[35] Although the initiation of vasoconstriction is probably due to release of renin and a subsequent increase in circulating angiotensin II, the majority of the response is due to local myogenic mechanisms activated by the rising pressure.[35] Elevated vasoconstriction continues over the following weeks in the 1K1C rat, but after 8 weeks, arteriolar vasoconstriction has returned nearly to control levels.[33] Vasoconstriction is elevated sufficiently during development of hypertension that small arterioles close to flow in skeletal muscle of both renal[33,34] and spontaneously hypertensive rats.[36] This phenomenon has been termed functional rarefaction and precedes structural rarefaction.[36] There is evidence in the SHR that the sympathetic nervous system contributes to the elevation and maintenance of blood pressure[37,38] and Bohlen[39] has shown that increased sensitivity of the arterioles to norepinephrine is at least partly responsible for functional rarefaction. Elevated levels of vascular tone continue in the established phase of hypertension in the SHR due to neural and local vascular control mechanisms.[36-38,40]

B. STRUCTURAL

1. Wall Area/Lumen Size

a. *Hypertrophy-hyperplasia*

In both human and animal models of hypertension, it is clear that structural changes in the vascular wall contribute to the maintenance of elevated vascular resistance. One of the major hypotheses is that of Folkow et al.[41] who proposed that increases in wall stress with the rising pressure leads to hypertrophy of the vascular wall, encroaching upon the lumen, increasing the wall/lumen ratio, and thereby giving a mechanical advantage which increases the responsiveness to vasoconstrictors. Wall hypertrophy has been readily confirmed in large and small mesenteric arteries of the SHR,[42-44] the result of cellular hypertrophy in large arteries and cellular hyperplasia in smaller resistance vessels.[44] Results obtained on arterioles in skeletal muscle have not been as clear with several studies indicating no decrease in lumen size in the SHR[2,36,45-48] nor hypertrophy of the arteriolar wall.[36,45,46] Recently obtained, unpublished data from 12-week-old SHR and WKY cremaster arterioles, however, indicate hypertrophy of the vascular media in 1As and 2As of the SHR, but no reduction in lumen size. These latter data were obtained on histological sections of perfusion-fixed tissue measured with a video image analysis system. Hypertrophy of vascular smooth muscle cells was obtained by scanning electron microscopy on larger arterioles of the SHR intestinal wall.[49] The lack of hypertrophy of the smaller arterioles (3A and 4A) may be due to the increase in tone which decreases wall stress, thus eliminating the stimulus for hypertrophy. Unlike skeletal muscle, hypertrophy and increases in wall/lumen ratio occur in the small cerebral arterioles of the stroke-prone SHR (SPSHR).[50]

b. *Remodeling*

Alternatively, medial thickness and the wall/lumen ratio of resistance vessels sometimes increase by structural reduction of the internal and external diameter, independently of changes in medial cross-sectional area. This has been termed remodeling of the vascular wall.[51] Although reported in human hypertensive subjects in 1959 by Short and Thomson,[52] remodeling has been overlooked in studies where the vessels were compared on the basis of diameter rather than branch order. In this case the increased wall/lumen ratio of the remodeled vessel leads to the mistaken interpretation of hypertrophy.[53]

According to Short and Thomson,[52] the mesenteric arterioles of subjects with chronic hypertension undergo a structural reduction in lumen size with no change in their wall cross-sectional area. Recent studies of subcutaneous small arteries of about 170 μm in diameter from human hypertensive subjects showed an increased medial thickness and media/lumen ratio, with a trend towards, but no statistically significant decrease in lumen size or increase in medial area.[54] These appear to be transition vessels midway between the hypertrophied larger arteries and the remodeled arterioles. Arterioles of the 1K1C[33] and 2K1C[34] hypertensive rats undergo remodeling which is very similar to that of human hypertensives.[52] That is, the lumens are reduced and the wall/lumen ratio is increased, with no increase in the wall cross-sectional area. Although DOCA-salt hypertensive rats undergo hypertrophy of the vascular wall during the first 8 weeks, remodeling was found in arterioles of rats with metacorticoid hypertension of 4-months duration.[55]

Although remodeling will result in the same hemodynamic changes of increased vasodilated resistance and responsiveness to vasoconstrictors as hypertrophy,[41] it requires a different hypothesis as to its origin. Rather than a stimulation of hypertrophy by the increased wall stress, it appears to be the result of sustained vasoconstriction leading to realignment of the smooth muscles and the extracellular matrix. The smooth muscles either slide over one another in a smaller circumference or shorten individually. If fibronectin and collagen reform around the smaller external diameter, the size of the vessel in the relaxed state would be limited. The cellular and molecular biology of this phenomenon must be explored to understand the mechanism.

2. Rarefaction

A reduction in the number of perfused vessels has been termed rarefaction. It is either functional — vessels nonperfused but present, or structural — vessels physically absent. Capillary rarefaction in the conjunctiva of hypertensive patients was reported as early as 1933 by Ruedemann[56] and again by Lack et al. in 1949.[57] Jackson[58] found the conjunctival arterioles to be in severe vascular spasm leading to a preponderance of nonperfusion of the capillary bed. More recent studies in the human conjunctiva confirmed arteriolar and capillary rarefaction in hypertensive subjects using quantitative methods.[59,60] Capillary rarefaction also occurs in skeletal muscle[61] and the nailfold of hypertensive subjects.[62] In all of these studies on live patients the difference between functional and structural rarefaction has never been assessed. Structural arteriolar rarefaction was well documented by Short and Thomson[52] in the postmortem mesenteric vascular bed of patients with chronic hypertension.

Arteriolar rarefaction was first noted in the cremaster muscle of the young SHR by Hutchins and Darnell[2] and confirmed by others.[39,63,64] At 6 to 8 weeks, no arteriolar rarefaction was found in the SHR gracilis muscle, at 12 to 14 weeks there was functional arteriolar rarefaction, and at 16 to 18 weeks there was structural rarefaction.[36] Rarefaction has also been found in the SHR mesentery,[65] skin,[66] and in the ciliary process and choroid of the eyes.[67] Arteriolar rarefaction has been documented in the cremaster muscle of 1K1C,[33] 2K1C,[34] and volume loading hypertensive rats.[68]

A study by Hansen-Smith et al.[69] is noteworthy because it documented for the first time the arterioles undergoing degeneration in the cremaster muscle. Thus the process appears to be the following. Vascular tone is great enough in the early stages of hypertension that arterioles close to flow — the period of functional rarefaction. Arterioles that remain closed eventually degenerate, producing the final result of structural rarefaction.

Bohlen[39] suggested that hyperresponsiveness to norepinephrine may contribute to arteriolar closure in the SHR and he found that acute denervation opened the closed arterioles. In other studies denervation did not open all the closed vessels and they opened only after application of a vasodilator.[36,63] Lombard et al.,[37] using tetrodotoxin to asses neural tone found no difference in the 4As between SHR and WKY, but the neural tone in the 3As was enhanced. Lombard et al.[70] also have shown a greater vasoconstrictor response of arterioles to elevations of oxygen tension in the SHR. They found that a greater percentage of arterioles closed completely in the SHR upon superfusion of a physiological salt solution equilibrated with 10% oxygen.

Another possible mechanism for closure of arterioles is altered function of the endothelial cells. Responses to the endothelial-dependent vasodilators, acetylcholine and bradykinin, but not to endothelium-independent sodium nitroprusside are reduced in arterioles of 1K1C hypertensive rats and the resting tone is higher than in controls.[71] Application of N^G-Monomethyl-L-Arginine (LNMMA) increased resting tone and inhibited the response to acetylcholine and bradykinin in controls, but not in 1K1C rats. A decreased vasodilator capability of the endothelial cells could be a mechanism contributing to arteriolar closure in the 1K1C rats. Thus functional rarefaction may result from a variety of mechanisms including autoregulatory mechanisms, increased responsiveness to vasoconstrictors, and altered endothelial function.

Although arteriolar rarefaction could contribute to the increase in vasodilated vascular resistance, it will not account for the increase in responsiveness to vasoconstrictors.[72] Its effects on vascular resistance are not as powerful as a change in vessel diameter, which has a fourth power relationship, but rarefaction may contribute to increased vascular resistance in muscles such as the cremaster where resting arteriolar diameters are not significantly smaller in the SHR than in controls.[2,45,63]

C. COMPENSATORY NATURE OF THE STRUCTURAL CHANGES

It is often suggested that hypertension is caused by an increase in peripheral vascular resistance and the structural changes in the arterioles serve a causative, or at least necessary, role in the development of hypertension. This ignores the dominant role of the kidney in long-term control of blood pressure as proposed by Guyton and Coleman[1] and supported in many studies which have recently been reviewed by Cowley.[73] Such studies include kidney transplants showing that hypertension follows the hypertensive kidney[74] and recently, the production of DOCA-salt hypertension in rats with arteriovenous fistulas which lower peripheral resistance below that of control rats.[75]

Recently, interest has developed in a genetic predisposition for vascular smooth muscle cells from SHR to grow faster than those of WKY, a characteristic that is maintained in tissue culture.[76] It should be kept in mind, however, that aortic smooth muscle cells from DOCA-salt hypertensive rats also proliferate faster in tissue culture.[77] In addition, a number of studies demonstrate that protecting vessels in the SHR hindquarter from the rising pressure prevents structural and functional changes in those vessels.[78-80] Elevated pressure possibly stimulates a growth response that, once switched on, cannot be regulated *in vitro*, but can be prevented or even reversed *in vivo*.[81]

These studies suggest that the structural changes in the vascular wall of peripheral resistance vessels are compensatory to control wall stress and autoregulate blood flow in spite of the elevated blood pressure. If structural changes in the afferent renal arterioles of young SHR can be shown to be responsible for the higher pressure needed by those kidneys to excrete a sodium load,[82] a case could be made for a role for resistance vessels in the development of hypertension.

III. POSSIBLE MECHANISMS UNDERLYING ALTERED VASCULAR REACTIVITY

Increased vascular reactivity in hypertension may result from either an increase in vessel wall/lumen ratio, as discussed above, and/or an overt hyperreactivity of the vascular smooth muscle. This section specifically examines mechanisms which may contribute to the latter situation.

A. VASCULAR SMOOTH MUSCLE

Alterations in microvascular reactivity could theoretically result from a disturbance at any level of the smooth muscle excitation-contraction coupling process (Figure 3). That is, from agonist/mechanical stimulation, through generation of membrane and intracellular messengers, to activation of the contractile proteins. At present there are few direct studies of the microvasculature which have examined such mechanisms. The following discussion, therefore, has considered data from a variety of vascular studies.

Many studies have indicated that an increased vascular responsiveness to norepinephrine occurs in hypertension. For example, Bohlen,[39] in studies of spontaneously hypertensive rats, demonstrated marked hyperresponsiveness of cremaster muscle arterioles (15 to 70 μm) to iontophoretically applied norepinephrine. Dennervation of the cremaster

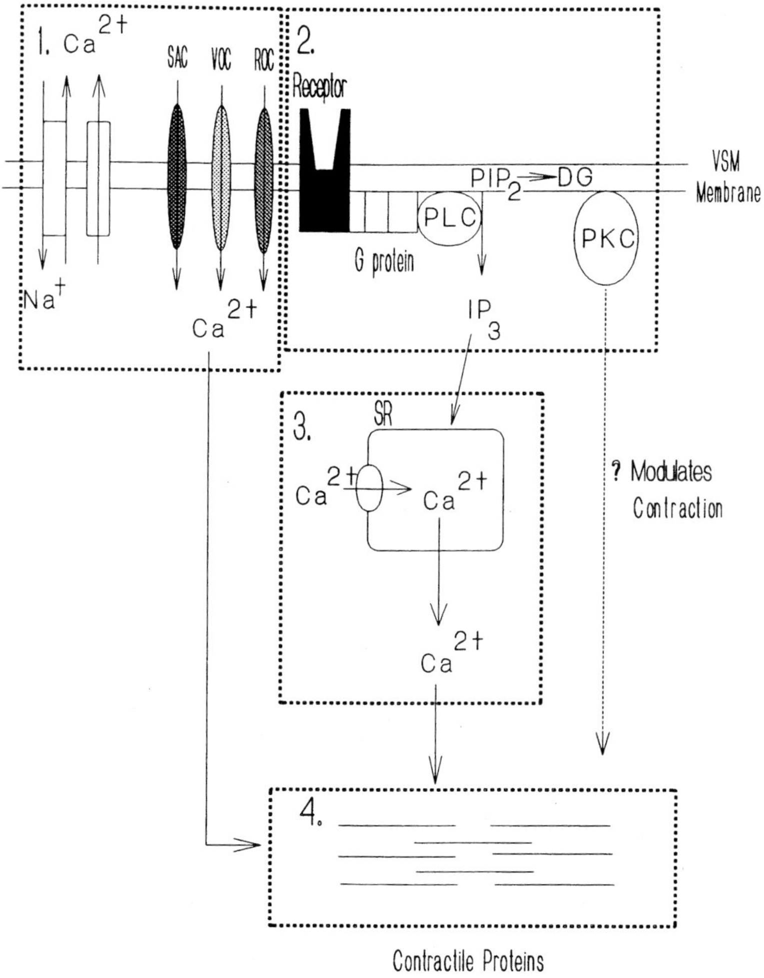

Figure 4-3 Schematic representation of contractile agonist signal transduction pathways in vascular smooth muscle. The four sections represent: (1) Ca^{+} influx/efflux, (2) membrane associated generation of second messengers, (3) SR Ca^{+} release/reuptake, and (4) contractile proteins. Abbreviations: (SAC) stretch-activated channel; (VOC) voltage-operated channel; (ROC) receptor-operated channel; (PLC) phospholipase C; (PIP_2) phoshphatidylinositol 4,5-bisphosphate; (DG) diacylglycerol; (PKC) protein kinase C; (IP_3) inositol trisphosphate, and (SR) sarcoplasmic reticulum.

muscle further suggested that hyperresponsiveness to endogenous norepinephrine contributed to vessel closure. The increased vascular reactivity in hypertension is not limited to norepinephrine but can also be seen in response to a variety of constrictor agents, such as, phorbol esters, Bay K 8644 and serotonin.[83] It is therefore unlikely that the enhanced reactivity reflects specific alterations in membrane receptor number and/or affinity. With respect to vascular α-adrenergic receptors, there is little evidence to support an alteration in receptor number or affinity in hypertension.[84] It is possible, however, that a nonspecific alteration to membrane structure may contribute to the altered reactivity. In this regard

Bohr[83] has suggested that changes in the lipid domain[85] (e.g., alterations in cholesterol: phospholipid ratio, degree of saturation) may lead to decreased membrane fluidity with subsequent impairment of the function of integral membrane proteins.

It is well accepted that the level of intracellular Ca^{2+} is a major determinant of vascular smooth muscle contraction and as such, disturbances in control of intracellular Ca^{2+} may contribute to alterations in reactivity and resistance. Intracellular Ca^{2+} concentrations are controlled by the net effect of a number of influx and extrusion pathways and intracellular release and sequestration mechanisms. Using electrophysiological techniques Hermsmeyer and Rusch[86] have demonstrated an increased proportion of L-type Ca^{2+} channels to T-type channels in smooth muscle cells isolated from the azygous vein of newborn SHRs. This model was chosen for the lack of exposure to increased intravascular pressure as the animals were at a stage regarded to be pre-hypertensive. The authors, therefore, suggested that a genetic abnormality in voltage-operated Ca^{2+} channel regulation may contribute to the genesis of hypertension. In a preliminary report Hermsmeyer[87] has indicated that a similar abnormality exists in smooth muscle cells from mesenteric resistance arteries of 6- to 8-week-old SHR. An abnormality in voltage-operated Ca^{2+} channels is also supported by the increased responsiveness of vascular smooth muscle, from spontaneously hypertensive rats, to the channel agonist Bay K 8644 while exposed to normal K^+ levels. In apparent contrast, data from Cauvin et al.[88] indicate that $^{45}Ca^{2+}$ influx into mesenteric resistance arteries of SHRs is increased in response to norepinephrine but not to KCl-induced depolarization.

In addition to alterations in Ca^{2+} entry via voltage-operated channels, other mechanisms could contribute to an increased intracellular Ca^{2+} concentration and enhanced reactivity to contractile stimuli, including impaired ion exchange mechanisms, an increased Ca^{2+} leak, or dysfunction of plasma and sarcoplasmic reticulum membrane Ca^{2+}-ATPases. Given the number of Ca^{2+} entry/efflux mechanisms, however, it would be surprising if hypertension were related to a specific defect in Ca^{2+} transport that could not be compensated for by the other mechanisms.

Several studies have considered the possible role of the phosphoinositide signaling pathway in hypertension.[89-91] This signal transduction mechanism is common to many contractile agonists including several of those which show an enhanced response in hypertension. Turla and Webb[89] reported an increased serotonin-induced phosphoinositide turnover, estimated by measurement of inositol phosphate accumulation in the presence of lithium chloride, in aorta of SPSHR as compared to WKY or Sprague Dawley control rats. Based on the known ability of inositol-1,4,5-trisphosphate to release intracellular Ca^{2+}, it was suggested that such data explain the increased reactivity to serotonin. Heagerty et al.[96] similarly demonstrated increased phosphoinositide turnover in aorta from SHR, both under basal conditions and in response to norepinephrine. In this latter study the increased activity was only apparent before a measurable increase in systemic pressure and structural changes had occurred, suggesting a possible role in the genesis of hypertension. Using more sensitive techniques to measure levels of individual inositol phosphates, this group[91] has since reported that inositol-1,4,5-trisphosphate production is increased, in subcutaneous resistance arteries (diameter approximately 150 μm), during developmental and established hypertension. While it is uncertain whether altered phosphoinositide metabolism is involved in the initial development of hypertension or represents a response to factors such as increased pressure, it does provide a mechanism for alterations in intracellular Ca^{2+}.

Breakdown of plasma membrane inositol phospholipids results from the activation of a specific phosphodiesterase, phospholipase C. Increased enzymatic activity of phospholipase C has been demonstrated in SHR aorta, both prior to an increase in systemic blood pressure and during established hypertension.[92] Interestingly, these authors reported that phospholipase A_2 was not similarly effected in the hypertensive animals and that cardiac phospholipase C activity was similar in the hypertensive and control animals, implying some specificity in the vascular alteration. Increased phospholipase C activity has also been demonstrated in platelets from a genetically salt-sensitive strain of rats while not being apparent in either the salt-resistant control animals or DOCA-salt hypertensive rats.[93]

In addition to leading to the production of inositol-1,4,5-phosphate, activation of this pathway results in the release of 1,2-diacylgylcerol, an activator of protein kinase C. As protein kinase C has been implicated in the control of microvascular tone,[94] possibly through regulation of contractile protein Ca^{2+} sensitivity, some interest has been shown in its role in hypertension. In this regard Storm et al.[95] demonstrated enhanced contractile responses of SHR aortas to a pharmacological activator of protein kinase C. Similar findings have been reported in a number of other studies. Interpretation of a role for protein kinase C in altered reactivity is made difficult by a lack of knowledge of the relevant substrates which it phosphorylates. As protein kinase C has been implicated in a number of growth processes, it is possible that any role it may have in hypertension is related to structural remodeling (see Section IV.B.1).

Little evidence currently exists for an alteration at the level of the contractile proteins in hypertension. Kamm et al.[96] reported that the hypertrophied carotid media from DOCA-induced hypertensive swine has normal mechanical properties considered in terms of maximal active stress and isotonic shortening velocity. Consistent with this Owens[97] found normal levels of actin and myosin and similar actin variants in hypertrophied vascular smooth muscle from SHR. Further, studies using skinned (Triton X-100) arterial preparations to study Ca^{2+} sensitivity of the contractile apparatus in the absence of Ca^{2+} influx and release have been unable to demonstrate an effect of hypertension at the level of the contractile apparatus.[98] Caution, however, must be exercised in extending these observations to resistance vessels. Indeed it has recently been shown that a difference exists between the Ca^{2+} sensitivity of triton skinned arteries and arterioles (diameter approximately 115 μm); with arterioles demonstrating an approximate three-fold increase in Ca^{2+} sensitivity.[99] Further, it appears that differences may exist, with respect to contractile protein isozyme composition, between different vessels.[99,100]

In addition to a disturbance in a specific step of the signal transduction process, it is possible that enhanced vascular reactivity results from the synergistic effects of one or more contractile mechanisms. For example, it has been demonstrated *in vivo* that myogenic constriction can account for a portion of the constrictor response to contractile agents such as phenylephrine and angiotensin II.[101] Further, arteriolar myogenic reactivity can be induced or potentiated by a number of situations including exposure to norepinephrine,[102] protein kinase C activation,[94] and cyclooxygenase inhibition.[103] Thus, activation of factors such as these, in hypertension, may increase vascular resistance via a myogenic mechanism. Enhanced myogenic reactivity, per se, would also be expected to contribute to increased resistance. In this regard it has been shown that isolated skeletal muscle arterioles from SHR (under conditions of no flow) show enhanced myogenic reactivity to increased intravascular pressure and an extended myogenic range compared to that of control animals.[104] The potentiated myogenic response was not simply related to altered wall structure, suggesting a more specific alteration in the signaling or regulatory pathways which underlie pressure/stretch activation.

B. INTERACTIONS BETWEEN CELL TYPES/CIRCULATING FACTORS

The above discussion has examined altered vascular reactivity in hypertension from the standpoint of an intrinsic disturbance in the vascular smooth muscle. It is conceivable, however, that such alterations in reactivity could result from interactions with other cell types, principally endothelial cells, or circulating factors.

1. Endothelial Cell Modulation of Reactivity

In recent years it has become apparent that the vascular endothelium is capable of modulating vascular tone through the production of vasoactive factors. Such substances, acting predominantly as paracrine factors, are involved in mediating or regulating the vasomotor responses to a variety of chemical (e.g., acetylcholine, bradykinin, histamine) and mechanical (e.g., shear stress) stimuli. Endothelial derived vasodilating substances include the endogenous nitrovasodilator nitric oxide, prostacyclin, and the yet to be characterized hyperpolarization factor. Those factors mediating constriction include thromboxane A_2, endoperoxide (PGH_2), and endothelin. The latter compound, unlike the other factors listed, is a peptide which shows long-lasting vasoactivity. While production and action of these substances has been characterized mainly in large conduit vessels it is evident that they perform similar roles in the microcirculation. For example, nitric oxide has been implicated in the *in vivo* response of skeletal muscle arterioles to vasodilators such as acetylcholine[105] and the flow-induced dilatation of isolated coronary arterioles.[106] Similarly, prostanoid vasodilators have been implicated in modulation of microvascular reactivity.[103,107]

The possibility that a defect in endothelial cell function leading to an alteration in the balance of vasoconstrictor and vasodilator substances which contributes to increased vascular resistance in hypertension is an attractive hypothesis. Whether such an alteration plays a primary role in the genesis of the disorder or occurs as a result of the hypertensive process is not entirely clear. Despite this, altered endothelial cell function, particularly in the microcirculation, could conceivably contribute to the maintenance of an elevated vascular resistance.

a. *Endothelial-Dependent Vasodilatation*

A number of studies have now indicated that experimental hypertension is associated with an impaired ability to vasodilate in response to endothelial-dependent vasodilators such as acetylcholine.[71,108-111] Similar results have been obtained from several models of hypertension including SHR, 1K1C, and 2K1C. Such findings are not limited to large arterial vessels but include resistance vessels from skeletal muscle,[71] kidney,[110] and mesentery.[111] The decreased capacity for relaxation was not a consequence of impaired ability to vasodilate, per se, as normal responses were found to endothelium-independent agents such as sodium nitroprusside. Nakamura and Prewitt,[71] however, found that the decreased capacity to vasodilate was not specific to those substances acting through the generation of nitric oxide but was also due to decreased ability to produce or respond to prostanoid vasodilators (e.g., prostacyclin). This latter study is suggestive of a more general impairment of endothelial cell function, possibly occurring as a result of the hypertensive process.

b. *Endothelial-Dependent Vasoconstriction*

In addition to a diminished ability of the endothelium to produce or release vasodilator paracrine factors, a similar scenario could result from the excess production of an endothelial-derived constricting factor (EDCF). In support of this suggestion, renal intralobar arteries (approximately 200 μm diameter) from SHRs produce a prostanoid constrictor factor in response to acetylcholine.[112] In the presence of indomethacin, such vessels dilated normally to acetylcholine. Similar results have been demonstrated in small mesenteric arteries from SPSHRs[113] and pial arterioles of SHR.[114] While the nature of this contracting factor is somewhat uncertain, it may be the arachidonic acid metabolite PGH_2, as its action can be blocked by a TxA_2/PGH_2 receptor blocker (e.g., SQ 29,548), but not by pretreatment with a TxA_2 synthetase inhibitor.

The recent discovery of the potent endothelial-derived constrictor peptide endothelin[115] has stimulated interest in its possible involvement in states of altered vascular resistance.

Studies aimed at measuring endothelin levels in hypertensive subjects have, to date, produced conflicting results. In a study by Naruse et al.[116] plasma immunoreactive endothelin levels were only elevated in subjects with established essential hypertension, suggesting that alterations in the level of the peptide may occur as a result of hypertension rather than being primary in the development of the disorder. As *in vitro* studies have shown that endothelial cells produce endothelin (as assessed by mRNA and immunoreactive endothelin) in response to shear stress,[117] it is conceivable that increased levels may result from alterations in hemodynamics. It is also possible that an increased production of endothelin participates in the adaptive vessel wall changes that characterize hypertension. It should be stated, however, that interpretation of plasma levels of this peptide is difficult as no information exists as to local biologically active levels, nor are specific antagonists widely available.

In addition to the production of increased quantities of endothelin, it is possible that vascular responsiveness to the peptide is altered in hypertension. In studies of mesenteric resistance arteries from renovascular and spontaneously hypertensive rats, Luscher's group[118] has demonstrated a normal or decreased reactivity to endothelin at the level of the smooth muscle. However, as endothelin-stimulated nitric oxide production is decreased in the vessels from hypertensive animals, the net constrictor response is similar to that of control animals. Studies performed in perfused isolated hearts from SHR have, however, demonstrated an increased vasoconstrictor response to endothelin, as estimated by changes in perfusion pressure, compared to WKY.[119] The increased response to endothelin could be attenuated by pretreatment of the hypertensive rats with the angiotensin converting enzyme inhibitor, enalapril, but not by pretreatment with hydralazine. These results are consistent with data suggesting that endothelin can act to potentiate the vasoconstrictor effects of the renin-angiotensin system.[120]

2. Contribution of Circulating Factors

Several studies have suggested that the elevated vascular resistance in some forms of hypertension is a consequence of a circulating inhibitor of the Na^+ pump.[121-123] This factor has been referred to as an endogenous digitalis-like substance and is thought to be produced in response to volume expansion. Reports from Hamlyn et al.[123] have characterized the compound as being structurally and functionally indistinguishable from ouabain. It is suggested that by blocking the Na^+ pump, intracellular Na^+ is increased leading to an elevation of intracellular Ca^{2+} by stimulation of Ca^{2+} entry via the Na^+-Ca^{2+} exchange mechanism. An increase in intracellular Ca^{2+}, with subsequent enhancement of tone and perhaps stimulation of growth processes, will also result in more Ca^{2+} taken up by the sarcoplasmic reticulum. This latter effect may then explain enhanced reactivity to vasoconstrictor agents such as norepinephrine and angiotensin II.

While a circulating inhibitor of the Na^+ pump may contribute to increased reactivity in certain forms of hypertension it is apparent that other mechanisms exist to increase resistance. In particular, local myogenic mechanisms act to elevate resistance when systemic pressure is initially increased. Using an acute model of renal hypertension in the rat Meininger et al.[124] demonstrated, by protecting the hindquarters from the increase in systemic pressure, that a component of vasoconstriction and increased resistance observed in cremaster muscle arterioles was pressure-dependent. Thus, this pressure-sensitive component would not appear to be dependent on circulating factors.

3. Summary

A number of potential sites exist for an intrinsic abnormality in reactivity in microvessels in hypertension. The available data, however, has not yet produced direct evidence for the involvement of an alteration in excitation-contraction coupling in the pathogenesis of hypertension. As a result it is critical to understand (1) whether the alterations described above reflect involvement in the genesis of the disorder or are secondary in nature, and (2) whether signal transduction mechanisms are similarly affected in macro- and microvessels. As such, direct studies are required to extend the data obtained from larger arterial vessels to actual resistance arterioles. The availability of isolated vessel techniques, Ca^{2+} imaging, patch-clamping, and the development of *micro*-biochemical procedures should provide the necessary tools.

IV. BIOLOGY OF THE MICROVASCULAR WALL

In recent years there has been an increasing number of laboratories focusing on cellular and molecular mechanisms underlying the functional and structural vascular changes in hypertension. Again, most of the information available has been obtained on large arteries or cultured cells, with only a small number of studies on arterioles and small resistance arteries. This information will be reviewed in the following sections with the expectation that techniques such as isolated arterioles and *in situ* hybridization will provide more direct information on arterioles in the immediate future.

A. REGULATION OF STRUCTURAL PROTEIN EXPRESSION

Predominant cell types in the microvascular wall are smooth muscle and endothelial cells. Both cell types have cytoskeletal proteins that serve to maintain the structural integrity of the cell, but the smooth muscle cells have contractile proteins as the major functional component. These structural proteins exist as groups of isoforms, which are expressed and regulated not only in a tissue-specific fashion and during developmental differentiation, but also in response to various pathophysiologic stimuli. Owens and Thompson[125] have demonstrated that a switch from nonmuscle to α-smooth muscle actin in aortic smooth muscle cells correlates with increases in force-generating capacity and suggested that the differential turnover of actin isoforms implies differences in structure and/or intracellular processing of these actins. Increases in actin synthesis and content accompanied by increases in actin mRNA expression was also observed in rat aortic smooth muscle cells treated with angiotensin (Ang II) or arginine vasopressin.[126] Regulated switching of actin isoforms in smooth muscle cells during hypertension may provide a mechanism whereby smooth muscle tissues could modulate their molecular structure in accordance with their work load.

It is also reasonable to hypothesize that increased wall tension in large vessels during hypertension is borne by an increased number of contractile units rather than the enhanced performance of each unit, so that adaptive hypertrophy of the wall could minimize changes in wall stress (wall tension/wall thickness). As reviewed above, however, vascular wall hypertrophy occurs only rarely in arterioles. Rather, remodeling which reduces the lumen without increased wall mass occurs in arterioles of human hypertensive subjects[52,54] and during experimental renal hypertension.[33,34] The exact mechanisms underlying the structural alterations of arterioles is unknown. It is conceivable, however, that various pathophysiologic factors may stimulate selective expression of proteins whose synthesis does not contribute to cellular hypertrophy. For example, certain trans-acting factors may be expressed in response to various stimuli and suppress the expression of the smooth muscle contractile protein gene. If this hypothesis holds true in the regulation of microvascular growth in hypertension, structural reduction of the arteriolar lumen following intense vasoconstriction could well be due to decreased longitudinal growth of smooth muscle cells, resulting from decreased and/or altered structural protein synthesis.

Another potential mechanism is trans-acting factors that may bind to regulatory elements of connective tissue protein genes, so that enhanced expression and synthesis of connective tissue proteins physically restrict dilation of the arteriole and reduce the relaxed diameter in hypertension. It has been shown that vascular tissues of young rats are sensitive to increased blood pressure, responding quickly with increased elastin and collagen production.[127,128] Additional studies will be required to determine which type of protein synthesis (regulatory or structural) or gene expression is altered in microvessels, and whether changes are controlled transcriptionally or posttranscriptionally.

B. EFFECTS OF AUTOCRINE AND PARACRINE SYSTEMS

1. Growth Factors

As discussed earlier, various types of stimuli may lead to structural alterations of vascular walls in hypertension. Platelet-derived growth factor (PDGF), the most well-characterized mitogen of vascular smooth muscle cells, is one of these stimuli. PDGF exists in three dimeric isoforms (PDGF-AA, -AB, and -BB) which interact with high-affinity receptors (a- and b-receptors) and generate different functional properties.[129,130] Although the AA homodimer has lower mitogenic activity, weaker chemotactic activity, and less ability to cause vasoconstriction and membrane ruffling than the BB form, the AA homodimer has a higher efficacy for activating protein kinase C.[129,130] Arterial smooth muscle cells not only bind and respond to PDGF but also are capable of secreting the mitogen themselves,[131-133] which may act locally to cause an autocrine or paracrine stimulation of cell proliferation under various pathophysiological conditions. With the availability of PDGF cDNA clones, it has become possible to determine which subunit gene of PDGF is expressed in vascular tissue. Smooth muscle cells from rat pups express both the A and B chains of PDGF,[134] while cells from adults express only the A chain of PDGF.[133,134] An increase in PDGF-A chain expression and an attendant smooth muscle cell proliferation have been found in the intimal hyperplastic lesion developed in the rat carotid artery after balloon injury and also in vascular cells isolated from human atheromatous lesions.[135,136] It would be of interest to determine which type of PDGF subunit is expressed in the proliferating wall of resistance arteries in SHR,[137] and whether PDGF contributes to the cellular hypertrophy of vascular smooth muscle cells. Although PDGF enhances expression of a group of genes including c-*fos* and c-*myc*,[138] PDGF induces a rapid and dramatic decrease in smooth muscle α-actin expression.[139,140] The repressive role of PDGF in smooth muscle α-actin synthesis may suggest an important function of PDGF that may be distinct from its mitogenic properties.

Besides PDGF, insulin-like growth factors (IGF) I and II, endothelial cell growth factor (ECGF), basic fibroblast growth factor (bFGF), and transforming growth factor-β (TGF-β) are made in aortic tissue and could cause autocrine or paracrine effects.[141] DOCA-salt hypertension increases the gene expression of TGF-β but not of the other growth factors listed above.[141] Recently, TGF-β has been shown to cause hypertrophy of smooth muscle cells in culture and to increase the number of polyploid cells,[142] suggesting that TGF-β may be involved in several important functions that may be associated with vascular injury and modulation of cell growth and connective tissue synthesis.[143]

2. Vasoactive Agents

There is now clear evidence demonstrating that vasoconstrictor agents such as Ang II, norepinephrine, and arginine vasopressin play a role in mediating growth responses of smooth muscle cells in hypertension as well as in developmental growth and maintenance of the vascular wall in normal animals. It has been shown that Ang II is capable of inducing cellular hypertrophy in cultured aortic smooth muscle cells[144] and hypertrophy and hyperplasia in cultured smooth muscle cells from mesenteric resistance arteries.[145] When Ang II is added to cultured rat aortic smooth muscle cells there is a rapid increase in mRNA levels of the proto-oncogenes, c-*fos*, c-*myc*, and c-*jun*, followed by a delayed increase in the level of PDGF A-chain, bFGF and TGF-β mRNA.[146-149] It appears that growth of smooth muscle cells in culture is regulated by Ang II through the balance of stimulation by PDGF A-chain and bFGF and inhibition by TGF-β, because the hypertrophic process is significantly attenuated by antisense oligonucleotides to PDGF A and bFGF mRNA while blockade of TGF-β with antisense oligomers increases DNA synthesis and cell proliferation.[149,150] *In vivo*, the evidence for local generation and subsequent secretion of Ang II by peripheral vascular tissue supports the idea that Ang II is likely to function in an autocrine and paracrine manner to regulate vascular growth.[151,152] In our study,[153] infusion of 200 ng/kg/min of Ang II by osmopump for 14 d caused an increase in the number of precapillary arterioles in spite of an elevation in vascular tone and a structural reduction in the arteriolar lumen. The hypertrophied aortic wall in this model shows the presence of PDGF by immunohistochemistry.[154] Aortic hypertrophy induced by Ang II infusion may be a direct response to Ang II rather than elevated pressure because it still occurs when hypertension is prevented by the addition of hydralazine to the drinking water.[155] Similarly, the suppression of Ang II levels with angiotensin converting enzyme inhibitor, captopril, attenuates the development of arteries and arterioles in normotensive and hypertensive rats.[156,157] Further, blockade of Ang II subtype-1 receptors with the antagonist losartan (DUP753) decreases the number of precapillary arterioles in the treated rats.[158] Additional examination of the mechanisms whereby Ang II alters expression of intracellular signaling should provide important insight regarding how Ang II acts as a vascular growth factor.

A number of studies have shown proliferative responses of smooth muscle as well as nonmuscle cells (e.g., fibroblasts) in response to a variety of vasoactive agents including arginine vasopressin,[159] bradykinin,[160] prostaglandin E_1,[161] and serotonin.[162] In general, the reported effects of these agents were relatively small as compared to growth factors such as PDGF. Given the considerable overlap in second messenger systems stimulated by vasoconstrictors and growth factors, it is not surprising that vasoconstrictors may show some growth-stimulating effects.

3. Sympathetic Nerves

It has been shown that sympathetic nerves exert long-term trophic influences on arterial smooth muscle mass,[163,164] and norepinephrine and epinephrine have been shown to increase the growth rate of cultured vascular smooth muscle cells.[165] Considerable progress has been made in understanding the cellular biochemical events subsequent to receptor stimulation by norepinephrine. It has been shown that the α_1-receptors are linked through a G-protein to phospholipase C, which when activated generates diacylglycerol and inositol-1,4,5,-trisphosphate.[166] As a consequence, the activation of protein kinase C by diacylglycerol and the mobilization of intracellular Ca^{2+} by inositol trisphosphate may cause the induction of c-*fos* mRNA.[167,168] In addition, phenylephrine produces dose-dependent stimulation of PDGF A-chain gene expression in rat thoracic aorta via agonist occupancy of α_1-adrenergic receptors.[169] It is therefore reasonable to speculate that the growth stimulation effect of norepinephrine may involve the induction of PDGF gene expression.

C. CELLULAR MECHANISMS ELICITED BY HEMODYNAMIC FACTORS

1. Pressure

There is considerable circumstantial evidence implicating a role for increased transmural pressure, through alterations in vascular wall stress, in the growth response of smooth muscle cells in hypertension. It has been shown that isolated arteries cultured under increased levels of wall stress increase their incorporation of ^3H-thymidine, indicative of replication of DNA[170] and cyclical stretching of cultured vascular smooth muscle cells stimulates the production of matrix components and hypertrophy.[171] These mechanical stimuli which produce cell stretch can activate intracellular pathways associated with growth.[172-175] The "receptor" for stretch may be a cell surface ion channel.[176] Furthermore, the fact that growth factors have been extracted from skeletal muscle with stretch-induced hypertrophy, as well as from hypertrophied cardiac muscle[177,178] suggests that genetic control of growth mediators might be a covariant of blood pressure. That is, a genetic alteration producing excess vascular growth factors in response to various stimuli might predispose an individual to hypertension by altering the structure of the vascular wall.

2. Flow

Changes in blood flow influence the size of blood vessels independently of changes in blood pressure. This has been demonstrated in the rabbit by Langille and O'Donnell,[179] who ligated the internal carotid artery to decrease blood flow in the common carotid without altering intraluminal pressure. Recently, we showed that reduced work load in an immature cremaster muscle, produced by unilateral orchidectomy, elicited growth reduction in lumen size, wall cross-sectional area, and number of microvessels.[16] A marked decrease in blood flow in this unloaded muscle was suggested as the most likely factor leading to the vascular growth regulation process.

The cellular mechanisms for the response for chronic, local adaptations to blood flow are not totally clear. However, accumulating evidence suggests that flow-induced shear stress is the principal hemodynamic force associated with the endothelium. Endothelial cells are known to respond to shear stress by a shape change which is accompanied by reorganization of the cytoskeleton.[180,181] The endothelial cell exposed to controlled levels of laminar shear stress in capillary flow tubes has demonstrated a K^+-selective, shear stress-activated ionic current.[182] Ultrastructural studies have demonstrated myoendothelial junctions in the microcirculation,[183,184] leading to the hypothesis that the endothelium and smooth muscle cells may act as a coupled system allowing smooth muscle responses to secondary signals generated in the endothelium and efficiently transferred through such junctions.[185,186] This mechanism is quite different from the release of endothelium-derived relaxing factor (EDRF) which mediates acute vasodilator responses to increased blood flow[187] and from other endothelial synthesized substances such as histamine,[188] prostacyclin,[189] and endothelin,[115] which respond to flow-related shear stress and might play a role in flow-induced growth regulation.

V. SUMMARY

The microcirculation has an important role in the maintenance of hypertension due to its major contribution to vascular resistance and regulation of blood flow. The structural changes in the arterioles appear to be compensatory to the rise in blood pressure, but also serve to maintain increased vascular resistance through a combination of rarefaction and reduction in lumen diameter, with or without hypertrophy of the wall. A number of alterations in reactivity are found in arteries of hypertensive subjects. At present it is unclear whether the alterations are intrinsic or compensatory and thus their role in the genesis and maintenance of increased resistance is uncertain. In addition, the number of structural and biochemical differences between arteries and arterioles is suggestive that many of the alterations may not be found in arterioles. Molecular and cellular mechanisms whereby mechanical or chemical stimuli result in functional and structural changes in the vasculature are being elucidated. The stimuli react with ion channels and/or specific receptors to initiate intracellular signalling mechanisms (IP_3, protein kinase C, and increased intracellular Ca^{++}). Through as yet incompletely understood pathways, protooncogenes become activated (c-*fos*, c-*myc*) and initiate transcription of DNA, leading to cell growth and proliferation. Continued studies along these lines may provide novel and specific approaches to prevent structural changes in arterioles and decrease peripheral resistance in hypertension.

REFERENCES

1. **Guyton, A. C. and Coleman, T. G.,** Quantitative analysis of the pathophysiology of hypertension, *Circ. Res.,* 24 (Suppl. I), I-1, 1969.
2. **Hutchins, P. M. and Darnell, A. E.,** Observations of a decreased number of small arterioles in spontaneously hypertensive rats, *Circ. Res.,* 34 (Suppl. I), I-161, 1974.
3. **Engelson, E. T., Skalak, T. C., and Schmid-Schönbein, G. W.,** The microvasculature in skeletal muscle. I. Arteriolar network in rat spinotrapezius muscle, *Microvasc. Res.,* 30, 29, 1985.
4. **Harper, S. L. and Bohlen, H. G.,** Microvascular adaptation in the cerebral cortex of adult spontaneously hypertensive rats, *Hypertension,* 6, 408, 1984.
5. **Chilian, W. H., Eastham, C. L., and Marcus, M. L.,** Microvascular distribution of coronary vascular resistance in beating left ventricle, *Am. J. Physiol.,* 251 (Heart Circ. Physiol. 20), H779, 1986.
6. **Dodd, L. R. and Johnson, P. C.,** Diameter changes in arteriolar networks of contracting skeletal muscle, *Am. J. Physiol.,* 260 (Heart Circ. Physiol. 29), H663, 1991.
7. **House, S. D. and Johnson, P. C.,** Microvascular pressure in venules of skeletal muscle during arterial pressure reduction, *Am. J. Physiol.,* 250 (Heart Circ. Physiol. 19), H838, 1986.
8. **Fronek, K. and Zweifach, B. W.,** Microvascular pressure distribution in skeletal muscle and the effect of vasodilation, *Am. J. Physiol.,* 228, 791, 1975.
9. **Bohlen, H. G., Gore, R. W., and Hutchins, P. M.,** Comparison of microvascular pressure in normal and spontaneously hypertensive rats, *Microvasc. Res.,* 13, 125, 1977.
10. **Hill, M., Simpson, B. E., and Meininger, G. A.,** Altered cremaster muscle hemodynamics due to disruption of the deferential feed vessel, *Microvasc. Res.,* 39, 349, 1990.
11. **DeLano, F. A., Schmid-Schönbein, G. W., Skalak, T. C., and Zweifach, B. W.,** Penetration of systemic blood pressure into the microvasculature of rat skeletal muscle, *Microvasc. Res.,* 41, 92, 1991.
12. **Baez, S.,** An open cremaster muscle preparation for the study of blood vessels by *in vivo* microscopy, *Microvasc. Res.,* 5, 384, 1973.
13. **Davis, M. J., Ferrer, P. N., and Gore, R. W.,** Vascular anatomy and hydrostatic pressure profile in the hamster cheek pouch, *Am. J. Physiol.,* 250 (Heart Circ. Physiol. 19), H291, 1986.
14. **Hertel, R. F. and Henrich, H.,** Arteriolar pressures, permeability and lymph flow rate in normotensive and spontaneously hypertensive rats: contribution to the subject of fluid balance in the microcirculation, in *Microvascular Aspects of Spontaneous Hypertension,* Henrich, H., Ed., Hans Huber, Bern, 1982, 125.
15. **Borders, J. L. and Granger, H. J.,** Power dissipation as a measure of peripheral resistance in vascular networks, *Hypertension,* 8, 184, 1986.
16. **Wang, D. H. and Prewitt, R. L.,** Microvascular development during normal growth and reduced blood flow: introduction of a new model, *Am. J. Physiol.,* 260 (Heart Circ. Physiol. 29), H1966, 1991.
17. **Fleming, B. P., Barron, K. W., Howes, T. W., and Smith, J. K.,** Response of the microcirculation in rat cremaster muscle to peripheral and central sympathetic stimulation, *Circ. Res.,* 61 (Suppl. II), II-26, 1987.
18. **Marshall, J. M.,** The influence of the sympathetic nervous system on individual vessels of the microcirculation of skeletal muscle of the rat, *J. Physiol.,* 332, 169, 1982.
19. **Furness, J. B. and Marshall, J. M.,** Correlation of the directly observed responses of mesenteric vessels of the rat to nerve stimulation and noradrenaline with the distribution of adrenergic nerves, *J. Physiol.,* 239, 75, 1974.

20. **Maspers, M., Björnberg, J., Grände, P.-O., and Mellander, S.,** Sympathetic a-adrenergic control of large-bore arterial vessels, arterioles and veins, and of capillary pressure and fluid exchange in whole-organ cat skeletal muscle, *Acta Physiol. Scand.,* 139, 509, 1990.
21. **Boegehold, M. A. and Johnson, P. C.,** Periarteriolar and tissue PO_2 during sympathetic escape in skeletal muscle, *Am. J. Physiol.,* 254 (Heart Circ. Physiol. 23), H929, 1988.
22. **Marshall, J. M. and Tandon, H. C.,** Direct observations of muscle arterioles and venules following contraction of skeletal muscle fibres in the rat, *J. Physiol.*, 350, 447, 1984.
23. **Björnberg, J., Maspers, M., and Mellander, S.,** Metabolic control of large-bore arterial resistance vessels, arterioles, and veins in cat skeletal muscle during exercise, *Acta Physiol. Scand.,* 135, 83, 1989.
24. **Meininger, G. A., Mack, C. A., Fehr, K. L., and Bohlen, H. G.,** Myogenic vasoregulation overrides local metabolic control in resting rat skeletal muscle, *Circ. Res,* 60, 861, 1987.
25. **Ekelund, U., Björnberg. J., Albert, U., Grände, P.-O., and Mellander, S.,** Myogenic vascular regulation in skeletal muscle in vivo is not dependent of endothelium-derived nitric oxide, *Acta Physiol. Scand.,* 144, 199, 1992.
26. **Meininger G. A.,** Responses of sequentially branching macro- and microvessels during reactive hyperemia in skeletal muscle, *Microvasc. Res.,* 34, 29, 1987.
27. **Björnberg. J., Albert, U., and Mellander, S.,** Resistance responses in proximal arterial vessels, arterioles and veins during reactive hyperaemia in skeletal muscle and their underlying regulatory mechanisms, *Acta Physiol. Scand.,* 139, 535, 1990.
28. **Ekelund, U. and Mellander, S.,** Role of endothelium-derived nitric oxide in the regulation of tonus in large-bore arterial resistance vessels, arterioles and veins in cat skeletal muscle, *Acta Physiol. Scand.,* 140, 301, 1990.
29. **Faraci, F. M.,** Role of endothelium-derived relaxing factor in cerebral circulation: large arteries vs. microcirculation, *Am. J. Physiol.,* 261 (Heart Circ. Physiol. 30), H1038, 1991.
30. **Cooke, J. P., Rossitch, E., Jr., Andon, N. A., Loscaizo, J., and Dzau, V. J.,** Flow activates an endothelial potassium channel to release an endogenous nitrovasodilator, *J. Clin. Invest.,* 88, 1663, 1991.
31. **Olesen, S.-P., Clapham, D. E., and Davies, P. F.,** Haemodynamic shear stress activates a K^+ current in vascular endothelial cells, *Nature*, 331, 168, 1988.
32. **Prewitt, R. L. and Dowell, R. F.,** Pressure-flow relationship during the development of spontaneous hypertension in the rat (SHR), in *Microvascular Aspects of Spontaneous Hypertension*, Henrich, H., Ed., Hans Huber, Bern, 1982, 11.
33. **Hashimoto, H., Prewitt, R. L., and Efaw, C. W.,** Alterations in the microvasculature of one-kidney, one-clip hypertensive rats, *Am. J. Physiol.,* 253 (Heart Circ. Physiol. 22), H933, 1987.
34. **Ono, Z., Prewitt, R. L., and Stacy, D. L.,** Arteriolar changes in developing and chronic stages of two-kidney, one clip hypertension, *Hypertension*, 14, 36, 1989.
35. **Meininger, G. A., Lubrano, V. M., and Granger, H. J.,** Hemodynamic and microvascular responses in the hindquarters during the development of renal hypertension in rats, Evidence for the involvement of an autoregulatory component, *Circ. Res.*, 55, 609, 1984.
36. **Prewitt, R. L., Chen, I. I. H., and Dowell, R.,** Development of microvascular rarefaction in the spontaneously hypertensive rat, *Am. J. Physiol.*, 243, H243, 1982.
37. **Lombard, J. H., Hess, M. E., and Stekiel, W. J.,** Neural and local control of arterioles in SHR, *Hypertension*, 6, 530, 1984.

38. **Smith, P. G., Poston, C. W., and Mills, E.,** Ontogeny of neural and non-neural contributions to arterial blood pressure in spontaneously hypertensive rats, *Hypertension*, 6, 54, 1984.
39. **Bohlen, H. G.,** Arteriolar closure mediated by hyperresponsiveness to norepinephrine in hypertensive rats, *Am. J. Physiol.*, 236, H157, 1979.
40. **Schmid-Schönbein, G. W., Zweifach, B. W., DeLano, F. A., and Chen, P. C. Y.,** Microvascular tone in a skeletal muscle of spontaneously hypertensive rats, *Hypertension*, 9, 164, 1987.
41. **Folkow, B., Hallback, M., Lundgren, Y., and Weiss, L.,** Background of increased flow resistance and vascular reactivity in spontaneously hypertensive rats, *Acta Physiol. Scand.*, 80, 93, 1970.
42. **Mulvany, M. J., Hansen, P. K., and Aalkjaer, C.,** Direct evidence that the greater contractility of resistance vessels in spontaneously hypertensive rats is associated with a narrowed lumen, a thickened media, and an increased number of smooth muscle cell layers, *Circ. Res.*, 43, 854, 1978.
43. **Lee, R. M. K. W., Garfield, R. E., Forrest, J. B., and Daniel, E. E.,** Morphometric study of structural changes in the mesenteric blood vessels of spontaneously hypertensive rats, *Blood Vessels*, 20, 57, 1983.
44. **Owens, G. K., Schwartz, S. M., and McCanna, M.,** Evaluation of medial hypertrophy in resistance vessels of spontaneously hypertensive rats, *Hypertension*, 11, 198, 1988.
45. **Bohlen, H. G. and Lobach, D.,** In vivo study of microvascular wall characteristics and resting control in young and mature spontaneously hypertensive rats, *Blood Vessels*, 15, 322, 1978.
46. **Schmid-Schönbein, G. W., DeLano, F. A., Chu, S., and Zweifach, B. W.,** Wall structure of arteries and arterioles feeding the spinotrapezius muscle of normotensive and spontaneously hypertensive rats, *Int. J. Microcirc. Clin. Exp.*, 9, 47, 1990.
47. **Zweifach, B. W., Kovalcheck, S., DeLano, F., and Chen, P.,** Micropressure-flow relationships in a skeletal muscle of spontaneously hypertensive rats, *Hypertension*, 3, 601, 1981.
48. **leNoble, J. L. M. L., Tangelder, G. J., Slaaf, D. W., vanEssen, H., Reneman, R. S., and Struyker-Boudier, H. A. J.,** A functional morphometric study of the cremaster muscle microcirculation in young spontaneously hypertensive rats, *J. Hypertension*, 8, 741, 1990.
49. **Miller, B. G., Connors, B. A., Bohlen, H. G., and Evan, A. P.,** Cell and wall morphology of intestinal arterioles from 4- to 6- and 17- to 19-week-old Wistar-Kyoto and spontaneously hypertensive rats, *Hypertension*, 9, 59, 1987.
50. **Hart M. N., Heistad, D. D., and Brody, M. J.,** Effect of chronic hypertension and sympathetic denervation on wall/lumen ratio of cerebral vessels, *Hypertension*, 2, 419, 1980.
51. **Baumbach, G. L. and Heistad, D. D.,** Remodeling of cerebral arterioles in chronic hypertension, *Hypertension*, 13, 968, 1989.
52. **Short, D. S. and Thomson, A. D.,** The arteries of the small intestine in systemic hypertension, *J. Pathol. Bacteriol.*, 78, 321, 1959.
53. **Short, D. S.,** The vascular fault in chronic hypertension, *Lancet*, 1, 1302, 1966.
54. **Aalkjaer, C., Heagerty, A. M., Petersen, K. K., Swales, J. D., and Mulvany, M. J.,** Evidence for increased media thickness, increased neuronal amine uptake, and depressed excitation-contraction coupling in isolated resistance vessels from essential hypertensives, *Circ. Res.*, 61, 181, 1987.
55. **Friedman, S. M., Nakashima, M., and Mar, M. A.,** Morphological assessment of vasoconstriction and vascular hypertrophy in sustained hypertension in the rat, *Microvasc. Res.*, 3, 416, 1971.

56. **Ruedemann, A. D.,** Conjunctival vessels, *JAMA,* 101, 1477, 1933.
57. **Lack, A., Adolph, W., Ralston, W., Leiby, G., Winsor, T., and Griffith, G.,** Biomicroscopy of conjunctival vessels in hypertension, *Am. Heart. J.*, 38, 654, 1949.
58. **Jackson, W. B.,** The functional activity of the human conjunctival capillary bed in hypertensive and normotensive subjects, *Am. Heart J.*, 56, 222, 1958.
59. **Harper, R. N., Moore, M. A., Marr, M. C., Watts, L. E., and Hutchins, P. M.,** Arteriolar rarefaction in the conjunctiva of human essential hypertensives, *Microvasc. Res.*, 16, 369, 1978.
60. **Sullivan, J. M., Prewitt, R. L., and Josephs, J. A.,** Attenuation of the microcirculation in young patients with high-output borderline hypertension, *Hypertension*, 5, 844, 1983.
61. **Henrich, H. A., Romen, W., Heimgärtner, Hartung, E., and Bäumer, F.,** Capillary rarefaction characteristic of the skeletal muscle of hypertensive patients, *Klin. Wochenschr.*, 66, 54, 1988.
62. **Gasser, P. and Bühler, F. R.,** Nailfold microcirculation in normotensive and essential hypertensive subjects, as assessed by video-microscopy, *J. Hypertension*, 10, 83, 1992.
63. **Chen, I. I. H., Prewitt, R. L., and Dowell, R. F.,** Microvascular rarefaction in spontaneously hypertensive rat cremaster muscle, *Am. J. Physiol.*, 241, H306, 1981.
64. **Roy, J. W. and Mayrovitz, H. N.,** Microvascular pressure, flow, and resistance in spontaneously hypertensive rats, *Hypertension*, 6, 877, 1984.
65. **Henrich, H., Hertel, R., and Assmann, R.,** Structural differences in the mesentery microcirculation between normotensive and spontaneously hypertensive rats, *Pflugers Arch.*, 375, 153, 1978.
66. **Haack, D. W., Schaffer, J. J., and Simpson, J. G.,** Comparisons of cutaneous microvessels from spontaneously hypertensive, normotensive Wistar-Kyoto and normal Wistar rats, *Proc. Soc. Exp. Biol. Med.*, 164, 453, 1980.
67. **Funk, R. and Rohen, J. W.,** Comparative morphological studies on blood vessels in eyes of normotensive and spontaneously hypertensive rats, *Exp. Eye Res.*, 40, 191, 1985.
68. **Lombard, J. H., Hinojosa-Laborde, C., and Cowley, A. W., Jr.,** Hemodynamics and microcirculatory alterations in reduced renal mass hypertension, *Hypertension*, 13, 128, 1989.
69. **Hansen-Smith, F., Greene, A. S., Cowley, A. W., Jr., and Lombard, J. H.,** Structural changes during microvascular rarefaction in chronic hypertension, *Hypertension*, 15, 922, 1990.
70. **Lombard, J. H., Hess, M. E., and Stekiel, W. J.,** Enhanced response of arterioles to oxygen during development of hypertension in SHR, *Am. J. Physiol.,* 250 (Heart Circ. Physiol. 19), H761, 1986.
71. **Nakamura, T. and Prewitt, R. L.,** Effect of N^G-monomethyl L-arginine on endothelium-dependent relaxation in arterioles of one-kidney, one-clip hypertensive rats, *Hypertension*, 17, 875, 1991.
72. **Hallbäck, M., Göthberg, G., Lundin, S., Ricksten, S.-E., and Folkow, B.,** Hemodynamic consequences of resistance vessel rarefication and of changes in smooth muscle sensitivity, *Acta Physiol. Scand.,* 97, 233, 1976.
73. **Cowley, A. W., Jr.,** Long-term control of arterial blood pressure, *Physiol. Rev.,* 72, 231, 1992.
74. **Bianchi, G., Fox, U., DiFrancesco, G. F., Giovanetti, A. M., and Pagetti, D.,** Blood pressure changes produced by kidney cross-transplantation between spontaneously hypertensive rats and normotensive rats, *Clin. Sci. Mol. Med.,* 47, 435, 1974.
75. **Huang, M., Hester, R. L., Guyton, A. C., and Norman, R. A., Jr.,** Hemodynamic studies in DOCA-salt hypertensive rats after opening of an arteriovenous fistula, *Am. J. Physiol.,* 262 (Heart Circ. Physiol. 31), H1802, 1992.

76. **Hadrava, V., Tremblay, J., and Hamet, P.,** Intrinsic factors involved in vascular smooth muscle cell proliferation in hypertension, *Clin. Invest. Med.,* 14, 535, 1991.
77. **Haudenschild, C. C., Grunwald, J., and Chobanian, A. V.,** Effects of hypertension on migration and proliferation of smooth muscle in culture, *Hypertension,* 7 (Suppl. I), I-101, 1985.
78. **Folkow, B., Gurèvich, Hallbäck, M., Lundgren, Y., and Weiss, L.,** The hemodynamic consequences of regional hypotension in spontaneously hypertensive and normotensive rats, *Acta Physiol. Scand.,* 83, 532, 1971.
79. **Hansen, T. R., Abrams, G. D., and Bohr, D. F.,** Role of pressure in structural and functional changes in arteries of hypertensive rats, *Circ. Res.,* 33 & 34 (Suppl. 1), I-101, 1974.
80. **Bund, S. J., Wesst K. P., and Heagerty, A. M.,** Effects of protection from pressure on resistance artery morphology and reactivity in spontaneously hypertensive and Wistar-Kyoto rats, *Circ. Res.,* 68, 1230, 1991.
81. **Stacy, D. L. and Prewitt, R. L.,** Effects of chronic hypertension and its reversal on arteries and arterioles, *Circ. Res.,* 65, 869, 1989.
82. **Roman, R. J.,** Altered pressure-natriuresis relationship in young spontaneously hypertensive rats, *Hypertension,* 9 (Suppl. 3), III-130, 1987.
83. **Bohr, D. F.,** Pathophysiology of the vasculature in hypertension, *Hypertension,* 18 (Suppl. III), III-69, 1991.
84. **Michel, M. C., Brodde, O.-E., and Insel, P. A.,** Peripheral adrenergic receptors in hypertension, *Hypertension,* 16, 107, 1990.
85. **Orlov, S. N., Gulak, P. V., Litinov, I. S., and Postnov, Y. V.,** Evidence of altered structure of the erythrocyte membrane in spontaneously hypertensive rats, *Clin. Sci.,* 63, 43, 1982.
86. **Hermsmeyer, K. and Rusch, N. J.,** Calcium channel alterations in genetic hypertension, *Hypertension,* 14, 453, 1989.
87. **Hermsmeyer, K.,** Ca^{2+} alterations in resistance arteries in hypertension, in *Resistance Arteries, Structure and Function,* Mulvany, M. J., et al., Eds., Elsevier, New York, 1991, 322.
88. **Cauvin, C., Gelband, C., and van Breemen, C.,** 45Ca fluxes in rat mesenteric resistance vessels, *J. Cardiovasc. Pharmacol.,* 10 (Suppl. 1), S44, 1987.
89. **Turla, M. B. and Webb, R. C.,** Augmented phosphoinositide metabolism in aortas from genetically hypertensive rats, *Am. J. Physiol.,* 258 (Heart Circ. Physiol. 27), H173, 1990.
90. **Heagerty, A. M., Ollernshaw, J. D., and Swales, J. D.,** Abnormal vascular phosphoinositide hydrolysis in the spontaneously hypertensive rat, *Br. J. Pharmacol.,* 89, 803, 1986.
91. **Durkin, H., Ollerenshaw, J. D., and Heagerty, A. M.,** Resistance artery phosphoinositide metabolism in genetic hypertension, *J. Hypertens.,* 8, 557, 1990.
92. **Uehara, Y., Ishii, M., Ishimitsu, T., and Sugimoto, T.,** Enhanced phospholipase C activity in the vascular wall of spontaneously hypertensive rats, *Hypertension,* 11, 28, 1988.
93. **Limon, I., Blanc, J., Koutouzov, S., Knorr, A., Meyer, P., and Marche, P.,** Platelet phospholipase C activity in salt-dependent hypertension, *Hypertension,* 15, 381, 1990.
94. **Hill, M. A., Falcone, J. C., and Meininger, G. A.,** Evidence for protein kinase C involvement in arteriolar myogenic reactivity, *Am. J. Physiol.,* 259 (Heart Circ. Physiol. 28), H1586, 1990.
95. **Storm, D. S., Turla, M. B., Todd, K. M., and Webb, R. C.,** Calcium and contractile responses to phorbol esters and the calcium channel agonist, Bay K 8644, in arteries from hypertensive rats, *Am. J. Hypertens.,* 3, 245S, 1990.

96. **Kamm, K. E., Gerthoffer, W. T., Murphy, R. A., and Bohr, D. F.,** Mechanical properties of carotid arteries from DOCA hypertensive swine, *Hypertension,* 13, 102, 1989.
97. **Owens, G. K.,** Mechanisms of smooth muscle growth: cellular hypertrophy vs. hyperplasia, in *Hypertrophic Response in Smooth Muscle*, Seidel, C. L., Ed., CRC Press, Boca Raton, FL, 1987, 1.
98. **Garwitz, McMahon, E. and Paul, R. J.,** Calcium sensitivity of isometric force in intact and chemically skinned aortas during the development of aldosterone-salt hypertension in the rat, *Circ. Res.,* 56, 427, 1985.
99. **Boels, P. J., Troschka, M., Ruegg, J. C., and Pfitzer, G.,** Higher Ca^{2+} sensitivity of triton-skinned guinea pig mesenteric microarteries as compared with large arteries, *Circ. Res.,* 69, 989, 1991.
100. **Fatigati, V. and Murphy, R. A.,** Actin and tropomyosin variants in smooth muscles: dependence on type, *J. Biol. Chem.,* 259, 14383, 1984.
101. **Meininger, G. A. and Trzeciakowski, J. P.,** Vasoconstriction is amplified by autoregulation during vasoconstrictor-induced hypertension, *Am. J. Physiol.,* 254 (Heart Circ. Physiol. 23), H709, 1988.
102. **Faber, J. E. and Meininger, G. A.,** Selective interaction of alpha-adrenoceptors with myogenic regulation of microvascular smooth muscle, *Am. J. Physiol.,* 259 (Heart Circ. Physiol. 29), H1126, 1990.
103. **Hill, M. A., Davis, M. J., and Meininger, G. A.,** Cyclooxygenase inhibition potentiates myogenic activity in skeletal muscle arterioles, *Am. J. Physiol.,* 258 (Heart Circ. Physiol. 27), H127, 1990.
104. **Falcone, J. C. and Meininger, G. A.,** The myogenic response of isolated arterioles from spontaneously hypertensive rats, in *Resistance Arteries, Structure and Function*, Mulvany, M. J., et al., Eds., Elsevier, New York, 317, 1991.
105. **Kaley, G., Koller, A., Rodenburg, J. M., Messina, E. J., and Wolin, M. S.,** Regulation of arteriolar tone and responses via L-arginine pathway in skeletal muscle, *Am. J. Physiol.,* 262 (Heart Circ. Physiol. 31), H987, 1992.
106. **Kuo, L., Chilian, W. M., and Davis, M. J.,** Interaction of pressure- and flow-induced responses in porcine coronary resistance vessels, *Am. J. Physiol.,* 261 (Heart Circ. Physiol. 30), H1706, 1991.
107. **Koller, A. and Kaley, G.,** Prostaglandins mediate arteriolar dilatation to increased blood flow velocity in skeletal muscle microcirculation, *Circ. Res.,* 67, 529, 1990.
108. **Luscher, T. F. and Vanhoutte, P. M.,** Endothelium-dependent responses in normotensive and hypertensive Dahl rats, *Hypertension,* 9, 157, 1987.
109. **Tesfamariam, B. and Halpern, W.,** Endothelium-dependent and endothelium-independent vasodilatation in resistance arteries from hypertensive rats, *Hypertension,* 11, 440, 1988.
110. **Ortenberg, J. M., Cook, A. K., Inscho, E. W., and Carmines, P. K.,** Attenuated afferent arteriolar response to acetylcholine in Goldblatt hypertension, *Hypertension* 19, 785, 1992.
111. **Dohi, Y., Theil, M. A., Buhler, F. R., and Luscher, T. F.,** Activation of endothelial L-arginine pathway in resistance arteries: effect of age and hypertension, *Hypertension,* 15, 170, 1990.
112. **Fu-Xiang, D., Skopec, J., Diederich, A., and Diederich, D.,** Prostaglandin H2 and Thromboxane A2 are contractile factors in intrarenal arteries of spontaneously hypertensive rats, *Hypertension*, 19, 795, 1992.
113. **Diederich, D., Yang, Z., Buhler, F. R., and Luscher, T. F.,** Impaired endothelium-dependent relaxations in hypertensive resistance arteries involve cyclooxygenase pathway, *Am. J. Physiol.,* 258 (Heart Circ. Physiol. 27), H445, 1990.

114. **Mayhan, W. G.,** Role of prostaglandin H2-thromboxane A2 in response of cerebral arterioles during chronic hypertension, *Am. J. Physiol.,* 262 (Heart Circ. Physiol. 31), H539, 1992.
115. **Yanagisawa, M., Kurihara, H., Kimura, S., Kobayashi, M., Mitsui, Y., Goto, K., and Masaki, T.,** A novel potent vasoconstrictor peptide produced by vascular endothelial cells, *Nature,* 332, 411, 1988.
116. **Naruse, M., Kawana, M., Hifumi, S., Naruse, K., Yoshihara, I., Oka, T., Kato, Y., Monzen, C., Kurimoto, F., Ohsumi, K., Hosoda, S., and Demura, H.,** Plasma immunoreactive endothelin, but not thrombomodulin, is increased in patients with essential hypertension and ischemic heart disease, *J. Cardiovasc. Pharmacol.,* 17 (Suppl. 7), S471, 1991.
117. **Yoshizumi, M., Kurihara, H., Sugiyama, T., Takaku, F., Yanagisawa, M., Masaki, T., and Yazaki, Y.,** Hemodynamic shear stress stimulates endothelin production by cultured endothelial cells, *Biochem. Biophys. Res. Comm.,* 161, 859, 1989.
118. **Dohi, Y., Criscone, L., and Luscher, T. F.,** Renovascular hypertension impairs formation of endothelium-derived relaxing factors and sensitivity to endothelin-1 in resistance arteries, *Br. J. Pharmacol.,* 104, 349, 1991.
119. **Takeshita, H., Nishikibe, M., Yano, M., and Ikemoto, F.,** Coronary vascular response to endothelin in isolated perfused hearts of spontaneously hypertensive rats, *Clin. Exp. Pharmacol. Physiol.,* 18, 661, 1991.
120. **Dohi, Y., Hahn, A. W., Boulanger, C. M., Buhler, F. R., and Luscher, T. F.,** Endothelin stimulated by angiotensin II augments contractility of spontaneously hypertensive rat resistance arteries, *Hypertension,* 19, 131, 1992.
121. **Haddy, F. J.,** Humoral factors in hypertension, NIPS 4, 202, 1989.
122. **Blaustein, M. P. and Hamlyn, J. M.,** Pathogenesis of essential hypertension: a link between dietary salt and high blood pressure, *Hypertension,* 18 (Suppl. 3), III-184, 1991.
123. **Hamlyn, J. M., Harris, D. W., and Ludens, J. H.,** Digitalis-like activity in human plasma: purification, affinity and mechanism, *J. Biol. Chem.,* 264, 7395, 1989.
124. **Meininger, G. A., Routh, L. K., and Granger, H. J.,** Autoregulation and vasoconstriction in the intestine during acute renal hypertension, *Hypertension,* 7, 364, 1985.
125. **Owens, G. K. and Thompson, M. M.,** Developmental changes in isoactin expression in rat aortic smooth muscle cells in vivo, *J. Biol. Chem.,* 261, 13373, 1986.
126. **Turla, M., Thompson, M., Corjay, M., and Owens, G.,** Angiotensin II and arginine vasopressin increase smooth muscle alpha-actin and nonmuscle beta-actin mRNA as well as actin synthesis and content in cultured rat aortic smooth muscle cells, *J. Cell Biol.,* 109, 244a, 1989.
127. **Keeley, F. W. and Alatawi, A.,** The response of aortic elastin synthesis and accumulation to developing hypertension. The inhibitory effect of colchicine on this response, *Lab. Invest.,* 64, 499, 1991.
128. **Keeley, F. W. and Johnson, D. J.,** The effect of developing hypertension on the synthesis and accumulation of elastin in the aorta of the rat, *Can. J. Biochem. Cell Biol.,* 64, 38, 1986.
129. **Nister, M., Hammacher, A., Mellstrom, K., Siegbahn, A., Ronnstrand, L., Westermark, B., and Heldin, C.-H.,** A glioma-derived PDGF A chain homodimer has different functional activities from a PDGF AB heterodimer purified from human platelets, *Cell,* 52, 791, 1988.
130. **Block, L. H., Emmons, L. R., Vogt, E., Sachinidis, A., Vetter, W., and Hoppe, J.,** Calcium-channel blockers inhibit the action of recombinant platelet-derived growth factor in vascular smooth muscle cells, *Proc. Natl. Acad. Sci. U.S.A.,* 86, 2388, 1989.

131. **Nilsson, J., Sjolund, M., Palmberg, L., Thyberg, J., and Heldin, C.-H.,** Arterial smooth muscle cells in primary culture produce a platelet-derived growth factor like protein, *Proc. Natl. Acad. Sci. U.S.A.,* 82, 4418, 1985.
132. **Seifert, R. A., Schwartz, S. M., and Bowen-Pope, D. F.,** Developmentally regulated production of platelet-derived growth factor-like molucules, *Nature*, 311, 669, 1984.
133. **Sjolund, M., Hedin, U., Sejersen, T., Heldin, C.-H., and Thyberg, J.,** Arterial smooth muscle cells express platelet-derived growth factor (PDGF) A chain mRNA, secrete, PDGF-like mitogen, and bind exogenous PDGF in a phenotype- and growth state-dependent manner, *J. Cell Biol.,* 106, 403, 1988.
134. **Majesky, M. W., Benditt, E. P., and Schwartz, S. M.,** Expression and developmental control of platelet-derived growth factor A-chain and B chain/Sis genes in rat aortic smooth muscle cells, *Proc. Natl. Acad. Sci. U.S.A.,* 85, 1524, 1988.
135. **Walker, L. N., Bowen-Pope, D. F., Ross, R., and Reidy, M. A.,** Production of platelet-derived growth factor-like molecules by cultured arterial smooth muscle cells accompanies proliferation after arterial injury, *Proc. Natl. Acad. Sci. U.S.A.,* 83, 7311, 1986.
136. **Libby, P., Warner, S. J. C., Salomon, R. N., and Birinyi, L. K.,** Production of platelet-derived growth factor-like mitogen by smooth-muscle cells from human atheroma, *Proc. Natl. Acad. Sci.,* 318, 1493, 1988.
137. **Mulvany, M., Baandrup, U., and Gundersen, H.,** Evidence for hyperplasia in mesenteric resistance vessels of spontaneously hypertensive rats using a three-dimensional dissector, *Circ. Res.,* 57, 794, 1985.
138. **Williams, L. T.,** Signal transduction by the platelet-derived growth factor receptor, *Science*, 243, 1564, 1989.
139. **Blank, R., Thompson, M., and Owens, G.,** Cell cycle versus density dependence of smooth muscle alpha actin expression in cultured rat aortic muscle cells, *J. Cell Biol.,* 107, 299, 1988.
140. **Corjay, M., Lynch, K., Thompson, M., and Owens, G.,** Differential effect of PDGF versus serum induced growth on SM alpha actin and beta non-muscle actin mRNA expression in cultured rat aortic smooth muscle cells, *J. Biol. Chem.,* 264, 10501, 1989.
141. **Sarzani, R., Brecher, P., and Chobanian, A. V.,** Growth factor expression in aorta of normotensive and hypertensive rats, *J. Clin. Invest.,* 83, 1404, 1989.
142. **Sporn, M. B. and Roberts, A. B.,** Transforming growth factor-B, multiple actions and potential clinical applications, *JAMA*, 262, 938, 1989.
143. **Owens, G. K., Geisterfer, A. T., Yang, Y. W., and Komoriya, A.,** Transforming growth factor-B-induced growth inhibition and cellular hypertrophy in cultured vascular smooth muscle cells, *J. Cell Biol.,* 107, 771, 1988.
144. **Geisterfer, A. A. T., Peach, M. J., and Owens, G. K.,** Angiotensin II induces hypertrophy, not hyperplasia, of cultured rat aortic smooth muscle cells, *Circ. Res.,* 62, 749, 1988.
145. **Lyall, F., Morton, J. J., Lever, A. F., and Gragoe, E. J.,** Angiotensin II activates Na^+-H^+ exchange and stimulates growth in cultured vascular smooth muscle cells, *Hypertension*, 6(4), 438, 1988.
146. **Naftilan, A. J., Gilliland, G. K., Eldridge, C. S., and Kraft, A. S.,** Induction of the proto-oncogene c-jun by angiotensin II, *Mol. Cell. Biol.,* 10(10), 5536, 1990.
147. **Naftilan, A. J., Pratt, R. E., and Dzau, V. J.,** Induction of PDGF A-chain and c-myc gene expression by angiotensin II in cultured rat vascular smooth muscle cells, *J. Clin. Invest.,* 83, 1419, 1989.
148. **Naftilan, A. J., Pratt, R. E., Eldridge, C. S., Lin, H. L., and Dzau, V. J.,** Angiotensin II induces c-fos expression in smooth muscle via transcriptional control, *Hypertension*, 13(6:2), 706, 1989.

149. **Itoh, H., Pratt, R. E., Gibbons, G., and Dzau, V. J.,** Angiotensin II modulates proliferation of vascular smooth muscle cells (VSMC) via dual autocrine loops of TGFb and bFGF, *Hypertension*, 18, 396, 1991.
150. **Itoh, H., Pratt, R. E., and Dzau, V. J.,** Antisense oligonucleotides complementary to PDGF mRNA attenuate angiotensin II-induced vascular hypertrophy, *Hypertension*, 116, 325, 1990.
151. **Nakamaru, M., Jackson, E. K., and Inagami, T.,** b-Adrenoceptor mediated release of angiotensin II from mesenteric arteries, *Am. J. Physiol.*, 250, H144, 1986.
152. **Mizuno, K., Nakamaru, M., Higashimori, K., and Inagami, T.,** Local generation and release of angiotensin II in peripheral vascular tissue, *Hypertension*, 11, 223, 1988.
153. **Wang, D. H. and Prewitt, R. L.,** Arteriolar proliferation in hypertension induced by infusion of angiotensin II (AngII), *Circulation*, 4(1), II-561, 1991.
154. **Wang, D. H., Keelan, C. A., and Prewitt, R. L.,** The induction of PDGF in vivo by infusion of Angiotensin II, *FASEB J.*, 6(5), M115, 1992.
155. **Griffin, S. A., Brown, W. C. B., MacPherson, F., McGrath, J. C., Wilson, V. G., Korsgaard, N., Mulvany, M. J., and Lever, A. F.,** Angiotensin II causes vascular hypertrophy in part by a non-pressor mechanism, *Hypertension*, 17, 626, 1991.
156. **Wang, D. H. and Prewitt, R. L.,** Captopril reduces aortic and microvascular growth in hypertensive and normotensive rats, *Hypertension*, 15, 68, 1990.
157. **Wang, D. H. and Prewitt, R. L.,** Longitudinal effect of captopril on aortic and arteriolar development in normotensive rats, *Am. J. Physiol.*, 260(6), H1956, 1991.
158. **Wang, D. H., Keelan, C. A., and Prewitt, R. L.,** The effect of DUP753, a nonpeptide angiotensin II antagonist, on arteries and arterioles in renal hypertensive rats, *FASEB J.*, 5(6), A1752, 1991.
159. **Rozengurt, E.,** Early signals in the mitogenic response, *Science*, 234, 161, 1986.
160. **Owen, N. and Villereal, M.,** Lys-bradykinin stimulates Na^+ influx and DNA synthesis in cultured human fibroblasts, *Cell*, 32, 979, 1983.
161. **Owen, N. E.,** Effect of prostaglandin E_1 on DNA synthesis in vascular smooth muscle cells, *Am. J. Physiol.*, 250, C584, 1988.
162. **Nemecek, G., Coughlin, S., Handley, D., and Moskowitz, M.,** Stimulation of aortic smooth muscle cell mitogenesis by serotonin, *Proc. Natl. Acad. Sci. U.S.A.*, 83, 674, 1986.
163. **Bevan, R. D. and Tsuru, H.,** Functional and structural changes in the rabbit ear artery after sympathetic denervation, *Circ. Res.*, 49, 478, 1981.
164. **Bevan, R. D. and Tsuru, H.,** Long-term influence of the sympathetic nervous system on arterial structure and reactivity: possible factor in hypertension, in *Disturbances in Neurogenis Control of the Circulation*, Abboud, F. M., Fozzard, H. A., Gilmore, J. P., and Reis, D. J., Eds., American Physiology Society, Bethesda, MD, 1981, 153.
165. **Blaes, N. and Boissel, J. P.,** Growth-stimulating effect of catecholamines on rat aortic smooth muscle cells in culture, *J. Cell Physiol.*, 116, 167, 1983.
166. **Heagerty, A. M. and Ollerenshaw, J. D.,** The phosphoinositide signalling system and hypertension, *J. Hypertension*, 5, 515, 1987.
167. **Taubman, M. B., Berk, B. C., Izumo, S., Tsuda, T., Alexander, R. W., and Bernardo, N. G.,** Angiotensin II induces c-fos mRNA in aortic smooth muscle: role of Ca^{2+} mobilization and protein kinase C activation, *J. Biol. Chem.*, 264(1), 526, 1989.
168. **Kawahara, Y., Sunako, M., Tsuda, T., Fukuzaki, H., Fukumoto, Y., and Takai, Y.,** Angiotensin II induces expression of the c-fos gene through protein kinase C activation and calcium ion mobilization in cultured vascular smooth muscle cells, *Biochem. Biophys. Res. Comm.*, 150(1), 52, 1988.

169. **Majesky, M. W., Daemen, M. J. A. P., and Schwartz, S. M.,** α_1-adrenergic stimulation of platelet-derived growth factor A-chain gene expression in rat aorta, *J. Biol. Chem.,* 265(2), 1082, 1990.
170. **Hume, W. R.,** Proline and thymidine uptake in rabbit ear artery segments in vitro increased by chronic tangential load, *Hypertension,* 2, 738, 1980.
171. **Leung, D. Y. M., Glagov, S., and Mathews, M. B.,** Cyclic stretching stimulates synthesis of matrix components by arterial smooth muscle cells in vitro, *Science,* 191, 475, 1976.
172. **Terracio, L., Miller, B., and Borg, T. K.,** Effects of cyclic mechanical stimulation of the cellular components of the heart: in vitro, *In Vitro Cell Dev. Biol.,* 24, 1988.
173. **Kent, R. L., Hoober, J. K., and Cooper, G.,** Load responsiveness of protein synthesis in adult myocardium: role of cardiac deformation linked to sodium influx, *Circ. Res.,* 64, 74, 1989.
174. **Kira, Y., Kochel, P. J., Gordon, E. E., and Morgan, H. E.,** Aortic perfusion pressure as a determinant of cardiac protein synthesis, *Am. J. Physiol.,* 246, C247, 1984.
175. **Vandenburgh, H. H. and Kaufman, S.,** Stretch-induced growth of skeletal myotubes correlates with activation of the sodium pump, *J. Cell. Physiol.,* 109, 205, 1981.
176. **Sachs, F.,** Biophysics of mechanoreception, *Membrane Biochem.,* 6, 173, 1986.
177. **Hammond, G. L., Lai, Y. K., and Markert, C. L.,** The molecules that initiate cardiac hypertrophy are not species-specific, *Science,* 216, 529, 1982.
178. **Vandenburgh, H. and Kaufman, S.,** In vitro model for stretch-induced hypertrophy of skeletal muscle, *Science,* 203, 265, 1979.
179. **Langille, B. L. and O'Donnell, F.,** Reductions in arterial diameter produced by chronic decreases in blood flow are endothelium dependent, *Science,* 231, 405, 1986.
180. **Franke, R. P., Grafe, M., Schnittler, H., Seiffge, D., Mittermayer, C., and Drenckhahn, D.,** Induction of human vascular endothelial stress fibers by fluid shear stress, *Nature,* 307, 648, 1984.
181. **Kim, D. W., Gotlieb, A. I., and Langille, B. L.,** In vivo modulation of endothelial F-actin microfilaments by experimental alterations in shear stress, *Arteriosclerosis,* 9, 439, 1989.
182. **Olesen, S. P., Clapham, D. E., and Davies, P. F.,** Haemodynamic shear stress activates a K^+ current in vascular endothelial cells, *Nature,* 331, 168, 1988.
183. **Rhodin, J. A.,** The ultrastructure of mammalian arterioles and precapillary sphincters, *J. Ultrastruct. Res.,* 18, 181, 1967.
184. **Rhodin, J. A.,** Ultrastructure of mammalian venous capillaries, venules and small collecting veins, *J. Ultrastruct. Res.,* 25, 452, 1968.
185. **Huttner, I., Boutet, M., and More, R. H.,** Gap junctions in arterial endothelium, *J. Cell. Biol.,* 57, 247, 1973.
186. **Sheridan, J. D. and Atkinson, M. M.,** Physiological roles of permeable junctions: some possibilities, *Annu. Rev. Physiol.,* 47, 337, 1985.
187. **Pohl, U., Holtz, J., Busse, R., and Bassenge, E.,** Crucial role of endothelium in the vasodilator response to increased flow in vivo, *Hypertension,* 8, 37, 1986.
188. **Deforrest, J. M. and Hollis, T. M.,** Shear stress and aortic histamine synthesis, *Am. J. Physiol.,* 236, H701, 1978.
189. **Frangos, J. A., Eskin, S. G., McIntire, L. V., and Ives, C. L.,** Flow effects on prostacyclin production by cultured human endothelial cells, *Science,* 227, 1477, 1985.

Chapter 5

Circulatory Shock

Lerner B. Hinshaw and Thomas E. Emerson, Jr.

CONTENTS

I. INTRODUCTION: RHEOLOGY OF THE MICROCIRCULATION

A review of basic principles of rheology of the microcirculation from the excellent review by Chien[1] will be of benefit in evaluating the mechanism and significance of microcirculatory changes occurring during circulatory shock.

Chien points out that the flow of blood in the microcirculation depends on the combination of the geometric features of the microvasculature and the flow properties of the blood. The flow components, "shear rate", expressed as the blood velocity gradient between adjacent fluid laminae, and "shear stress", the force parallel to the direction of blood flow, are related to the viscosity of blood as follows:

$$\frac{\text{Shear Stress}}{\text{Shear Rate}} = \text{Viscosity} \qquad \textbf{(5-1)}$$

Blood viscosity decreases to low levels under conditions of very high shear rates and elevated shear stresses (as in the normal flow state) which occurs because red blood cells are deformed by shear. In contrast, blood viscosity increases during low blood flow conditions (as present in shock) because of a decrease in shear stress and resultant relative absence of red cell deformation and disaggregation.

Resistance to blood flow is another important factor influencing the behavior of the microcirculation. It is a calculated value and is expressed as follows:

0-8493-4547-2/94/$0.00+$.50

$$\text{Vascular Resistance} = \frac{\text{Arterial Pressure} - \text{Venous Pressure}}{\text{Blood Flow}} \quad \textbf{(5-2)}$$

Blood viscosity and a new term, blood vessel geometry ("hindrance") are related to vascular resistance as follows:

$$\text{Vascular Resistance} = \text{Vascular Hindrance} \times \text{Blood Viscosity} \quad \textbf{(5-3)}$$

Vascular hindrance in the microcirculation has been found to vary with the number, diameter (to the fourth power), and length of blood vessels. The diameter relationship is as follows:

$$\text{Vascular Hindrance} \propto \frac{1}{\text{diameter}^4} \quad \textbf{(5-4)}$$

The low hematocrit observed in the microcirculation lowers the blood viscosity component of resistance and thus offsets the effect of narrowness of the blood vessels in raising vascular hindrance as shown in the formula above. The increase in resistance due to the small diameter of the microvessels is therefore compensated for by the decrease in hematocrit which progressively decreases linearly from arterioles to capillaries, rising again in the large venules.[1] The result of these changes in hematocrit is that blood flow through the microvessels is increased.

Chien points out certain unfavorable occurrences in a low flow (shock) state: under conditions of severe vasoconstriction, vascular resistance remains high because of a marked increase in vascular hindrance. Low blood flow may result from either, or both, an increase in resistance and a decrease in arterial perfusion pressure (shock). Whether a reduction in blood flow results from systemic hypotension, vasoconstriction, or a rheological disturbance, the consequent decrease in shear stress could cause a further increase in blood viscosity and retardation of flow, thus leading to a vicious cycle.

Another serious derangement may result from the shear-dependent behavior of blood viscosity: under normal conditions, the shear rates are high in arterioles and venules so that blood viscosity is low. However, in contrast during low blood flow states the arteriolar shear rate may still be high enough to allow blood viscosity to be low, but the shear rate of venules may be reduced sufficiently to elevate blood viscosity to a marked degree. Under this unfortunate hemodynamic condition, postcapillary resistance (venous resistance) is elevated over precapillary resistance (arterial resistance) thus increasing mean capillary pressure resulting in transcapillary fluid leakage (edema).[1] This effect would subsequently decrease the plasma volume, increase both the circulating hematocrit and blood viscosity, leading to another vicious cycle.

Chien's careful evaluation of factors influencing the rheology of the microcirculation underscores the importance of analyzing the pathophysiological disturbances in shock and designing means of improving the state of microcirculatory rheology.

II. MICROCIRCULATION AND SHOCK: THE PROBLEM

Pathophysiological changes in the microvasculature of regional vascular beds may have profound influences on the morbidity and mortality of shock. According to Sibbald,[2] the sepsis syndrome is a disease characterized by a diffuse increase in microvascular permeability within the lung and systemic microcirculation. Such damage to the microvasculature occurs before clinical evidence of multiple organ failure (MOF) by creating diffuse cellular ischemia. Devising an adequate therapy necessitates an understanding of the precise etiology of microvascular injury and the development of methods to reduce or prevent the injury.

Wang and colleagues[3] point out that severe hemorrhage remains one of the major causes of morbidity and mortality in patients with trauma and that in those who survive an initial injury there is a risk of sepsis, MOF, and eventual death. In addition, these patients may suffer immunosuppression which further compromises their ability to survive. Since cardiovascular changes occur early, including suppression of cardiac output, circulating blood volume, and decreased organ blood flow, attention should be given to the resulting regional microcirculatory disturbances which may lead to MOF and death. Such studies should include measurements and behavior of regional microvascular blood flow in various organs during both the untreated shock period and attempted therapy.

It has long been recognized that the traumatized or infected patient shows a variety of dysfunctions including, among others, decrease in tissue perfusion, acidosis, cardiovascular collapse, and ultimately multiple organ failure and death.[4] It is important to determine how microvascular responses in various organs contribute to these serious sequelae.

Clinicians have believed for many years that the basic metabolic defect in shock follows as a result of a disturbance of blood flow rate and blood flow distribution within the microvasculature.[5] It has been emphasized that the distribution of blood flow to individual vascular beds is determined in large part by neurohumoral factors and local autoregulatory mechanisms. According to Haljamae,[5] a serious disparity may exist in flow distribution to central vital organs (brain, liver) vs. other more peripheral organs (skin, skeletal muscle), the latter being "target organs" for neurohumoral compensatory vascular adjustments. In relation to our lack of understanding of the cause of inadequate blood perfusion of regional beds, the mechanisms of the underlying microcirculatory disturbances have not been revealed by adequately performed microcirculatory studies. A part of the problem of interpreting the seriousness of clinically observed shock is that the cellular metabolic consequences of microcirculatory deterioration in "peripheral" tissues, e.g., skeletal muscle, during shock are only partially reflected by changes in "central" tissues, e.g., liver, and therefore may conceal the impact of a "peripheral defect", e.g., skeletal muscle, the largest cell mass of the body and the major source of lactate.[5] Information on local vascular changes and blood-tissue gradients of oxygen, pH, and potassium in skeletal muscle may have considerable value in the management of critically ill patients.[5]

Badonnel et al.[6] provide insight into the importance of studying the role of the microcirculation in the central nervous system (CNS) during shock. They discuss the century-old question, "Is shock the result of a failure of cerebrovascular compensatory mechanisms or vice versa?" Some authors have suggested that CNS injury may antecede damage to other tissues and lead to irreversible shock through a central neurogenic influence on the systemic circulation, the brain thereby being one of the first organs to fail in the sequence of MOF. A current view proposes that the central nervous system is injured in shock through the development of an impaired microcirculation.

Robb and Jabs[7] stress the importance of two microvascular beds, the pulmonary microcirculation and the peripheral microcirculation, each perfused by separate pumps which develop pressure and provide flow. It is suggested that there is a common dysfunction, i.e., hypercoagulation defect, which may occur in each of the microcirculations of lung and periphery leading to shock.

Cryer et al.[8] point out that arteriolar dilatation, loss of venous tone, and a decrease in circulating and tissue pH all contribute to the decompensated state of hemorrhagic shock. The mechanisms accounting for these dysfunctions may be learned from studies of the microcirculation. At the present time, there exists a concept that acidosis reduces microvascular reactivity to catecholamines, contributing in a significant way to peripheral vascular failure in shock. Peripheral vascular failure may result from combinations of losses in vascular sensitivity to vasoconstrictor hormones, or increased sensitivity to vasodilator hormones, or increased local tissue production of vasodilator hormones and/or tissue metabolites.[8]

III. MICROVASCULAR RESPONSES OF REGIONAL VASCULAR BEDS DURING SHOCK

The object of this review is to consider the role of the microcirculation in shock by reviewing various microvascular responses in regional vascular beds and to identify pathophysiological mechanisms occurring in the microcirculation during shock.

Microvascular responses of organs most frequently studied during shock are pulmonary, splanchnic, and skeletal muscle while less discussed organs/tissues are heart, central nervous system, and skin. A survey of the literature reveals significant findings in the microcirculatory systems of all of the above and they will be discussed briefly in this section.

A. PULMONARY SYSTEM

It has long been recognized that the lungs perform a critical role in hemorrhagic shock, especially during the period of transfusion therapy when maldistribution of pulmonary blood flow is apparent.[9] Attempts have been made to study the microvascular circulation of the lung during shock and following recovery.[7] Fluorometry, comprised of fluorescence-photographic techniques[9] and cinephotomicrography[7] have been employed in pulmonary microvascular studies. Observations of the microcirculation in experimental shock models have been made during reactions to blood loss, trauma, burns, endotoxin, and antigen, and in all these, platelet and red cell aggregations are major occurrences. Platelet aggregates and their entrapment in the pulmonary capillary system are compatible with the development of disseminated intravascular coagulation (DIC). In addition to aggregates formed within the microcirculation of the lung during shock, platelet and red blood cell (RBC) aggregates from all vascular beds in all forms of experimental shock may be "washed" into the pulmonary microcirculation where they obstruct flow through the pulmonary arterioles. The resulting blockage of flow causes elevated right heart (pulmonary) pressures and low left heart (left atrial and systemic) pressures. It appears that blockage of the pulmonary microcirculation is a basic defect in shock which may lead to a "vicious cycle", including the progressive development of pulmonary edema and poor systemic peripheral perfusion of blood to vital organs and finally terminating in an irreversible condition of shock.[7]

Platelets, white blood cells (WBCs), RBCs, miscellaneous particulate material, and "sludge" aggregates have been observed in various microcirculatory studies since the time of Krogh in 1922. Robb and Jabs emphasize that these effects occur in all forms of shock while others point out that the primary adverse pulmonary changes in the microcirculation occur during transfusion therapy.[7,9]

Robb and Jabs, using cinephotomicrography, demonstrated remarkable obstructive changes in the pulmonary microcirculation in many forms of shock.[7] The dynamic effects of a platelet aggregate are described as it becomes lodged within the pulmonary microcirculation: "shifting and shunting of blood flow occurs as the embolus slides into one branch of a bifurcation." In direct response to pulmonary microvascular blockage, other events occur, including elevated pulmonary and right-heart pressures, rising vascular resistances, and electrocardiographic (ECG) changes, and this series of events if sustained, usually terminates in irreversible shock.[7] Perbeck et al.,[9] using photographic fluorescence techniques, describe severe pathophysiologic changes after transfusion therapy including pulmonary and endothelial injury, presence of microthrombi, edema, hemorrhage, and maldistribution of pulmonary blood flow. Large areas of the lungs do not receive any blood during transfusion therapy while some small areas show increased permeability, suggesting damage to lung capillaries: It appears that the progressive development of pulmonary vascular blockage, caused by the accumulation of multiple small microemboli in the pulmonary microcirculation is the basis for the primary pathogenetic events leading to sustained shock and death.

B. SPLANCHNIC BED

The role of intestinal ischemia leading to death in shock has been seriously considered for over 30 years. Scalia et al.[10] have pointed out circumstantial evidence favoring this view: (1) many of the circulating mediators released in most experimental forms of shock, including cytokines and eicosanoids among others, are associated with intestinal vasoconstriction or ischemia; (2) infections in the peritoneal cavity and infections at remote sites are due to intestinal-derived organisms; (3) leakage of endotoxin from the huge endogenous intestinal reservoir is considered to be a precursor for the leakage of bacteria (translocation), and (4) bacterial translocation from the intestine to the blood has been demonstrated in experimental shock models.[10,11]

Recent observations in experimental models seem to coalesce into a growing body of evidence implicating the intestine in the pathogenesis of the state of "hyperdynamic" sepsis, and the subsequent pathophysiology leading to MOF.[10]

Experimental animal models have yielded important information about the role of the splanchnic microcirculation in shock. Guth and Morishita[12] developed an *in vivo* microscopical technique to study the microvasculature of rats during hemorrhagically induced systemic hypotension (shock). A decrease in gastric mucosal blood flow was observed using this technique: a significant correlation (n = 0.92) was found between RBC velocity and mean systemic arterial blood pressure. Microvessel diameters did not change with reduction of blood pressure in these experiments and RBC velocity measured by microscopy reflected changes in blood flow. A linear correlation was found between mucosal blood flow and graded systemic pressures progressively down to shock levels (30 mmHg), which was unexpected in as much as this is an organ considered by some to be nonessential to survival during the course of shock.[12]

Whitworth and others observed hypoperfusion of the intestinal microcirculation without decreased cardiac output during live *Escherichia coli*-induced sepsis in rats.[11] They studied the microcirculation of a loop of small intestine with intact neurovascular connections by means of *in vivo* video microscopy and optical Doppler velocimetry at a magnification of × 1500. Cardiac output measured by a transpulmonary thermodilution procedure increased with infusion of 10^9 colony forming units (CFU) *E. coli* while microvascular flow to the small intestine decreased by nearly 30% in 1 h and 60% in 2 h. Progressive arteriolar constriction occurred during the high cardiac output (hyperdynamic) stage at all levels of blood flow in the intestinal microcirculation.[11] It was considered that this degree of hypoperfusion could contribute to intestinal mucosal injury and intestinal mucosal barrier dysfunction during shock. The importance of this work was in its human relevance since a state of relatively compensated normotension could be titrated by adjustment of the *E. coli* dose. It is possible that intestinal mucosal lesions occurring during sepsis in the presence of systemic arterial hypotension could be due to extravascular shunting of oxygen between parallel arterioles and venules. It has been shown that animals who developed mucosal lesions experience a short period of intense intestinal vasoconstriction and hypoperfusion in the early phase of bacteremia while they are normotensive: intestinal vasoconstriction occurs in spite of a normal total peripheral vascular resistance with normal or elevated cardiac outputs and suggests that a distinct sustained vascular response, i.e., local vasoconstriction, could ultimately be seriously detrimental to the host. Furthermore, in this study, while vasoconstriction occurred at all levels of the premucosal microcirculation, vasoconstriction of third-order arterioles (small microvessels), which terminate as central villous arterioles, was intense and therefore mucosal blood flow was particularly compromised.[11] Of interest, venules showed only early mild vasoconstriction. These findings of previllous arteriolar constriction during high cardiac output bacteremia suggest that the resulting decreased intestinal mucosal microvascular blood flow may contribute to the development of mucosal barrier dysfunction and translocation of bacteria to the blood.

C. SKELETAL MUSCLE

Microcirculatory changes occurring in skeletal muscle during shock are of major importance since muscle represents the largest tissue mass in the body and is a target for compensatory vascular adjustments. Recent improvements in techniques used to study the microcirculation have provided useful information on skeletal muscle microvascular responses during shock. Studies of hemorrhagic shock have revealed important responses of the skeletal muscle circulation. During blood loss, a period of microcirculatory arrest is seen followed by reperfusion of 30 to 50% of the capillaries perfused during the resting state.[5] Many capillaries remain unperfused while in others slow, intermittent blood flow is seen. This heterogenous perfusion behavior results in various degrees of hypoxic injury to the tissue, and the blood-tissue exchange of substances is impaired because of the reduction of capillary surface area and various changes within the interstitial compartment.

Haljamae has summarized the generally observed microcirculatory responses during hemorrhagic shock.[5] He points out that the capillaries in skeletal muscle are not even continuously perfused under *resting* conditions; there is intermittent blood flow through groups of capillaries supplied by the same terminal arterioles. Blood loss results in intense vasoconstriction of the arterioles which leads to complete cessation of flow within the tissue; however, this initial period is short (minutes). Intermittent flow usually occurs quickly thereafter and there are variations of vasoconstriction in pre- and postcapillary (arterial and venous) vessels. However, this early "compensatory" period is again soon followed by a period of intense vasoconstriction, and complete microcirculatory arrest is seen lasting up to 20 min. Then when tissue perfusion ultimately reappears, the intermittent pattern of flow has disappeared and the number of perfused capillaries has decreased by 50 to 70% compared with that of the resting state.[5]

Many variations in blood flow perfusion have been reported in the skeletal muscle microcirculation during shock: three levels, between positive flow and no flow, have been observed. Some arterioles remain intensely constricted providing no blood flow; unperfused terminal arterioles are commonly seen but with some perfusion of tissue occurring from adjacent arterioles; some capillaries are constantly perfused with flow rates exceeding control flow; many capillaries remain constantly unperfused, while in postcapillary vessels the blood flow is sluggish, relatively absent, or normal, even during late shock. Although these observations underscore the complex heterogeneous patterns of perfusion of skeletal muscle microvasculature during shock, net flow is uniformly reduced by 50 to 70% of control values during shock.

Results from two skeletal muscle preparations, the rat cremaster muscle and rabbit tenuissimus muscle, have yielded interesting microcirculatory findings during shock.[4,13] Garrison and Cryer performed a number of experiments in outlining the role of the skeletal muscle microcirculation during hemorrhage and sepsis.[4] They explained the transition from the compensated to the decompensated state in hemorrhagic shock on the basis of loss of vascular smooth muscle tone in small precapillary arterioles. In contrast, in their *E. coli*-induced *hyperdynamic* sepsis model they observed a mild constriction of large arterioles but a marked dilation of small arterioles, the latter response contributing to the decreased calculated systemic vascular resistance seen during sepsis. Of great interest was their observation that the microvessels reacted similarly in the *hypodynamic* state; however, the marked vasoconstriction of large arterioles seen in hemorrhage was not present in sepsis, indicating a possible vasodilator influence, or loss of vasoconstrictor reactivity, during sepsis. Similar findings were noted in both hyper- and hypodynamic endotoxemia.

Garrison and Cryer's experimental preparation yielded a model devoid of drug anesthesia, yet being under continual microscopic view by utilizing *in vivo* videomicroscopy. The microvascular anatomy of the cremaster muscle was defined by vessel branch order:[4] the major inflow arteriole was termed a first-order arteriole (A_1) and was accompanied by an adjacent venule (V_1). Smaller second-order arterioles (A_2) and venules (V_2) were perpendicular branches while successive arteriolar branches were termed A_3 and A_4 vessels which did not have accompanying venules, and were terminal arterioles directly feeding muscular capillaries.

Mazzoni et al.[13] investigated capillary microvascular responses during hemorrhagic shock in the rabbit tenuissimus muscle. They measured lumenal diameters of capillaries during shock by use of intravital microscopy. Capillary networks were identified under low power and studied under high magnification (×100). A muscle capillary with circulating RBCs in single-file passage could be clearly observed. They examined luminal diameters of capillaries during shock for a 1-h (40% hemorrhage) period (mean pressure, 30 mmHg) using RBCs as "intraluminal markers." In their studies, reduced and intermittent blood flows were observed during hemorrhage with complete cessation of flow in about 20% of the capillaries, while luminal diameters of capillaries were substantially reduced.[13] These results were essentially similar to those of Garrison and Cryer.[4]

In summary, the various altered microcirculatory responses in skeletal muscle are impressive in the degree of their intensity, heterogeneity of responses, and complex contributions to both compensatory and decompensatory stages of shock. Of special concern is their impact and influence on the development of the "irreversible state" of shock and subsequent 100% lethality, in as much as restoration of this huge bed to the normal state may be permanently impaired and prevented by a long-standing insult of subnormal perfusion.

D. CENTRAL NERVOUS SYSTEM

Badonnel et al. studied the intracerebral microcirculation of the rat in hemorrhagic shock, and proposed that the nervous system is injured through an early development of vascular permeability which led to impaired blood flow and cell death.[6] Protective mechanisms of the cerebral circulation include the well-recognized autoregulatory phenomenon which maintains blood flow within normal limits in spite of large varieties of cerebral perfusion pressures. During severe shock however, arterial perfusion pressures may drop below the range of autoregulatory protection (<40 mmHg) and cerebral blood flow thereafter decreases in direct proportion to a further fall in mean arterial blood pressure. Death may rapidly result as a consequence. Short of this drastic lowered perfusion state, but in the lower range of autoregulatory control (>40 mmHg) during shock, there is still a question of whether the cerebral microcirculation may suffer derangement.

In addition to autoregulatory influences on cerebral microcirculatory blood flow, one must also consider the effect of endothelial injury on altering the dilator and constrictor responses of brain microvessels to vasoactive agents.[14]

Hemorrhagic shock is a frequent complication of traumatic injury and changes in cerebral consciousness and the presence of electrical abnormalities during this state open the possibility that the cerebral microcirculation may be seriously altered and thus cause depressed cerebral function.[6] Furthermore, it is possible that deranged CNS function resulting from a depressed/damaged microcirculation may in turn contribute to the lethality of shock through failure of central regulatory neurogenic influences on the systemic circulation. In any event, an adequate study of the microcirculation of the CNS is long overdue and requires urgent attention.

Badonnel et al. studied the intracerebral microcirculation of the isocortex of unanesthetized rats during hemorrhagic shock by utilizing three markers, Evans blue for fluorescence microscopic visualization, India ink for gross and light microscopy, and Horseradish peroxidase for light and electron microscopic study.[6] The conditions causing severe shock were 50 to 65% blood loss and a mean systemic arterial pressure of 30 to 40 mmHg. With these conditions, absence of India ink in the microcirculation suggested the presence of adequate cerebral blood flow, while Evans blue fluorescence and peroxidase activities demonstration on the luminal surfaces of endothelial cells by light microscopy indicated abnormal retention of these markers. These findings and ultrastructural confirmations document that regional alterations of the endothelium have indeed occurred during shock.

The microcirculation of the cat cerebral cortex has been studied in acute hemorrhagic hypotension. In these studies a small transilluminated area of the cerebral cortex were observed directly, and blood cells flowing through the capillary network were recorded on cinefilm using a high-speed cinecamera.[15] Cell motion was analyzed frame-by-frame. The time during which a single WBC remains at a capillary branching is termed "stagnant time" (ST). It was found that ST was much longer during hemorrhagic hypotension than that seen in the normal state.[15] WBC plugging occurred at capillary branches, a nonuniform flow pattern (plasma-WBC-RBC) occurred in perfused capillaries, and RBC velocity was reduced in capillaries. These findings indicate that hemorrhagic hypotension, induced by withdrawing approximately 40% of the blood volume resulting in a markedly lowered mean systemic arterial blood pressure (45 mmHg) for a 5-min period, induces blood flow maldistribution in the cerebral microcirculation.

E. OTHER TISSUES

Minimal changes in the microcirculation of the rat heart, using the fluorescence microscopy technique, have been observed during hemorrhagic shock (3 h at 35 mmHg mean systemic arterial pressure.)[9] This finding is consistent with the great capacity of the coronary vasculature for blood flow autoregulation.

Microvascular diameter measurements in the skin have been made during hemorrhagic shock in unanesthetized hamsters.[16] The skin-fold window technique was employed which permits the visualization of the microvasculature without the effects of acute surgery, anesthesia, and tissue exposure. The hemorrhage was nonlethal and was produced by slow blood withdrawal for 50 min to sustain a mean arterial blood pressure of 40 mmHg. During the shock period, vasomotion disappeared in all arterial vessels. The small arteries and arterioles, A_1 (70 to 100 μm, mean diameter), A_2 (40 to 70 μm), and A_3 (15 to 40 μm) contracted significantly. A_4 terminal arterioles (<15 μm) dilated, their rhythmic diameter changes stopped, and their diameter increased significantly. V_1, small veins (150 to 200 μm mean diameter) contracted while V_2 (35 to 55 μm) and V_3 (25 to 30 μm) did not show changes in mean diameters.

An advantage of this study[16] was the avoidance of anesthesia and acute surgery, which would have complicated the findings. These well designed and executed studies provide the following summary: The response of the arterial microvasculature of the skin to hemorrhage is specific to the branching order and size of vessels. A_1, A_2, and A_3 microvessels constricted and vasomotion disappeared when the mean arterial pressure was reduced to 40 mmHg. A_4 terminal arterioles remained dilated throughout the hypotensive period and lost their rhythmic diameter changes when the mean systemic arterial pressure fell to 90 mmHg. A_4 arterioles dilated to their maximum but the flow was sluggish and aggregation of blood cellular components occurred. Large veins constricted uniformly. Capillary blood varied in different vessels from absence of flow to slow but constant flow.

IV. PATHOPHYSIOLOGICAL MECHANISMS OF THE MICROCIRCULATION

The pathophysiological mechanisms of the microcirculation comprise those factors originating from without each microvascular unit (e.g., neurohumoral, temperature, and nutritional factors), and those contributed by local influences, e.g., anatomical (microvascular dimensions, endothelium) and rheological (microvascular hindrance, white and red blood cell behavior) factors. The ultimate (net) pathophysiological condition is the result of the interplay between, and combination of, "external" and "internal" factors, imposing adverse influences on each "microvascular unit."

The purpose of this section is to address the separate components of the influences which convert a "normal" physiologic status of the microvasculature to a so-called "compensatory" stage (i.e., for the benefit of the total organism) followed by a "noncompensatory" stage (i.e., noncompensatory because of the imposed morbidity and mortality effects on the total organism).

A. ROLE OF THE WHITE BLOOD CELL, PLATELET, AND RED BLOOD CELL

It is apparent that WBCs may even temporarily obstruct blood flow during their passage through capillaries perfused at normal blood pressures. It is now also obvious that WBCs may perform a major role in promoting a pathophysiological state of shock by more drastically affecting the distribution of the blood flow in the microcirculation. The presence of a very heterogenous distribution of blood within the microvasculature as a result of WBC "plugging" (obstructing vessels) may result in local variations in tissue oxygen tension and adverse changes in blood-tissue exchange processes. In sustained shock, failure to deliver cellular nutritive requirements, interstitial accumulation of metabolites, hydrogen ions, potassium, and other ions may initiate the "decompensatory" phase because of local interference with the function of vascular smooth muscle cells.[5]

When shock occurs and capillary perfusion pressure falls, further problems may arise: energy is lost that is required to dislodge WBCs from sequestered sites in the microcirculation and energy is lost that is also needed to deform WBCs in promoting their successful passage through the microvasculature.

Schmid-Schönbein[17] has discussed the relationship between granulocyte (WBC) activation and capillary obstruction, and proposed that granulocytes are involved in ischemic organ injury at the very beginning of a perfusion pressure reduction. It was pointed out that granulocytes start to accumulate in the microvasculature at the instant pressure is reduced and that these cells by adhering to both capillary and postcapillary segments contribute substantially to the increased vascular resistance. Granulocyte accumulation is usually accompanied by cell injury. Activated granulocytes, in their roles of chemotaxis and phagocytosis, release of elastase, oxygen radicals, lysosomes, and adhesion energies to other cells or substrates following their vascular wall attachment, aggregate formation, and impaired motion in the microcirculation.[17] The net effect of these actions is a loss of the cells from the circulating pool, elevation of vascular resistance, and depression of organ function.

It was found that the number of activated neutrophils per unit volume of blood is a predictor for survival of the host in hemorrhagic shock: animals having a high activated neutrophil density and animals releasing activated cells from storage pools into the circulation during hemorrhagic shock did not survive.[17]

Chien determined the influence of WBCs on the viscous resistance of the microcirculation by observing single arteriolar vessels after hemorrhage in the cat.[1] Following reduction of blood pressure to 50 mmHg by hemorrhage, the viscous resistance increased 70% above control, and at the same time many WBCs were seen adhering to the vascular endothelium. Narrowing of the microvessels by the adhered WBCs accounted for the elevation of vascular resistance.[1] The adhesive force between the WBCs and endothelium was calculated to be approximately 400 dynes/cm^2 and with this large adhesive force the white blood cells could not be dislodged from the endothelium because the low blood flow state did not provide sufficient shear stress.

Bagge et al.[18] reported that WBC plugging was primarily due to pressure-flow alterations in the microcirculation and was a major cause of capillary blood flow maldistribution in skeletal muscle during hemorrhagic shock. They found no qualitative differences in WBC "stiffness" after shock but suggested that the stiffest portion of the leukocyte (WBC) population had already been removed from the circulation.[18] In contrast to these results, Chung et al.[19] reported decreases in RBC deformability correlated with decreased survival in dogs administered live *E. coli* organisms.

Bagge[20] proposed that leukocyte plugging of the capillaries was the primary cause of a heterogenous microcirculation. In addition to capillary plugging by WBCs, Bagge described the adherence of large numbers of cells to the microvascular endothelium during hemorrhagic shock, including primarily the postcapillary venules. The significance of adherence either in arterioles or venules is that stiff leukocytes protruding into the lumina of the microvessels constituted a significant hindrance to blood flow. Possibly offsetting this adverse effect is the observation that the adhering cells may have disappeared from the circulation by migrating through the endothelium into the extravascular region in a time-dependent fashion.[20]

Sepsis is associated with MOF and endotoxin is considered to perform an important role in the development of MOF by inducing microvascular injury. It is not known whether endotoxin alters microvascular responses directly or whether other cells or mediators are also responsible for the injury. Matsuda et al.[21] have examined the role of circulating neutrophils in inducing increases in microvascular permeability after endotoxin administration. It was found that the increases in permeability are dependent in part on the presence of circulating neutrophils and that the induction of neutropenia attenuated the extent of the induction of microvascular hypermeability.

A recent review evaluated the role of phagocytes (WBCs) in health and disease.[22] In addition to their ability to engulf or phagocytose bacteria, they produce powerful enzymes, elastase, cathepsin G, highly reactive metabolic by-products of molecular oxygen (oxygen free radicals) capable of destroying organisms, and metabolic mediators, including tumor necrosis factor (αTNF) and interluekin-1.[22] These characteristics testify to a highly developed and efficient defense system designed for the protection of the patient threatened by pathogenic bacteria. In contrast, however, recent research indicates that substances produced by activated WBCs may actually contribute significantly to patient morbidity and mortality: cells of the defense system appear to cause significant morbidity in their efforts to defend against disease. At first glance, WBC activation and stimulation of the acute phase response to injury and sepsis seems to be a beneficial response. However, the time has come to question whether the immune system is acting in the best interest of the host or whether it has "lost direction".[22]

A brief summary of the roles of the platelet and RBC is appropriate: platelets have been observed to aggregate in the microcirculation in response to many stimuli including endotoxin, antigen, and burns. These aggregates embolize to block pulmonary and hepatic microcirculations. Beyond the emboli, blood vessels collapse. This phenomena has been excellently demonstrated by Robb and Jabs utilizing cinephomicrography in which sequential frames clearly demonstrate the dynamic changes occurring during platelet aggregation:[7] as a platelet aggregate becomes lodged within the pulmonary microcirculation its sudden obstructive effect is readily visualized. The sequestration of platelet aggregates and consumption of other clotting factors are directly related to the fact that platelets have been caught in the microcirculation.

During anaphylaxis, which represents a rapid sequence of events similar to those in endotoxin shock and during hemorrhagic shock in a delayed fashion, a drop in platelet concentrations occurs in sensitized rabbits from approximately 250,000 to 20,000/mm^3 in the blood,[7] and platelet aggregates are observed to lodge in the pulmonary arterioles. In the mesentery of the sensitized rabbit, platelet aggregation occurs at the junction of two venules as a result of topical application on the intestinal wall.

During endotoxin shock in rabbits, two phases are recognized: the first phase is similar in its development to anaphylactic shock and a drop in platelet concentration occurs. During this early phase, platelet aggregates accumulate at the arteriolar bifurcations in the lung.[7] Recovery of platelet concentrations eventually occurs followed by a much later phase when the animal is in severe hypotensive shock. During this later period, platelet concentrations in the blood may decrease to 10,000/mm^3. Animals with typically lower concentrations of platelets die while those who recover from thrombocytopenia survive, although both groups experience the early initial decreases in platelet concentrations. Large clumps and aggregations circulate and accumulate in the microcirculation of the lungs during both the first (early) and later phases of shock.[7]

During hypovolemic shock, vasoconstriction is visible in the microcirculation both in arterioles and venules, and RBCs, WBCs, and platelets aggregate in the intestinal wall of the rabbit, and are hence "washed" into the lung. Pulmonary microembolism thus formed occurs at a lower rate than in endotoxin or anaphylactic shock. Mottling and cyanosis is associated with the aggregation of RBCs, WBCs, and platelets.[7]

Robb and Jabs[7] point out that infection in burn patients results in microvascular platelet aggregation leading to pulmonary microembolism. They postulate that the drop in platelet concentration and DIC seen in burn patients is due to sequestration of platelets both at the peripheral burn site and in the pulmonary microcirculation. In addition to shock produced by hemorrhage, endotoxin, anaphylaxis, and burns, release of a tourniquet after several hours can also result in the release of thrombotic material which may obstruct the pulmonary circulation.

RBCs can influence the behavior of WBCs at a branch point in the microcirculation.1 If a WBC arrives at a junction from one branch and a RBC is not arriving from the other branch, the WBC will tend to stay in the stream and move forward with minimal contact with the vessel wall. If however, RBCs are entering from the other branch, the RBCs tend to press the WBC against the vascular endothelium beyond the point of convergence. When there is a sufficient number of RBCs in the microvasculature the WBCs tend to remain in close contact with the venular endothelium.

B. ROLE OF THE ENDOTHELIUM

It has been noted previously that early after endotoxin shock in rats, the endothelial cells which line the splanchnic precapillary vessels are contorted, often swollen, and have lost their normal wetable surfaces.[23] Of importance is the observation that the most striking cellular alteration of the "shock lung" is swelling of the endothelial cells, although the cause is obscure. During hypovolemic shock in dogs, localized rather than diffuse swelling of capillary endothelial cells occur in the lungs, liver, and skeletal muscle.[24] Endothelial cell swelling in rabbits is reported to occur in skeletal muscle during hemorrhagic shock.[13] Swollen endothelial cells with leakage between the cells in rats is seen in the intracerebral microcirculation during hemorrhagic shock.[6]

Several theories have been proposed regarding the mechanism(s) of the morphologic/pathologic changes in endothelial cells during shock of various etiologies. White cell accumulation in microvessels is not always a prerequisite for the changes since endothelial swelling is observed in skeletal muscle in the absence of WBC accumulation.[23] However, the authors propose that WBCs may have been responsible for endothelial cell damage in lung and liver tissue which led to increased permeability and interstitial edema. The authors propose different mechanisms for endothelial cell damage in skeletal muscle: hypoxia with depletion of energy-rich phosphates and mediators, e.g., toxic oxygen radicals. Others have proposed that the cause of endothelial cell swelling in skeletal muscle during hemorrhagic shock is lowered capillary perfusion pressure,[13] but only if the cells lose control of their volume so that solute moves with water into the cell in order to maintain osmotic equilibrium.

Functional derangements in the capillaries observed during shock, including swollen endothelial cells, could be contributing factors in causing mechanical obstruction to blood flow in the microcirculation, a condition which is not necessarily reversible and often a harbinger of organ deterioration and death.[13] This view is supported by a report on the cerebral microcirculation in hemorrhagic shock, in which impaired blood flow was presumably caused by swollen endothelial cells acting as a microcirculatory obstruction.[6]

Significant changes have been described in cerebral endothelial cells subjected to the effects of hemorrhagic shock: surface changes of the endothelium of a pathologic nature have been reported, including alterations of the endothelial surface, leakage between endothelial cells (suggesting necrosis of the cells), and changes in the normal endothelial electrical charge brought about by injury to the endothelium during shock.[6] "Contour changes" of the endothelium have been discovered by electron microscopy. In the pathological state of shock, the caliber of the endothelial cell is altered which should have a significant effect on blood perfusion. A decrease in blood flow is produced by extravascular compression (due to tissue edema) of the microvessels. This compression action will increase the degree of ischemia and cause further swelling of the extravascular tissue ("neuropils"), creating a "vicious cycle".[6] A report of lethal septic shock in the baboon utilizing electron microscopy, showed that the vascular endothelium is not disrupted but remains structurally intact; only the loss of fenestrae was observed. The endothelium however, was considered to be functionally altered and appeared to propagate the initial inflammatory process.[25]

C. NEUROHUMORAL FACTORS

Shock is characterized by the emergence of a "compensatory" period which involves an integrated vasoconstrictor response mediated by catecholamines, particularly norepinephrine.[26] "Decompensation" occurs when arteriolar vasodilation displaces vasoconstriction even in the face of continued hypovolemia and high circulating levels of catecholamines. During this latter phase there is a loss of an integrated cardiovascular response with maldistribution of circulating blood volume, and muscle blood flow increases in spite of decreased cardiac output. Flint et al. point out that numerous studies have shown decreased microvascular resistance during decompensated shock,[26] and pose possible explanations: (1) loss of vasoconstrictor effects of catecholamines, (2) the unmasking of a vasodilator (beta) effect of these substances, and (3) vasodilator effects of humoral mediators or tissue metabolites at the microcirculatory level, possibly due to leakage of dilator substances from injured/dying cells.

1. Hemorrhagic Shock

The decompensatory phase of hemorrhagic hypotension has continued to be the subject of intense investigation because of the high mortality rate in the presence of severely depressed cardiac output, profound metabolic acidosis,[9] decreased arterial pressure, and arteriolar hyposensitivity. Zhao et al.[27] found that the single feature consistently associated with nonsurvival was that vascular responsiveness to epinephrine and norepinephrine administration was diminished, with all types of arterioles becoming refractory to these agents. Depressed sensitivity to epinephrine, in the microcirculation, was observed in rat skeletal muscle several hours before death of the animal from hemorrhagic shock, and therefore the altered responsiveness was not considered to be a terminal event. In contrast, arteriolar responsiveness in surviving animals was well maintained.[24]

Cryer and others found that acidosis reduced microcirculatory reactivity to catecholamines.[8] Their studies showed that a decreased pH attenuated the vasoconstrictor responses of the larger arterioles (A_1 and A_2) and venules (V_1 and V_2) during both the compensatory and decompensatory phases of hemorrhage. Their work supports the concept that tissue acidosis contributes significantly to peripheral vascular failure in shock. They suggest that acidosis counteracts mechanisms that induce vasoconstriction of the larger arterioles during hemorrhage but does not alter the dilator responses of the smaller arterioles. Flint et al.[26] concluded that differential microcirculatory responses to shock occur at different levels of the arteriolar and venular circulations: dilatation of A_3 and A_4 arterioles (smaller microvessels) occurs during the late phase of hemorrhagic shock and venoconstriction decreases. Concomitantly, constrictor responses to norepinephrine are retained in A_3 and A_4 arterioles and V_1 and V_2 venules while sensitivity of A_1 and A_2 vessels to norepinephrine may be depressed in shock.

2. Endotoxin Shock

A comprehensive search of the literature suggests the existence of two conflicting views concerning the microvascular responses to endotoxin: arteriolar constriction vs. arteriolar dilation. Bond[28] describes results from studies of the microcirculation in which arteriolar constriction and venular dilation were observed shortly (minutes) after endotoxin administration to hamsters, guinea pigs, and rabbits. Topical application of endotoxin results in dilation of arterioles and constriction of venules while systemic administration of endotoxin causes uniform constriction of arterioles and venules with decreased blood flow to the capillary bed. It has been noted that dilation of larger arterioles and constriction of smaller arterioles, along with a progressive dilation of venules, occurs in the splanchnic bed after endotoxin administration.[29] These observations suggest that endotoxin possesses both local and systemic actions which may explain differential microvascular responses.

Functions of microvascular circuits from first-order arterioles to first-order venules are complicated by variations in hemodynamic, rheologic, and dimensional parameters.[29] Endotoxin causes significant changes in these circuits, particularly by curtailing blood flow, thereby reducing the supply of oxygen and nutrients to tissues. Baker and Wilmoth[30] point out that the responses of the microcirculation to endotoxin are variable according to the species of animals and tissues studied. The rat cremaster muscle was selected by Baker's group since this tissue allows the study of responses of several branching orders of arterioles and venules in a single microscopic field, thereby allowing analysis of the relative contributions of the series-coupled segments of the microvascular response to endotoxin.

Microvascular studies of rat skeletal muscle during endotoxin shock demonstrate altered adrenergic responses. After a 1-h period of endotoxin infusion, Baker and Wilmoth observed a gradual and progressive constriction of both arterioles and venules.[30] The threshold dosage for norepinephrine administered to test a given level of adrenergic responsiveness was found to progressively increase with time. It was concluded that microvessel sensitivity to norepinephrine is markedly reduced during endotoxin shock[30] and the question was posed whether the decrease in sensitivity was due to (1) a decrease in the active state of vascular smooth muscle, (2) a reduction in length of the smooth muscle fibers, or (3) other factors such as receptor sensitivity. It was noted that as time progressed during shock, the adrenergic system was eventually incapable of maintaining constriction of the microvessels. It was concluded that there are alterations in sympathetic adrenergic activities throughout the response to endotoxin which initially cause microvessel constriction. Finally, it was suggested that the increase in microvessel diameter occurring concomitantly with the change in norepinephrine sensitivity indicated a reduction in sympathetic adrenergic activity. In conclusion, reduction of microcirculatory sensitivity to catecholamine during endotoxin shock was due to alterations in the active state of vascular smooth muscle and to changes in muscle fiber length or alterations in sympathetic α-adrenergic activity.[30]

The effects of endotoxin have been studied in two types of tissue for comparative purposes: in the mesentery of cats, dilation of larger arterioles and constriction of smaller arterioles occurred together with a gradual progressive dilation of venules after endotoxin administration. In contrast to these results, it was found that there were distinctly different responses of the cremaster muscle, in which there is a gradual and progressive constriction of arterioles and venules after endotoxin.

3. Histamine: Role in Shock

A long-standing question still remaining today is: "Is histamine an important mediator of the shock syndrome and what is its role in the microcirculation?" The significance of histamine in shock has been studied for more than 75 years. Histamine lowers blood pressure, dilates small blood vessels, increases capillary permeability, and can result in lethal shock if administered in large amounts. According to a 1982 review by Altura,[31] histamine:

(1) is not present in animals that are not in shock at concentration levels that exert deleterious effects,
(2) can be produced and released in a variety of types of shock,
(3) can be isolated in large quantities from animals and patients in shock,
(4) can exert severe pathophysiologic effects on vital organs,
(5) is present in the blood of humans and animals in shock.

Histamine may act on two distinct receptors on small blood vessels to promote vasodilation; it can attenuate arteriolar constriction induced by a variety of neurohumoral agonists, and acts on different receptors, H_1-receptors mediating contraction and H_2-receptors mediating relaxation.[31]

It has been demonstrated that histamine can induce concentration-dependent and potent vasodilatation of rat mesenteric terminal arterioles. Histamine when applied locally to arterioles in doses as little as 10^{-5} μg can evoke dilator responses. Histamine is no doubt a "true" physiologic dilator of the microcirculation, and can provoke widespread arteriolar vasodilation in at least the splanchnic region.[31] H_1 histamine receptors mediate contraction of vascular smooth muscle, whereas H_2 histamine receptors mediate its relaxation. Altura's group has documented evidence for a role of histamine in shock: pretreatment of animals with H_1-receptor antagonists protect them against shock due to hemorrhage and bowel ischemia. Rats and mice pretreated with H_2-receptor antihistamines demonstrated an increased mortality after induction of shock. The hemodynamic parameters that were assessed paralleled the beneficial H_1-antihistamines and detrimental H_2-antihistamines actions of the histamine antagonists.

V. THERAPEUTIC CONSIDERATIONS

As emphasized in the early portion of this chapter, pathophysiological changes in the microvasculature of regional vascular beds may have profound influences on the morbidity and mortality of shock. It has been emphasized that the sepsis syndrome is a disease characterized by increases in microvascular permeability in both pulmonary and systemic circulations,[2] actions which also appear to be true in other forms of shock, especially in terms of microcirculatory obstruction of blood flow.[6]

Most alarming, in terms of human patient significance is that shock carries with it a high probability of death from MOF.[32] The probability of death from MOF appears to be a linear function of the number of organ systems involved. In a series of clinical reports, the frequency and clinical significance of end-organ failure (MOF) in nearly 1200 patients at risk from emergency operations, intraabdominal abscess, bacteremia, and trauma were as follows:[32]

Number of Organ Systems Failing	Number of Patients	Deaths (Mortality %)
One organ	143	36 (25%)
Two organs	72	39 (54%)
Three organs	74	56 (76%)
Four organs	19	19 (100%)
Two or more organs	165	114 (69%)

When evaluating clinical variables responsible for the development of MOF, uncontrolled infection was clearly the most consistently associated factor of this syndrome.[32]

Messmer and Kreimeier[33] discuss microcirculatory therapy during shock. They point out that the normal microvascular perfusion pattern is characterized by temporal and spatial variations of capillary blood flow. Local driving pressure, arteriolar vasomotion, and endothelial cells are key factors for local regulation of hydraulic resistance and fluid balance between the blood and tissue compartments. In shock, both the central and local mechanisms controlling microvascular perfusion are impaired. The microvascular perfusion pattern becomes inhomeogenous due to lack of arteriolar vasomotion, changes of blood flow properties, endothelial cell swelling, and blood cell-endothelium interactions.

It is emphasized that definite objectives must be met in conducting an effective therapy of the microcirculation during shock: establishment of precapillary blood pressure, reestablishment of arteriolar vasomotion, and opening of obstructed microvascular pathways to permit passage of blood for nourishment of cells and removal of metabolic waste products.

A prominent view is that therapy aimed at improving the microcirculatory status in recovery from shock must primarily include a rapid restoration of the circulating blood volume. Benefits cannot be achieved by administration of vasoactive drugs unless blood volume has been restored and blood fluidity improved by hemodilution. A popular view for therapy of the microcirculation in shock is the use of hypertonic/hyperoncotic solutions because they directly affect the endothelial cell, rather than the smooth muscle of the microvascular segments. The uses of vasoactive drugs to improve cardiac function and systemic perfusion are best employed together with the administrations of hypertonic/hyperoncotic solutions. The employment of vasoactive agents, including among others, vasodilators, adrenergic agents, and calcium agonists, will influence the microcirculation more efficiently if volume homeostasis of the cellular environment is supported by adequate volume replacement.[33]

Cryer et al. (1988)[34] have studied means of maintaining renal microvascular blood flow during bacteremia in rats. They determined the specific role of prostaglandins in maintaining renal perfusion during hyperdynamic live *Escherichia coli* bacteremia. They used *in vivo* videomicroscopy and optical doppler velocimetry to quantitate changes in renal microvascular blood flow to determine if endogenously released prostaglandins participated in these responses. Their findings suggested that renal prostaglandin production is an important factor in the maintenance of renal microvascular blood flow during hyperdynamic sepsis. As final evidence, inhibition of renal prostaglandin production with mefenamate after *E. coli* infusion caused renal arteriolar constriction and decreased renal blood flow.

The efficacy of pentoxifylline in restoring intestinal microvascular blood flow during hemorrhagic shock and its recovery has been described by Flynn et al.[35] They considered the problem of sustained splanchnic hypoperfusion to be of major importance in that persistent splanchnic blood flow deficits may contribute to MOF in patients following resuscitation from hemorrhagic shock. They pointed out that substantial reduction of splanchnic blood flow observed even during the resuscitation period should lead to intestinal mucosal ischemic damage, impairment of intestinal barrier function, and translocation of bacteria or endotoxin. The purpose of their work was to observe the effects of pentoxifylline, a methylxanthine derivative, on resuscitation from hemorrhagic shock by employment of *in vivo* videomicroscopy. Hemorrhage caused intestinal microvascular blood flow to decrease to 15% of control values and it remained at 30% of baseline levels even during resuscitation in the group not receiving pentoxifylline. Interestingly, addition of pentoxifylline to the resuscitation regimen resulted in an immediate hyperemic response with an increase in intestinal microvascular blood flow to greater than control values followed by return to baseline levels. They observed that arteriolar dilation was not responsible for the improvement of blood flow. The mechanism of the improved blood flow implicated an interaction between RBCs, WBCs, and the microvascular endothelium.[35] In summary, it was found that intestinal microvascular blood flow is not improved by resuscitation with blood and crystalloid despite return of mean arterial blood pressure and cardiac output to normal levels. Addition of pentoxifylline to the resuscitation infusate results in a uniform return of microvascular blood flow to control or above control values.

VI. AIDS: A NEW MICROVASCULAR PROBLEM?

Findings have implicated microcirculatory dysfunction in AIDS patients.[36] A substantial involvement of the microcirculation in the AIDS syndrome in human subjects was discovered using close-circuit television observations of the microcirculation of the nail fold of AIDS patients. A striking pattern of severe microvascular disturbance was demonstrated by the observation of (1) suppression of the spontaneous rhythmic adjustments of capillary blood perfusion and (2) damage to the endothelium of the capillary wall. Findings suggest a substantial involvement of the microcirculation in the pathogenetic development of the AIDS syndrome, as well as a close relationship between microvascular perfusion and the immune condition of the host.[36] This finding is not considered unusual in as much as the status of the microcirculation is one of the key factors contributing to the development of important systemic diseases.

Findings from the above study suggested that the autoregulatory vasomotion of arteriolar vessels is impaired in severe AIDS infection on the basis of slow filling and emptying of capillary loops. In addition, in the majority of the microvessels, the outer wall of the endothelial tissue was found to be covered by a "pericapillary sheath," which is a condensation of extracellular matrix containing collagen and reticular fibrils. The finding of a heterogenous mass within the wall of the microvessels suggests that there may be a migration of HIV virus-infected products, or the virus proper, into the endothelial cell cytoplasm. Another possible microvascular dysfunction is the extravasation of megablasts of RBCs through a widening of the interendothelial cell-cell junctions. Although significant microcirculatory perturbations have been found in AIDS patients, it is not known if the dysfunctions are causal in the pathogenesis of the disease in terms of tissue damage/injury of other organs.[36]

A 1991 report[37] on the status of bacteremia in persons with HIV infection points out that individuals with HIV infection are susceptible to the development of severe bacterial infections. Severe staphylococcal infections are seen, perhaps resulting from detrimental effects of HIV on neutrophil function.[37] Bacteremia is probably the most challenging problem in the treatment of HIV-infected patients; it is difficult to diagnose clinically and can be associated with serious sequelae such as sepsis. The increase in the rate of septicemia in the U.S. has been attributed to concomitant bacteremia and HIV infections.[38] An increase in septicemia-associated mortality among HIV-infected patients has been noted.[39]

VII. SUMMARY

Abnormal rheologic behavior of the microcirculation may have serious consequences in the pathogenesis of many forms of shock. Examples are (1) the effects of sustained low blood flow in which the decrease in shear stress elevates blood viscosity, which lowers blood flow, leading to a vicious cycle, and (2) the condition of a low blood flow state in which the arteriolar shear rate is still high enough to allow blood viscosity to be low but the shear rate of venules may be reduced sufficiently to elevate blood viscosity to a marked degree, so that venous resistance is elevated over precapillary resistance, leading to transcapillary fluid leakage. It is apparent that evaluation of the state of the microcirculations of various organ systems is vital in order to properly understand the pathophysiological disturbances during shock.

Pathophysiological changes in the microvasculature of regional vascular beds may have profound influences on the morbidity and mortality of shock. Further, damage to the microvasculature during circulatory shock may occur in advance of evidence of MOF, so that an early diagnosis of the state of the microcirculation could provide helpful "markers" for the pathogenesis of the disease process which should aid in the choices of therapeutic interventions. Research on animal "shock models" which are designed to resemble the human clinical entity are crucial in gaining a solid understanding of the microcirculatory pathophysiology. *In vitro* systems may also serve an important role in understanding intricate mechanisms occurring in the various subcellular systems.

For years, clinicians have suspected that the basic metabolic defect in circulatory shock is a result of a disturbance of blood flow rate and blood flow distribution in the microcirculation. Much work needs to be done in designing definitive studies of the microcirculation, in particular those in the brain, adrenal gland, lung, liver, and kidney, where crucial changes are taking place which may be in the pathogenic mainstream of the disease. A current view, not yet fully substantiated, is that the central nervous system, including the brain, is damaged in shock through the development of an impaired microcirculation. Of the numerous factors undoubtedly performing chief roles in the pathogenesis of shock are the degrees of microvessel constrictions and dilatations due to active and passive changes, the obstructive effects of WBCs and platelets in the microvasculature, the effects of the release of numerous mediators including the cytokines, histamine, prostaglandins, among others, and neurohumoral agents including the catecholamines, and finally the effects of disturbances of the microcirculation of one organ system on another, e.g., "washing" of microthrombi from a peripheral organ into the lung.

There is a great need to study microcirculatory responses of many organ systems during various shock states, including especially hemorrhage, sepsis, and burns. This chapter focused on certain critical beds in which research has been conducted to a considerable degree, primarily emphasizing the pulmonary system, the splanchnic bed, skeletal muscle, and the central nervous system. Of chief importance appears to be the entrapment of platelet aggregates in the pulmonary microcirculation. Blockage of the pulmonary microcirculation may lead to a "vicious cycle" including the progressive development of pulmonary edema and poor systemic peripheral perfusion of blood to vital organs, finally possibly terminating in the condition of irreversibility. Other pulmonary microcirculatory dysfunctions include edema, hemorrhage, and maldistribution of blood flow which may also lead to a serious status of shock and possibly the development of MOF and death.

The splanchnic bed has occupied a central role in shock pathogenesis for many years, yet its participation in the development of multiple organ failure is still uncertain. Exciting research now includes the associations of the various cytokines and eicosanoids and other circulating mediators, and the possible presence of translocation of bacteria, endotoxins, or other agents into the general circulation. There is now a growing consensus which implicates the intestine in the pathogenesis of "hyperdynamic sepsis" and MOF. Recent experimental animal models have yielded important information concerning the role of the splanchnic microcirculation in shock. Of particular interest is the observation that severely depressed intestinal microvascular blood flow can be sustained during the hyperdynamic (high cardiac output) stage of sepsis. This observation provides important information concerning the mechanism of the development of mucosal barrier dysfunction and translocation of bacteria to the blood.

Microcirculatory changes occurring in skeletal muscle during shock are of major importance since muscle represents the largest tissue mass in the body and is a target for compensatory vascular adjustments. The various microcirculatory responses in skeletal muscle are impressive in the degree of their intensity, heterogeneity of responses, and complex contributions during the compensatory and decompensatory stages of shock.

The central nervous system, including the cerebral circulation, appears to be an early target in various kinds of shock. Changes occurring in its microcirculations include early development of vascular permeability leading to impaired blood flow and death. Endothelial injury is a major "player" in the pathologic response.

There are many mechanisms causing pathophysiological changes in the microcirculation. Emphasized in this chapter are the chief factors documented by investigators to perform important pathophysiological roles in shock. These are the roles of the WBC, the platelet, and the RBC, the endothelium, and the various neurohumoral factors. A strong case has been made for major roles of WBCs and platelets in the development of serious derangements of the microcirculations in many organ systems, plugging of microvessels being the most serious event by virtue of ultimately diminishing blood flow and causing an abnormal distribution of blood in the microcirculation. These factors may provide antecedent warning of subsequent adverse changes, including endothelial damage, cell swelling, accumulation of metabolites, failure to provide nutritive requirements, abnormal accumulation of ions, and development of severe tissue edema. Altered sensitivity to circulating neurohumoral agents in the microcirculation may seriously change blood flow dynamics and intra- and extravascular fluid balances, thereby contributing to MOF and cell death.

REFERENCES

1. **Chien, S.,** Rheology in the microcirculation in normal and low flow states, *Adv. Shock Res.,* 8, 71, 1982.
2. **Sibbald, W. J.,** Circulatory responses to the sepsis syndrome, in *Second Vienna Shock Forum,* Alan R. Liss, New York, 1989, 1075.
3. **Wang, P., Hauptman, J. G., and Chaudry, I. H.,** Hemorrhage produces depression in microvascular blood flow which persists despite fluid resuscitation, *Circ. Shock,* 32, 307, 1990.
4. **Garrison, R. N. and Cryer, H. M., III,** Role of the microcirculation to skeletal muscle during shock, in *Perspectives in Shock Research: Metabolism, Immunology, Mediators, and Models,* Alan R. Liss, New York, 1989, 43.
5. **Haljamae, H.,** Microcirculation and hemorrhagic shock, *Am. J. Emerg. Med.,* 2, 100, 1983.

6. **Badonnel, M. C., De Girolami, U., Joris, I., and Guido, M.,** The intracerebral microcirculation of the rat in hemorrhagic shock, *J. Neuropathol. Exp. Neurol.,* 42, 561, 1983.
7. **Robb, H. J. and Jabs, C. M.,** Microcirculation in shock, in *Shock: the Reversible Stage of Dying,* Hardaway, R. M., Ed., PSG, Littleton, MA, 1988, 140.
8. **Cryer, H. M., Kaebnick, H., Harris, P. D., and Flint, L. M.,** Effects of tissue acidosis on skeletal muscle microcirculatory responses to hemorrhagic shock in unanesthetized rats, *J. Surg. Res.,* 39, 59, 1985.
9. **Perbeck, L., Lund, F., and Thulin, L.,** Intrathoracic microvascular circulation in haemorrhagically shocked rats. Studies by fluorescence techniques, *Clin. Physiol.,* 9, 567, 1989.
10. **Scalia, S., Burton, H., Van Wylen, D., Steinberg, S., Hoffman, A., Roche, F., and Flint, L.,** Persistent arteriolar constriction in microcirculation of the terminal ileum following moderate hemorrhagic hypovolemia and volume restoration, *J. Trauma,* 30, 713, 1990.
11. **Whitworth, P. W., Cryer, H. M., Garrison, R. N., Baumgarten, T. E., and Harris, P. D.,** Hypoperfusion of the intestinal microcirculation without decreased cardiac output during live *Escherichia coli* sepsis in rats, *Circ. Shock,* 27, 111, 1989.
12. **Guth, P. H. and Morishita, T.,** The gastric microcirculation in shock, *Ann. N.Y. Acad. Sci.,* 597, 282, 1990.
13. **Mazzoni, M. C., Borgstrom, P., Intaglietta, M., and Arfors, K. E.,** Lumenal narrowing and endothelial cell swelling in skeletal muscle capillaries during hemorrhagic shock, *Circ. Shock,* 29, 27, 1989.
14. **Rosenblum, W. I.,** Control of brain microcirculation by endothelium, *Keio. J. Med.,* 39, 137, 1990.
15. **Yamakawa, T., Yamaguichi, S., Niimi, H., and Sugujama, I.,** White blood cell plugging and blood flow maldistribution in the capillary network of cat cerebral cortex in acute hemorrhagic hypotension, *Circ. Shock,* 22, 323, 1987.
16. **Colantuoni, S., Bertuglia, S., and Intaglietta, M.,** Microvessel diameter changes during hemorrhagic shock in unanesthetized hamsters, *Microvasc. Res.,* 30, 133, 1985.
17. **Schmid-Schönbein, G.,** Granulocyte activation and capillary obstruction, in *Blood Flow in Large Arteries: Applications to Atherogenesis and Clinical Medicine,* Liepsch, D. W., Ed., Karger, Basel, 1990, 150.
18. **Bagge, U., Amundson, B., and Lauritzen, C.,** White blood cell deformability and plugging of skeletal muscle capillaries in hemorrhagic shock, *Acta. Physiol. Scand.,* 180, 159, 1980.
19. **Chung, T. W., O'Rear, E. A., Whitsett, T. L., Hinshaw, L. B., and Smith, M. A.,** Survival factors in a canine septic shock model, *Circ. Shock,* 33, 178, 1991.
20. **Bagge, U.,** Leukocytes and capillary perfusion in shock, in *White Cell Mechanisms: Basic Science & Clinical Aspects,* Alan R. Liss, New York, 1984, 285.
21. **Matsuda, T., Rubinstein, I., Robbins, R. A., Koyama, S., Joyner, W. L., and Rennard, S. I.,** Role of neutrophils in endotoxin-mediated microvascular injury in hamsters, *J. Appl. Physiol.,* 71, 307, 1991.
22. **Gough, D. B.,** Educate the phagocyte!, *Br. J. Surg.,* 78, 1, 1991.
23. **Altura, B. M., Gabrewold, A., and Burton, R. W.,** Failure of microscopic metarterioles to elicit vasodilator responses to acetylcholine, bradykinin, histamine and substance P after ischemic shock, endotoxemia and trauma: possible role of endothelial cells, *Microcirc. Endothelium Lymphatics,* 2, 121, 1985.
24. **Schlag, G. and Redl, H.,** Morphology of the microvascular system in shock: lung, liver, and skeletal muscles, *Crit. Care Med.,* 13, 1045, 1985.
25. **Voss, B. L., DeBault, L. E., Blick, K. E., Chang, A. C. K., Stiers, D. L., Hinshaw, L. B., and Taylor, F. B.,** Sequential renal alterations in septic shock in the primate, *Circ. Shock,* 33, 142, 1991.

26. **Flint, L. M., Cryer, H. M., Simpson, C. J., and Harris, P. D.,** Microcirculatory norepinephrine constrictor response in hemorrhagic shock, *Surgery,* 96, 240, 1984.
27. **Zhao, K. S., Junker, D., Delano, F. A., and Zweifach, B. W.,** Microvascular adjustments during irreversible hemorrhagic shock in rat skeletal muscle, *Microvasc. Res.,* 30, 143, 1985.
28. **Bond, R. F.,** Peripheral circulatory responses to endotoxin, in *Handbook of Endotoxin,* Vol. 2, Hinshaw, L. B., Ed., Elsevier, Amsterdam, 1985, chap. 3, p. 64.
29. **Baker, C. H., Wilmoth, F. R., and Sutton, E. T.,** Reduced RBC versus plasma microvascular flow due to endotoxin, *Circ. Shock,* 20, 127, 1986.
30. **Baker, C. H. and Wilmoth, F. R.,** Microvascular responses to *E. coli* endotoxin with altered adrenergic activity, *Circ. Shock,* 12, 165, 1984.
31. **Altura, B. M.,** Reticuloendothelial system function and histamine release in shock and trauma: relationship to microcirculation, *Klin. Wochenschr.,* 60, 882, 1982.
32. **Fry, D. E.,** Splanchnic perfusion and sepsis, in *Prospectives in Shock Research: Metabolism, Immunology, Mediators, and Models,* Alan R. Liss, New York, 1989, 9.
33. **Messmer, K. and Kreimeier, U.,** Microcirculatory therapy in shock, *Resuscitation,* 18, S51, 1989.
34. **Cryer, H. M., Unger, L. S., Garrison, R. N., and Harris, P. D.,** Prostaglandins maintain renal microvascular blood flow during hyperdynamic bacteremia, *Circ. Shock,* 26, 71, 1988.
35. **Flynn, W. J., Cryer, H. G., and Garrison, R. N.,** Pentoxifylline restores intestinal microvascular blood flow during resuscitated hemorrhagic shock, *Surgery,* 110, 350, 1991.
36. **Xui, R.-J., Jun, C., and Berglund, O.,** Microcirculatory disturbances in AIDS patients — a first report, *Microvasc. Res.,* 42, 151, 1991.
37. **Northfelt, D. W. and Polsky, B.,** Bacteremia in persons with HIV infection, *Aids Clin. Rev.,* 459, 1991.
38. **Centers for Disease Control,** Increase in national hospital discharge survey rates for septicemia-United States, 1979–1987, *Morbid. Mortal. Weekly Rep.,* 39, 31, 1990.
39. **Buekler, J., Berkelman, R., Devine, O., and Chevarley, F.,** Impact of the HIV epidemic on mortality trends in men 25–44 years of age, United States, in *Proc. Int. Conf. AIDS,* 16(Abstr.), 16, 1989.

Chapter 6

Ischemia/Reperfusion Injury

Paul Kubes, Peter R. Kvietys, and D. Neil Granger

CONTENTS

I. INTRODUCTION

Approximately a decade ago, it was first postulated that xanthine oxidase-derived oxidants play an integral role in the microvascular injury associated with reperfusion of ischemic tissues.[1,2] Since that time, much work has been done to test the xanthine oxidase hypothesis and to further characterize the pathophysiological alterations associated with ischemia/reperfusion (I/R). The prevailing view that has resulted from this expanded body of literature is that both reactive oxygen metabolites and granulocytes contribute to the process of reperfusion injury. The objective of this chapter is to summarize the available evidence that relates to the possible role of reactive oxygen metabolites and granulocytes in reperfusion-induced microvascular dysfunction. The intestine has undergone extensive scrutiny as a target organ that is particularly vulnerable to the deleterious effect of I/R. Thus, in this treatise, the intestine will be used as a model system for describing the mechanisms involved in I/R injury.

0-8493-4547-2/94/$0.00+$.50

II. CONCEPTS OF REPERFUSION INJURY

When a tissue is subjected to ischemia, a sequence of chemical reactions is initiated which may ultimately lead to cellular dysfunction and necrosis. Although no single process can be identified as the critical event in ischemia-induced tissue injury, it is generally believed that depletion of cellular energy stores and accumulation of toxic metabolites may contribute to cell death. If the ischemic episode is sufficiently severe and/or prolonged, no therapeutic intervention can reverse the cell dysfunction incurred and tissue necrosis is inevitable. If, however, the ischemic episode is mild and/or of short duration the intervention of choice has been the reestablishment of tissue perfusion, since this allows for the regeneration of cell charge and the washout of toxic metabolites. Studies evaluating the efficacy of this approach have uncovered the paradoxical phenomenon of reperfusion-induced tissue injury. Based on physiological and morphological criteria it appears that reperfusion of ischemic tissues exacerbates the deleterious effects of the ischemic episode itself (Table 1).

Parks and Granger[3] have evaluated the relative contributions of ischemia and reperfusion to the intestinal mucosal injury incurred in a common model of regional hypotension. The morphologically demonstrable injury to the intestinal mucosa observed after 3 h of regional ischemia (blood flow reduced to 20% of normal) and 1 h of reperfusion is much greater than that observed after 4 h of ischemia (no reperfusion). This observation implicates some reaction initiated by the return of blood to the ischemic tissue as the cause of the reperfusion-induced injury. Further studies showed that if de-oxygenated solutions were used to reperfuse ischemic tissues very little damage is incurred,[3-5] suggesting that the return of oxygen to ischemic tissue plays a pivotal role in reperfusion-induced injury.

Shorter durations of ischemia, while not producing morphological injury, do induce microvascular dysfunction manifested by increases in microvascular permeability to plasma proteins.[2] If the cat small bowel is subjected to 1 h of ischemia (blood flow reduced to 20% of control) without reperfusion, a doubling in microvascular permeability occurs (Table 1). However, the same period of ischemia followed by reperfusion results in a five-fold increase in microvascular permeability. *In vitro* studies[6] using cultured endothelial cell monolayers to assess the effects of hypoxia (pO_2 20 mmHg) and reoxygenation (pO_2 145 mmHg) on monolayer permeability to albumin have yielded similar results. Exposure of the monolayers to hypoxia increased albumin permeability 1.5-fold and upon reoxygenation albumin permeability increased further (2.3-fold). These studies provide further support that reintroduction of oxygen to hypoxic tissue is the initiating factor in reperfusion-induced tissue injury.

The reactions initiated upon reperfusion which lead to tissue injury appear to involve the formation of cytotoxic oxidants derived from molecular oxygen. Oxidant formation has been demonstrated during reperfusion of the ischemic bowel by electron-spin resonance spectrometry[7] and chemiluminescence.[8,9] These studies indicate that there is a burst of oxidant formation immediately after reperfusion. Evidence supporting the notion that these oxidants are responsible for tissue injury is based on studies which use agents that

Table 6-1 **Physiological and morphological indices of mucosal injury produced by ischemia and reperfusion**

	Vascular Permeability ($1-\sigma$)	Mean Villus Height (μm)
Control	0.08 ± 0.01	631 ± 7
Ischemia	0.15 ± 0.03*	637 ± 25
Ischemia/reperfusion	0.40 ± 0.01*§	239 ± 9*

Note: *Indicates $p < 0.05$ relative to control. §Indicates $p < 0.05$ relative to ischemia.

either restrict the production of these cytotoxic oxidants or act as scavengers after the oxidants are produced. The administration of these antioxidants attenuate only the component of the increased permeability that occurs upon reperfusion of a vascular bed *in vivo*[10] or reoxygenation of endothelial cells *in vitro*.[6] Furthermore, these antioxidants are just as effective in preventing mucosal injury when given either just prior to reperfusion or before the induction of ischemia.[8]

III. CHEMISTRY OF FREE RADICALS

A. SUPEROXIDE ANION

The univalent reduction of molecular O_2 gives rise to the superoxide anion (O_2^-), which may act as a reductant (reduces ferric ions and heme proteins) or an oxidant (oxidized sulfhydryl compounds and catecholamines). O_2^- is a relatively weak oxidant, but it can be cytotoxic by virtue of its ability to inactivate specific enzymes that are essential to cell function (e.g., RNase and glyceraldehyde-3-phosphate dehydrogenase). The cellular toxicity associated with O_2^- is usually attributed to its role as a precursor of more reactive radical species, i.e., ·OH.[11,12]

B. HYDROGEN PEROXIDE

H_2O_2 may be formed as a result of two types of reactions: (1) divalent reduction of O_2 (e.g., via monoamine oxidase), or (2) dismutation of O_2^-, i.e.,

$$2O_2^- + 2H^+ \rightarrow H_2O_2 + O_2 \qquad \textbf{(6-1)}$$

Because the spontaneous dismutation of O_2^- proceeds relatively rapidly in aqueous solutions, the production of O_2^- *in vivo* is always accompanied by production of H_2O_2. The dismutation of O_2^- can be enhanced by a factor of 10^{10} by the enzyme superoxide dismutase.[12]

Unlike O_2^-, H_2O_2 is stable in the absence of trace metals. It is a powerful but sluggish oxidant in biologic systems and cytotoxic only at concentrations that are orders of magnitude greater than the normal intracellular flux. Like O_2^-, the cytotoxic effects of H_2O_2 are generally ascribed to its role as a precursor of ·OH.

C. HYDROXYL RADICAL

·OH is an extremely powerful oxidant. Unlike O_2^- and H_2O_2, it will react with almost all biologic substrates. This suggests that it only reacts with substrates close to its site of generation; to exert long-range effects it must rely on the formation of more stable secondary species.

The major danger of accumulation of O_2^- and H_2O_2 in a cell is the potential for production of ·OH in the presence of certain transition metals (notably iron):

$$O_2^- + Fe^{3+} \rightarrow O_2 + Fe^{2+} \qquad \textbf{(6-2A)}$$

$$H_2O_2 + Fe^{2+} \rightarrow \cdot OH + OH^- + Fe^{3+} \qquad \textbf{(6-2B)}$$

$$\text{net } O_2^- + H_2O_2 \rightarrow \cdot OH + OH^- + O_2 \qquad \textbf{(6-2C)}$$

This iron catalyzed Haber-Weiss reaction (Equation 2, also called O_2^--driven Fenton reaction) can occur *in vivo* by the interaction of H_2O_2 with iron-containing compounds such as transferrin, lactoferrin, ferritin, and hemoglobin.[11,13]

There are no known endogenous systems that can scavenge ·OH. Therefore, when ·OH is generated, cellular injury may be extensive via various reactions. A notable characteristic of ·OH is its ability to abstract methylene hydrogen atoms from polyunsaturated fatty acids, which initiates lipid peroxidation. Membrane peroxidation can lead to changes in membrane fluidity and permeability, enhanced rates of protein degradation, and, ultimately, cell lysis. ·OH also depolymerizes hyaluronic acid, degrades collagen, inactivates essential enzymes and transport proteins via sulfhydryl oxidation, and nicks DNA. It has been suggested that intracellular generation of ·OH may be an important cause of intrinsic mutagenesis.[14]

Others[15,16] have suggested that another radical species, the ferryl iron $(FeOH)^{+3}$ formed when Fe^{+2} reacts with H_2O_2, may be responsible for all or some of the cytotoxicity generally attributed to the ·OH.

$$Fe^{+2} + H_2O_2 \rightarrow (FeOH)^{+3} + OH^- \qquad \textbf{(6-3)}$$

The ability to test the physiological importance of both ·OH and $(FeOH)^{+3}$ is hampered by the lack of specific scavengers for these oxidants.

The ubiquity and reactivity of oxidant-generating systems in mammalian tissues is matched by the presence of complex sets of protective mechanisms that prevent or limit oxidative damage. The antioxidant enzymes that provide the first line of defense against oxygen radical-mediated cellular injury include superoxide dismutase (SOD), catalase, and glutathione peroxidase. SOD represents a family of metalloproteins that catalyze the dismutation of O_2^- to H_2O_2 (Equation 1). The enzyme is almost exclusively confined to the cytosolic and mitochondrial compartments of the cell. In the presence of SOD, the ability of O_2^- to react with potential substrates (other than itself) or to drive O_2^--dependent reactions that lead to formation of ·OH are virtually eliminated. Because only trace amounts of SOD activity are found in plasma and lymph, extracellular substrates are not as well protected against O_2^-.

Catalase and glutathione peroxidase (GPO) both remove H_2O_2 from the cell. Catalase is a heme protein that catalyzes the dismutation of H_2O_2:

$$2H_2O_2 \xrightarrow{\text{catalase}} O_2 + 2H_2O \qquad \textbf{(6-4)}$$

Catalase is localized in the cytosolic or peroxisomal fractions of most mammalian cells.

GPO catalyzes the oxidation of reduced glutathione (GSH) by H_2O_2 to form oxidized glutathione (GSSG) and water:

$$2GSH + H_2O_2 \xrightarrow[\text{peroxidase}]{\text{GSH}} 2H_2O + GSSG \qquad \textbf{(6-5)}$$

GPO is localized in the cytosol and mitochondria of most cells, with erythrocytes and hepatocytes having large amounts of it.

Although both catalase and GPO prevent or minimize an increase in intracellular H_2O_2, the latter enzyme appears to play a greater role in protecting cells from low fluxes of H_2O_2. Much higher concentrations of H_2O_2 are required for maximal activity of catalase relative to GPO. There are only trace amounts of catalase in the extracellular compartment; however, extracellular H_2O_2 may be rapidly metabolized by circulating erythrocytes because H_2O_2 rapidly crosses the erythrocyte membrane and therefore can be destroyed by the erythrocyte catalase-GSH peroxidase system.[17]

The second line of defense against oxidant-induced cellular injury is provided by nonenzymatic scavengers. The term "free radical scavenger" is frequently used to describe substances that readily donate a hydrogen atom (H·) to free radicals to become a less-reactive radical species. Of biologic significance are substances that act as easily

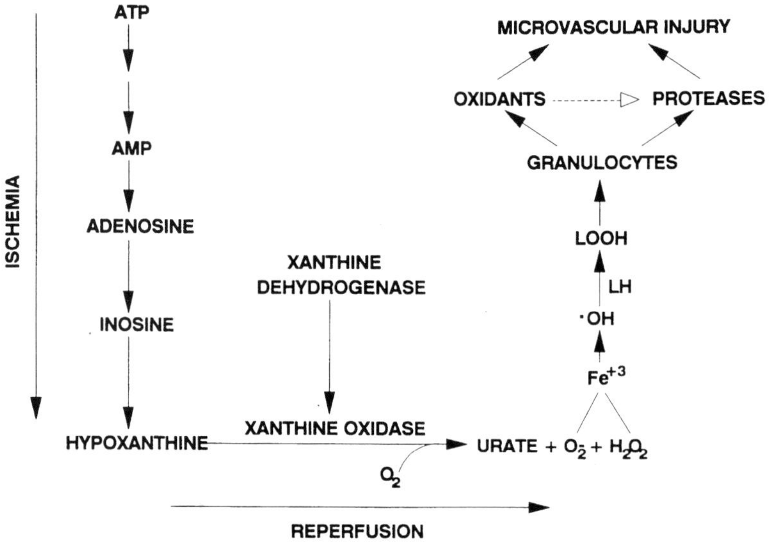

Figure 6-1 Proposed sequence of events leading to the microvascular injury observed upon reperfusion of ischemic tissue.

oxidizable substrates (scavengers) at physiologic concentrations, such as GSH, α-tocopherol, carotenoids, ascorbate, uric acid, and methionine. There are a number of pharmacologic agents that can be administered to animals for free radical scavenging. Mannitol and dimethylsulfoxide (DMSO) are frequently used as ·OH scavengers.[11,18]

IV. MICROVASCULAR PERMEABILITY

A. ROLE OF XANTHINE OXIDASE

Xanthine oxidase appears to be a major source of the oxy-radicals produced in postischemic tissues. The mechanism of xanthine oxidase-mediated radical production following reperfusion was first proposed by Granger et al.[1] They proposed that the hypoxic stress of ischemia initiates the conversion of xanthine dehydrogenase to xanthine oxidase and promotes ATP catabolism to yield hypoxanthine. When O_2 is reintroduced into the tissue at the time of reperfusion, it reacts with hypoxanthine and xanthine oxidase to produce a burst of O_2^- and H_2O_2. In the presence of Fe^{3+}, O_2^- and H_2O_2 react via the Haber-Weiss reaction (Equations 2A through 2C) to form ·OH, which appears to play a pivotal role in microvascular and parenchymal cell injury (Figure 1).

A role for xanthine oxidase in reperfusion-induced oxidant production is supported by the observation that substances that either inhibit (allopurinol, pterin aldehyde) or inactivate (tungsten-supplemented diet) the enzyme afford protection against reperfusion injury similar to that noted with radical scavengers.[19] Some reports contend that the beneficial effects of allopurinol and oxipurinol in I/R are due to direct free radical-scavenging properties of the agents rather than to their ability to inhibit xanthine oxidase. However, we have recently demonstrated that the regimen of allopurinol treatment used in most I/R studies does not lead to a significant increase in the antioxidant properties of extracellular fluid.[20]

A growing body of evidence supports the assumption that ischemia leads to hypoxanthine accumulation and a concomitant conversion of xanthine dehydrogenase to xanthine oxidase. The total activity of the enzyme (dehydrogenase and oxidase) varies greatly between tissues and animal species.[21] In most species, the small bowel and liver are the richest sources of the enzyme, whereas muscle (heart and skeletal muscle), lung, and brain contain low to negligible activities. Although xanthine oxidase is absent in the intestinal mucosal of human and pig neonate, significant activities are detected in adults.[22]

Studies[23] have cast some doubt on localization of the enzyme using immunologic approaches, since it is difficult to prepare antibodies against purified xanthine oxidase (i.e., free of immunoglobulins). This explains why immunofluorescence studies localize xanthine oxidase in myocardial capillaries,[24] whereas other approaches indicate a lack of detectable activity in this tissue.[25]

An important aspect of xanthine dehydrogenase to xanthine oxidase conversion relative to reperfusion-induced tissue injury is the rapidity of the conversion process. Roy and McCord[26] have reported that a dramatic conversion of xanthine dehydrogenase-to-oxidase (D-to-O) activity occurs in rat intestine subjected to only 1 min of global ischemia. They also noted that little (<10%) enzyme conversion occurs after 1 h of global ischemia in liver, lung, and kidney. Recent work by Parks et al.[27] indicates that D-to-O conversion in ischemic rat intestine proceeds at a much slower rate (50% conversion after 2 h of ischemia) than originally predicted by Roy and McCord.[26] Engerson et al.[28] have demonstrated that 50% conversion in liver, kidney, and lung requires 3.6 h, 6 h, and 14 h of isothermic ischemia, respectively (Figure 2). It is difficult to relate the extent of D-to-O conversion to the extent of reperfusion injury, since the relationship between XO activity and tissue injury *in vivo* is not known.

Relatively little attention has been devoted to the mechanisms responsible for D-to-O conversion. In the small intestine, limited proteolysis appears to account for the irreversible conversion induced by ischemia. D-to-O conversion in ischemic liver and kidney involves both reversible and irreversible modifications of the enzyme. The reversible conversion is initiated by sulfhydryl modification, whereas limited proteolysis leads to

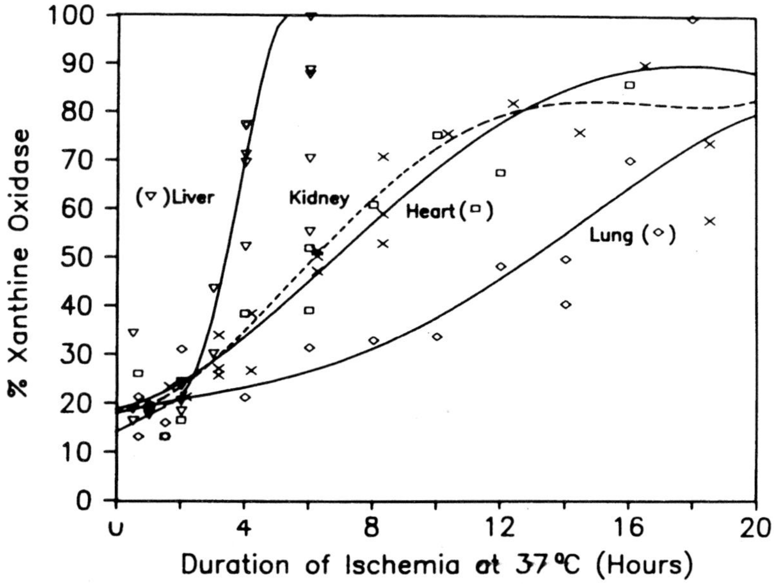

Figure 6-2 Time course of ischemia-induced conversion of xanthine dehydrogenase to xanthine oxidase from four different tissues.

the formation of an irreversible oxidase derived from either the native dehydrogenase or the reversible oxidase.[29] Proteolytic conversion of dehydrogenase-to-oxidase does not appear to involve the calcium-dependent thiol proteases called calpains.[30]

A number of investigators have observed that allopurinol provides protection against I/R injury even in tissues that have essentially undetectable levels of xanthine oxidase. One explanation for this observation is that the xanthine oxidase activity required for cytotoxicity in *in vitro* studies (2 mU per ml) is well within the range or much lower than the enzyme activity measured in most organs in various species, including humans. Therefore, it is conceivable that the low xanthine oxidase levels noted in some tissues are sufficient to produce enough oxidants to mediate cell injury. Another explanation for the protective effect of allopurinol in tissues with low xanthine oxidase activity is that the enzyme is concentrated in a small population of cells (i.e., microvascular endothelium). Indeed, Jarach et al.[31] have prepared antibodies against xanthine oxidase from bovine milk. They used immunolocalization techniques to demonstrate that the enzyme is localized primarily in the cytoplasm of milk-secreting epithelial cells. In other tissues, including the liver, small and large intestines, skeletal muscle, lung, and heart, they found the enzyme located primarily, if not exclusively, in capillary endothelial cells. Assuming the enzyme activity in endothelial cells is sufficiently high to produce cytotoxic quantities of oxidants, then xanthine oxidase-mediated oxidant injury should be initiated at the level of the microvasculature.

Several studies[32-34] indicate that all of the components for free radical generation by xanthine oxidase are present in cultured endothelial cells derived from a variety of sources. Ratych et al.[32] observed a fivefold increase in endothelial cell xanthine oxidase activity (D-to-O conversion) after exposure to 45 min of anoxia followed by reoxygenation (Figure 3). An increase in the activity of xanthine oxidase should optimize conditions for formation of oxygen radicals upon reoxygenation. Indeed, electron paramagnetic resonance measurements indicate that cultured endothelial cells exposed to anoxia and then reoxygenated produced oxygen radicals upon reoxygenation.[33] The reoxygenation-induced burst in oxygen radical formation is largely prevented by oxypurinol, an inhibitor of xanthine oxidase. In these experiments the oxidant stress (anoxia for 30 min) was sufficient to produce cell lysis. The endothelial cell injury incurred upon reoxygenation is largely prevented by the oxygen radical scavengers SOD and catalase, as well as inhibitors of xanthine oxidase.

In addition to acting locally to produce tissue injury via generation of oxygen radicals, xanthine oxidase can be released from ischemic tissue into the general circulation and thereby may produce tissue damage at distant, nonischemic sites. Xanthine oxidase is released into the circulation from ischemic livers[35] and skeletal muscle[36] in concentrations sufficient to produce endothelial cell injury when provided with substrate. The endothelial cell injury incurred by exposing endothelial cells to hypoxanthine and xanthine oxidase (HX/XO) is very similar to that observed after reoxygenation of previously anoxic cells. The HX/XO-induced injury can be prevented by catalase[32,37] and mimicked by addition of H_2O_2 (in concentrations which would be generated by HX/XO). These findings would suggest that H_2O_2 is the cytotoxic radical produced by xanthine oxidase. However, H_2O_2 is not generally considered cytotoxic per say, but has cytotoxic potential by virtue of its ability to interact with iron to form the highly cytotoxic radical, such as the hydroxyl radical. Pretreating the endothelial cells with deferoxamine, a potent iron chelator, prevented the cytotoxicity induced by either HX/XO or H_2O_2 (Figure 4). Pretreatment with deferoxamine bound to a high molecular weight dextran (cell impermeant) was ineffective. These findings support the hypothesis that xanthine oxidase-derived H_2O_2 interacts with intracellular iron to form a cytotoxic radical which subsequently produces endothelial cell injury. The intracellular source of iron for this reaction does not appear to be ferritin, but may be the intracellular low molecular weight

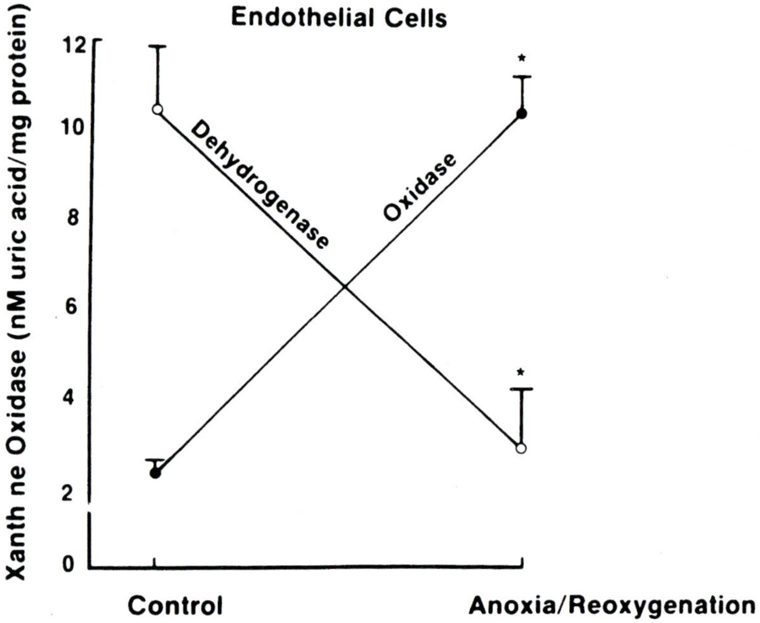

Figure 6-3 Conversion of xanthine dehydrogenase to xanthine oxidase produced by anoxia/reoxygenation of cultured pulmonary artery endothelial cells.

iron pool. The recent observation that xanthine oxidase reversibly binds to vascular endothelium,[38] suggests that xanthine oxidase released from ischemic tissue could attach to vascular endothelium at a distal site and produce injury to the microvasculature.

B. ROLE OF SUPEROXIDE ANION

If indeed oxygen radicals do mediate the tissue injury observed during reperfusion of ischemic tissue, rather than a delayed manifestation of injury incurred during the ischemic period, then antioxidants and inhibitors of oxy-radical formation should offer protection against reperfusion-induced microvascular injury. Figure 5 illustrates that pretreatment of animals with SOD, the superoxide radical-scavenging enzyme previously discussed, significantly attenuated the permeability changes induced by regional ischemia followed by reperfusion.[1] Furthermore, a small lipophilic compound that is known to have SOD-like activity Cu(II)-3,5-diisopropylsalicylic acid (DIPS) also attenuates the I/R-induced increase in capillary permeability as noted in Figure 5.[39] These data suggest that oxidants generated during I/R do indeed mediate the microvascular injury. Moreover, if oxidants are generated at the time of reperfusion then antioxidants should afford protection irrespective of whether they are administered just prior to reperfusion or before the induction of ischemia. Indeed Morris et al.[8] clearly demonstrated that SOD was equally beneficial in protecting against intestinal I/R injury if given prior to or at the end of the ischemic period.

Finally, if superoxide mediates the microvascular injury in postischemic vessels, then generation of oxygen radicals using a superoxide-generating system (xanthine oxidase and hypoxanthine) should promote microvascular dysfunction in nonischemic intestine similar to that observed following I/R. Figure 5 demonstrates that the increase in microvascular permeability associated with local intra-arterial infusion of xanthine and xanthine oxidase mimics that seen following I/R.[40] This permeability increase is largely

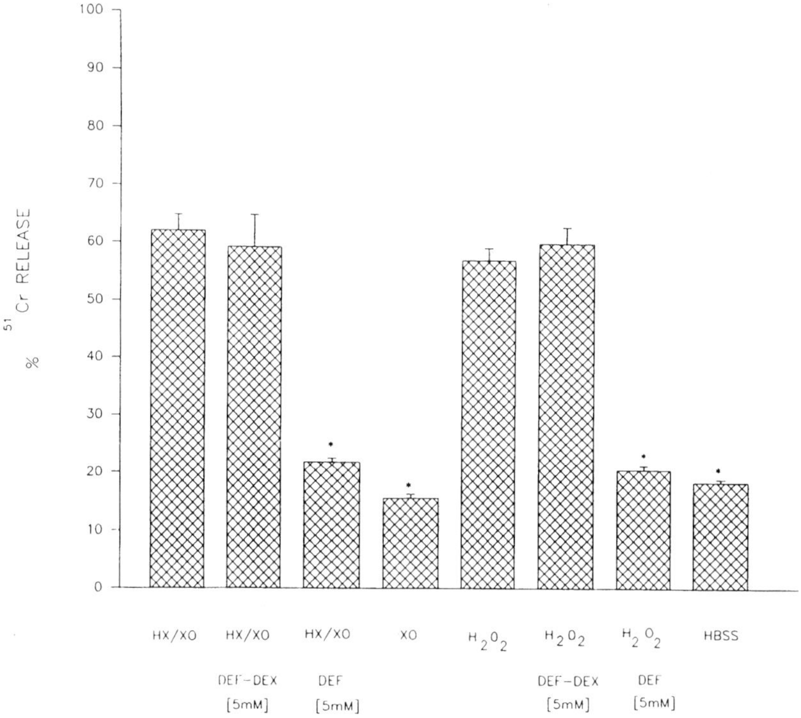

Figure 6-4 Effect of pretreatment (5 h) of endothelial cells with either free deferoxamine (DEF) or deferoxamine bound to dextran (mol wt 40,000) (DEF-DEX) on endothelial cell injury (^{51}Cr release) induced by either hypoxanthine-xanthine oxidase (HX/XO) reaction mixture or 800 μM H_2O_2.

prevented if SOD is infused along with xanthine oxidase and hypoxanthine.[40] While it is indirect evidence, the latter experiments further implicate superoxide in the I/R-induced increase in microvascular permeability.

Until recently, the only available evidence of radical production was the effect of radical scavengers on physiological or morphological parameters. The difficulty associated with measuring the O_2^- radical is related to its unstable nature with a lifetime of milliseconds. Two new techniques, chemiluminescence[41] and electron-spin resonance spectroscopy[7] were developed which permitted investigators to demonstrate elevated levels of oxy-radicals following reperfusion of the ischemic bowel. Nevertheless, some incongruities exist between these new measurements of superoxide and the work reported using superoxide radical scavengers. Nilsson et al.[7] used electron-spin resonance spectroscopy and noted an increase in oxidant formation at the onset of reperfusion (2 h of ischemia). However, the activity returned to pre-ischemic control values by 10 min of reoxygenation. In contrast, Suzuki et al.[42] reported that SOD administration following even 1 h of reperfusion was still effective in attenuating certain oxy-radical-mediated responses suggesting that oxy-radicals still play a role at this time.

Using chemiluminescence, Roldan et al.[41] observed a 40% increase in the emission of chemiluminescence following 3 to 5 min of ischemia in the rat small bowel supporting the notion of Roy and McCord[43] that oxy-radical production can occur within a short ischemic period. One point of concern regarding this study was the absence of an increase in XO activity over the short interval of ischemia. At the time of reperfusion, hypoxan-

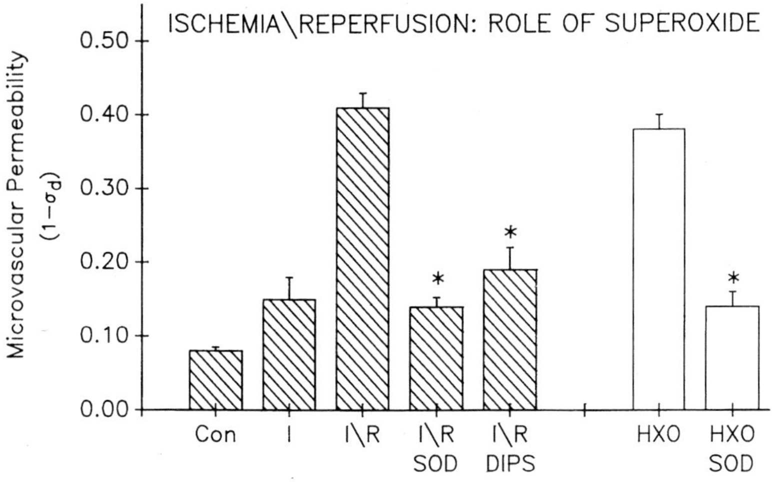

Figure 6-5 Effect of superoxide dismutase (SOD) and copper diisopropylsalicylate (DIPS) pretreatment on the increased microvascular permeability induced by ischemia/reperfusion (I/R).[1,39] For comparative purposes the effect of local intra-arterial infusion of hypoxanthine and xanthine oxidase (HXO) (superoxide generating system) are included in the absence and presence of SOD.[4] σ = osmotic reflection coefficient of the intestinal microvasculature to total plasma proteins. *$p < 0.05$ relative to I/R or HXO.

thine and O_2 are certainly not limiting factors, and since xanthine oxidase activity did not increase following 5 min of ischemia one would not expect an enhanced oxy-radical formation as predicted by the chemiluminescence response. Therefore, either xanthine oxidase is not the source of the oxidant production, or there are some underlying difficulties associated with the measurement of superoxide that must await the development of new and more sensitive techniques for monitoring oxidant production.

C. ROLE OF HYDROGEN PEROXIDE

Although there is some strong evidence for the involvement of superoxide in I/R-induced microvascular injury, this anion per se is a relatively weak oxidant. The low reactivity of this compound makes it an unlikely candidate as the final mediator of I/R injury. However, O_2^- may be a precursor to a more potent oxidant that eventually mediates I/R injury. Although superoxide is formed by xanthine oxidase, much of the O_2 consumed by the enzyme (80%) is divalently reduced to H_2O_2. Moreover, the superoxide that is generated will also spontaneously and rapidly dismutate to produce H_2O_2 and O_2. To determine the role of H_2O_2 in the postischemic vasculature, some animals were pretreated with catalase. If H_2O_2 is detoxified with catalase as noted in Figure 6, the increased microvascular permeability was again greatly reduced during I/R.[44] These data suggest that H_2O_2 is also an important mediator of the I/R-induced microvascular dysfunction. There is an apparent inconsistency in these findings, in that superoxide dismutase scavenges superoxide and produces H_2O_2 yet superoxide dismutase provided protection. A possible explanation for this enigma is that superoxide and H_2O_2 are needed simultaneously to perhaps produce a final mediator of the I/R injury observed.

A naturally occurring scavenging enzyme, GPO converts H_2O_2 to O_2 and H_2O with the formation of GSSG from GSH. It has recently been reported that exogenous glutathione can protect cells against oxidative injury.[45] Clearly, during I/R, the oxidative stress is of sufficient magnitude to far outweigh the protective effects of GPO. Nevertheless, in-

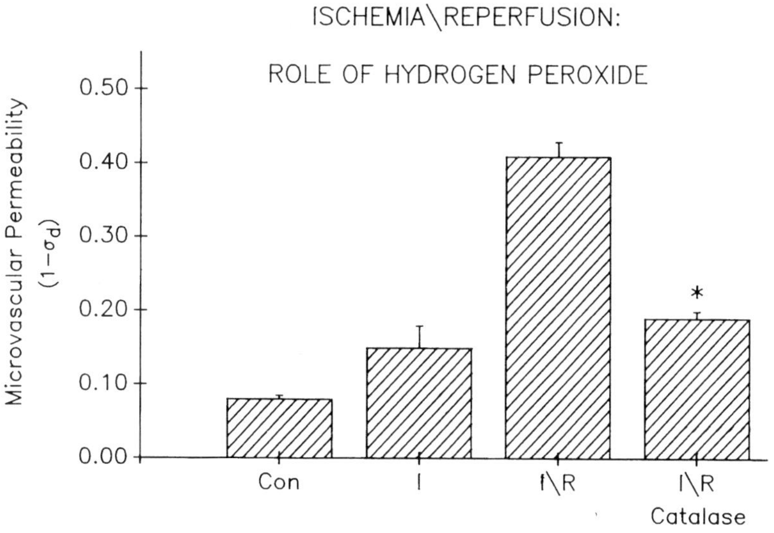

Figure 6-6 Effect of catalase pretreatment on the increased microvascular permeability induced by I/R.[44] Ischemia (I) is also included. σ = osmotic reflection coefficient of the intestinal microvasculature to total plasma proteins. *$p < 0.05$ relative to I/R.

creased concentrations of GSSG have been observed during reperfusion of the ischemic bowel.[46] Levels of GSSG are considered to be a fairly accurate index of H_2O_2 release, indicating that H_2O_2 is produced in the postischemic intestine.

D. ROLE OF HYDROXYL RADICAL

H_2O_2 is a rather stable and unreactive molecule in the absence of trace metals and has been shown to be a sluggish oxidant in its reactivity toward biological compounds. In the presence of certain transition metals, particularly iron, H_2O_2 yields (Haber-Weiss reaction) the hydroxyl radical (·OH), a potent oxidizing agent. Normally, iron is stored in enterocytes in the form of ferritin micelles. However, superoxide can react with Fe^{3+} in ferritin to liberate Fe^{2+}.[12,47] Thus, xanthine oxidase-generated superoxide provides ferrous iron which would then react with H_2O_2 to form ·OH in the postischemic intestine. To evaluate the role of iron in I/R-induced microvascular dysfunction, an iron chelator (deferoxamine) and an iron-binding protein (apotransferrin) were tested to determine whether they afford protection against the increased intestinal microvascular permeability produced by I/R. Figure 7 clearly demonstrates that both deferoxamine and apotransferrin provided significant protection in our I/R model.[48] However, if deferoxamine or apotransferrin were iron-loaded prior to administration, then no protection was observed (Figure 7), suggesting that iron binding accounts for the beneficial effects of these substances.

The hydroxyl radical, considered to be the most reactive free radical produced *in vivo*, is capable of damaging many biological compounds including proteins, lipids, carbohydrates, and nucleotides.[49-51] The principal mechanism proposed to explain radical-mediated increases in permeability involves peroxidation of lipid components of cellular membranes. The formation of lipid-derived free radicals such as conjugated dienes, lipid hydroperoxide radicals, and fragmentation products (e.g., malondialdehydes) alters the structural integrity and biological function of cell membranes.[52]

Evidence for reperfusion-induced lipid peroxidation in the intestinal mucosa was reported by Younes et al.,[53] who observed that tissue levels of conjugated dienes more

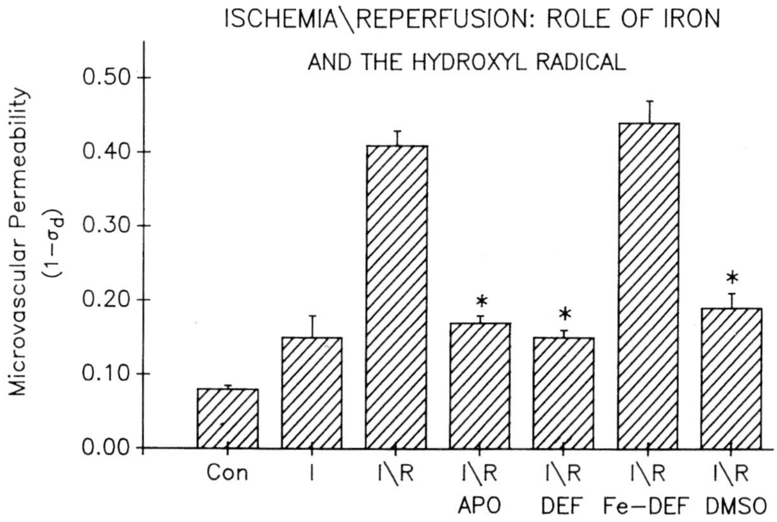

Figure 6-7 Effects of apotransferrin (APO), deferoxamine (DEF), iron-loaded deferoxamine (Fe-DEF), and dimethylsulfoxide (DMSO) pretreatment on the increased microvascualr permeability associated with I/R.[48,54] σ = osmotic reflection coefficient of intestinal microvasculature to total plasma proteins. *$p < 0.05$ relative to I/R.

than doubled 10 min following reperfusion of the ischemic bowel. Furthermore, the assumption that the hydroxyl radical plays a critical role in I/R injury is supported by studies[54] in which cats were treated with DMSO, a hydroxyl radical scavenger (Figure 7). Microvascular permeability was greatly attenuated in these animals. Therefore, the protective effects of DMSO, catalase, deferoxamine, and apotransferrin and elevated levels of conjugated dienes are consistent with the view that the cytotoxic hydroxyl radical is formed during reperfusion by the Haber-Weiss reaction and it plays a role in the injury to intestinal cells induced by I/R.

E. ROLE OF PEROXYNITRITE

Recently, Beckman et al.[55] have proposed an alternative hypothesis to explain the results associated with superoxide dismutase, deferoxamine, and DMSO. Based on the fact that there is very little free iron available *in vivo*, making the iron-catalyzed Haber-Weiss reaction an unlikely occurance, Beckman et al. postulated that superoxide reacts with nitric oxide (NO), a stable free radical, to yield secondary cytotoxic species including the hydroxyl radical. An intermediary step would be the production of peroxynitrite anion ($ONOO^-$), independent of iron catalysis. Interestingly, deferoxamine is a strong scavenger of the peroxynitrite molecule suggesting that scavenging of peroxynitrite may be an alternative antioxidant mechanism of deferoxamine in addition to iron chelation. Furthermore, it should be noted that if deferoxamine is loaded with iron, then deferoxamine becomes ineffective at inhibiting the actions of peroxynitrite, suggesting that the same functional groups on deferoxamine are responsible for iron chelation and peroxynitrite inactivation. Beckman et al.[55] also proposed that generation of peroxynitrite may be considerably more toxic than the hydroxyl radical because the hydroxyl radical reacts almost instantaneously with whichever molecule it contacts, whereas $ONOO^-$ has a half-life of sufficient duration to permit diffusion over several cell diameters before it decomposes to produce the hydroxyl radical. Therefore, the latter scenerio allows for more far-reaching damage than the former, where the movement of the toxic molecule is greatly restricted.

Evidence to support or refute a role for $OONO^-$ in I/R is limited inpart because peroxynitrite is stable at rather high pH so that *in vivo* testing is not feasible. Additionally, there is no specific inhibitor of peroxynitrate available at this time, so that it is impossible to make any conclusive remarks regarding its role in I/R. Lefer et al.[56] have shown that nitric oxide-induced relaxation is impaired in postischemic vessels via a superoxide-mediated mechanism. These data suggest that superoxide and NO do indeed react in postischemic tissue; however, they do not provide evidence to suggest that the resultant molecule is the mediator of the microvascular injury.

Moreover, data from other studies raise some inconsistencies regarding the peroxynitrite hypothesis. Firstly, exogenous sources of NO have been shown to greatly increase I/R-induced animal survivability.[57] If indeed NO and superoxide react to form a mediator of the I/R injury, one might predict that adding more of the substrate should not be beneficial. On the other hand, Mulligan et al.[58] have demonstrated that LNAME, an inhibitor of NO production, reduced vascular protein leakage in an oxidant-dependent, immune complex model of lung injury. Based on these data, the investigators implicated a role for the peroxynitrite molecule. In contrast, Antunes et al.[59] have demonstrated that the apparent beneficial effects regarding protein leakage observed with NO inhibitors could be completely reversed if in addition to LNAME, iloprost, a vasodilator was given. These investigators concluded that LNAME rather than being beneficial simply reduces blood flow to the inflamed organ to such a degree that it reduces protein leakage. Clearly there is a lack of direct evidence to support the view that peroxynitrate per se plays an important role in I/R injury, yet this novel idea warrants further attention.

V. ROLE OF NEUTROPHILS IN ISCHEMIA/REPERFUSION INJURY

A. MEDIATORS OF NEUTROPHIL-INDUCED CYTOTOXICITY

It is now recognized that activated neutrophils can undermine vascular integrity by releasing a variety of cytotoxic products into extracellular fluid. Reactive oxygen metabolites and granule constituents are liberated from neutrophils following the interaction of inflammatory mediators (e.g., leukotriene B_4, platelet-activating factor, complement fragments) with specific receptors on the neutrophil plasma membrane.[60] Activated neutrophils undergo a dramatic increase in oxygen consumption (respiratory burst) which is associated with the generation of reactive oxygen metabolites. Approximately 90% of the extra oxygen consumption in the activated neutrophil can be attributed to the generation of superoxide via a plasma membrane-associated NADPH oxidase (which is also found in monocytes, eosinophils, and macrophages):

$$NADPH + 2O_2 \rightarrow NADP^+ + 2O_2^- + H^+ \qquad \textbf{(6-6)}$$

The NADPH required for this reaction is generated by glucose metabolism in the activated hexose monophosphate shunt of the stimulated neutrophil. The superoxide generated by the NADPH oxidase system undergoes spontaneous dismutation to form H_2O_2. Some investigators have proposed that neutrophil-derived superoxide and H_2O_2 may interact with low molecular iron to yield the highly reactive hydroxyl radical ($\cdot OH$). However, recent data suggest that neutrophils produced very little (if any) $\cdot OH$ *in vivo*.

Once activated, neutrophils also release the contents of azurophilic granules, which contain the hemoprotein myeloperoxidase (MPO). This enzyme utilizes the H_2O_2 generated by neutrophils to oxidize Cl^- to form hypochlorous acid (HOCl). HOCl is approximately 100 to 1000 times more toxic than either superoxide or H_2O_2.[12] The hypohalous acid is a nonspecific oxidizing and chlorinating agent that reacts rapidly with a variety of biological compounds, including sulfhydryls, thioethers (methionine), DNA, aliphatic and aromatic amino acids, and nitrogen-containing compounds. HOCl reacts rapidly with the unprotonated form of primary amines (RNH_2) to yield N-chloroderivatives (RNHCl) which have the oxidizing equivalence of H_2O_2 and HOCl. Two classes of neutrophil-derived RNHCl have been identified: one class may be represented by taurine monochloramine, the reaction product derived from the interaction between HOCl and taurine. Inasmuch as the sulfonic acid residue is negatively charged at physiological pH, taurine monochloramine is very hydrophilic (membrane impermeable), long-lived, and relatively nontoxic. A second class of RNHCl are lipophilic in nature and quite cytotoxic. These RNHCl are very short-lived owing to their ability to rapidly penetrate the membrane bilayer and react with intracellular components. An example of this class of oxidants is monochloramine ($NHCl_2$). The lipophilic N-chloramines are likely causes of cellular injury associated with HOCl production. The cytotoxicity associated with HOCl and N-chloramines may be mediated via oxidation of sulfhydryls, inactivation of heme protein and cytochrome, chlorination of purine bases on DNA, and degradation of amino acids and proteins. Furthermore, MPO-generated oxidants have been shown to degrade and depolymerize important components of the extracellular matrix such as hyaluronic acid and collagen.[60]

Another consequence of neutrophil activation is release of lysosomal granules. Neutrophil granules contain a number of enzymes and other proteins that are capable of mediating vascular injury. The most potent of the enzymes released by neutrophils are elastase, gelatinase, and collagenase. Each of these proteases is capable of attacking the key components of the interstitial matrix and the capillary basement membrane, including elastins, collagens, fibronectin, and proteoglycans. These matrices serve to maintain normal tissue architecture and act as an interactive substratum that modulates the shape, growth, migration, and differentiation of cells.

Elastase is a serine protease that reacts with a broad spectrum of substrates, i.e., it can attack cross links in the nonhelical portions of interstitial collagens (types I, II, III) as well as the helical portions of collagen types III and IV and fibronectin. Neutrophil-derived elastase will hydrolyze certain glycoproteins, proteoglycans, immunoglobulins, complement components, and clotting factors. Collagenase and gelatinase are metalloproteinases that can cleave the interstitial collagens (types I, II, III) and basement membrane collagen (type IV), respectively.[61]

Although the neutrophilic proteases possess tremendous destructive potential, evidence implicating these enzymes in the neutrophil-mediated tissue injury has been difficult to obtain. This difficulty results in part from the fact that extracellular fluid (plasma and interstitial fluid) contains powerful antiproteinases (α_1 proteinase inhibitor and α_2 macroglobulin) that can rapidly and irreversibly inhibit serine proteases. Although metalloproteinases (collagen, gelatinase) are generally not as susceptible to inactivation by α_1 antiproteinase as is elastase, their role as mediators of tissue injury has been questioned because they are released from the neutrophil in a latent, inactive form. However, recent work indicates that oxidants play an important role in activating neutrophil-derived proteases in the presence of extracellular fluid.[12] It has been shown that the HOCl produced by activated neutrophils can inactivate α_1 proteinase inhibitor (and α_2 macroglobulin) thereby allowing for uncontrolled proteolysis by elastase. HOCl also has been shown to activate the latent collagenase and gelatinase secreted by neutrophil. The results of all of the aforementioned studies suggests that oxidative inactivation of protease inhibitors, coupled to the oxidant-mediated activation of latent proteases, creates an environment for the neutrophil that allows elastase, collagenase, and gelatinase to injure endothelial cells and to degrade the vascular basement membrane and interstitial matrix.

B. LEUKOCYTE-ENDOTHELIAL CELL ADHESIVE INTERACTIONS

One of the early events in an inflammatory response is adhesion of granulocytes to the endothelial cells lining the walls of small venules. Granulocyte adhesion begins as a rolling movement such that the leukocytes move slower than erythrocytes in the stream of blood bathing the vascular endothelium. As inflammation progresses, the number of rolling leukocytes increases and the velocity of leukocyte rolling decreases. These changes increase the probability for a strong adhesive interaction between the leukocyte and endothelium, which ultimately leads to an elevated number of stationary (adherent) leukocytes and emigration of the phagocytes into the adjacent interstitial compartment. Although the importance of these events in the overall process of inflammation has been recognized for well over a century, only recently has it become clear that leukocyte-endothelial cell adhesion is a well controlled physiological phenomenon that is influenced by both physical and chemical forces acting on cell (leukocyte and endothelium) surfaces. Physiologic factors that appear to make a significant contribution to leukocyte-endothelial cell adhesion during inflammation include: (1) adhesion molecules expressed on the surface of activated neutrophils and/or endothelial cells, (2) reactive oxygen metabolites and granule-associated proteins released by activated neutrophils, (3) electrostatic charge interactions between the neutrophil and endothelial cell surfaces, and (4) hydrodynamic dispersal forces (e.g., wall shear stress) that tend to sweep leukocytes away from the vascular wall.

Several studies have been undertaken to assess the leukocyte-endothelial cell interactions that occur in tissues (e.g., cat mesentery, hamster cheek pouch) subjected to ischemia followed by reperfusion. Using a low-flow (blood flow reduced to 20% of baseline for 1 h) model, we demonstrated[62] that the number of adherent and emigrated leukocytes in cat mesenteric venules increases significantly during the ischemic period and that there is a pronounced exacerbation of these responses within 10 min following reperfusion (Figure 8). The reperfusion-induced increment in leukocyte adhesion is sustained for as long as 2 h (the longest time period studied). During the first hour following reperfusion, we estimate that the rates of leukocyte adherence (R_{LA}) and emigration (R_{LE}), which are expressed as the number of leukocytes per min per 100 μm length of venule, are 2.3 and 0.5, respectively. The ratio of R_{LE} to R_{LA} indicates that approximately 20% of the leukocytes that adhere to venular endothelium during the reperfusion period are destined to emigrate into the mesenteric interstitium. The magnitude of the reperfusion-induced leukocyte accumulation predicted by intravital microscopic estimates of adherence and emigration is comparable to that predicted by measurements of tissue myeloperoxidase (an enzyme which is largely confined to granulocytes) in intestinal mucosa.[63] It has been shown using light and electron microscopy that neutrophils are the predominant (>85%) population of leukocytes that adhere and emigrate in mesenteric venules following reperfusion.[64]

1. Adhesion Molecules

An important factor that determines whether a leukocyte adheres to microvascular endothelium is the pro-adhesive force generated by leukocyte adhesion molecules. A variety of proinflammatory mediators (fMLP, PAF, LTB_4, C5a) are known to act directly on the neutrophil to enhance its adherence to endothelium and to biologically inert surfaces (e.g., plastic). The pro-adhesive action of these mediators occurs quickly (within 1 to 2 min) and is dependent on the mobilization of specific adhesion molecules to the surface of the leukocyte. The bulk of available evidence implicates the leukocyte adhesion glycoprotein complex termed CD11/CD18 (or Mac-1, LFA-1, p150,95) as the primary mediator of adhesion of activated neutrophils to endothelial cells.[65] This adhesive glycoprotein complex is composed of a family of three structurally and functionally

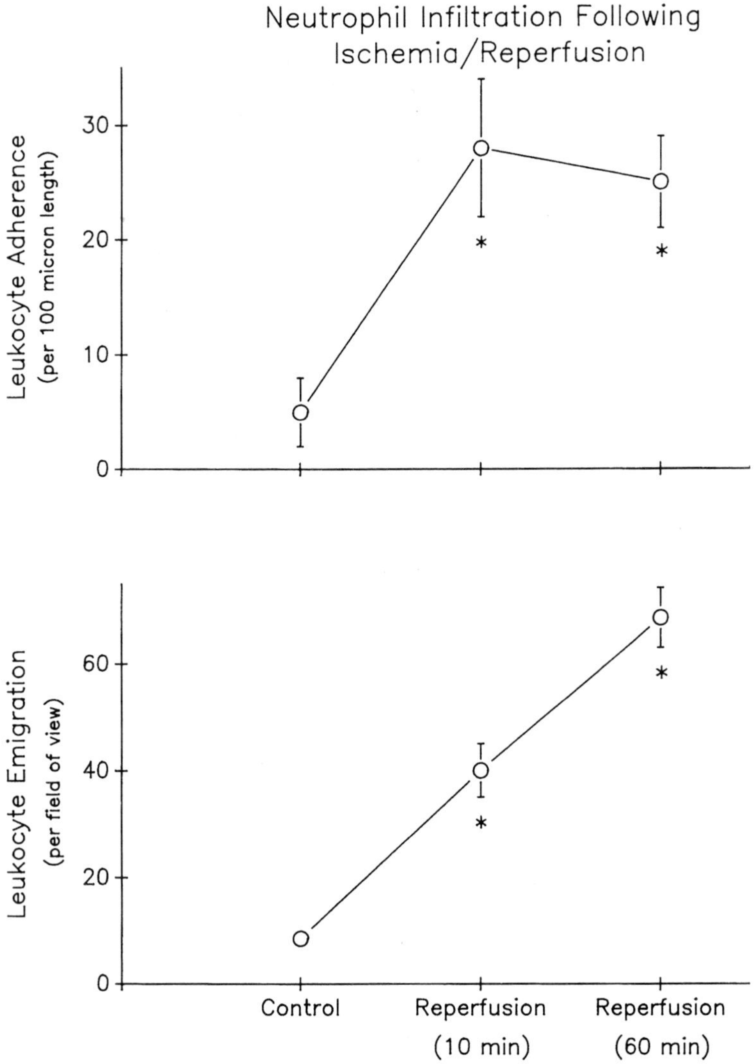

Figure 6-8 Leukocyte adherence and emigration during control and at 10 and 60 min following the reperfusion of postischemic vessels. *$p < 0.05$ relative to control values.

related glycoprotein heterodimers, each consisting of an immunologically distinct α-subunit (CD11) that is noncovalently associated with a common β-subunit (CD18). LFA-1 (CD11a/CD18) is present in all leukocytes, while Mac-1 (CD11b/CD18) and p150,95 (CD11c/CD18) are primarily expressed on granulocytes and monocytes. Leukocyte adhesion deficiency (LAD) is an inherited disorder of leukocyte function characterized by markedly reduced or absent cell surface expression of the three CD11/CD18 glycoproteins on leukocytes. *In vitro* studies have demonstrated that neutrophils from patients with LAD exhibit markedly diminished adherence to endothelial cell monolayers in response to LTB_4, PAF, and fMLP.[65] The critical role of the common β-subunit (CD18) in neutrophil adherence to endothelium has also been demonstrated using monoclonal antibodies (MoAbs) to CD18 (e.g., MoAbs 60.3 and IB_4), which inhibit neutrophil adherence stimulated by a variety of chemotactic peptides and lipid mediators. Antibodies against CD18 effectively reduce neutrophil adhesion without influencing other (adhesion-independent) neutrophil functions, such as protease release and superoxide formation.

Suzuki et al.[42] have assessed the role of CD18 in mediating the leukocyte adherence observed in mesenteric venules subjected to 1 h of ischemia, followed by reperfusion. Their results indicate that reperfusion-induced leukocyte adherence (which is 19 times greater than control adherence) can be reduced by approximately 80% within 10 min after immunoneutralization of CD18 with 1 mg/kg MoAb IB_4. We have obtained similar results with MoAb 60.3, which is directed against the same epitope on the adhesive glycoprotein (unpublished observations). In addition, we have shown that pretreatment with either MoAb 60.3 or MoAb IB_4 largely prevents the increased microvascular permeability induced by reperfusion of the ischemic bowel.[66] Finally, it was demonstrated that MoAb IB_4 largely abolishes the rise in leukocyte adherence in mesenteric venules induced by local intra-arterial infusion of PAF.[67]

Although there are several reports that implicate the common β-subunit (CD18) of the leukocyte adhesion complex in neutrophil adherence, less is known about the importance of CD18 in modulating leukocyte **emigration** in *in vivo* models of acute inflammation. Recently, it was demonstrated that pretreatment of cat mesentery with the CD18-specific antibody IB_4 entirely prevented the leukocyte emigration elicited by I/R (Figure 9).[64] A comparable inhibitory action of IB_4 on leukocyte emigration has been observed in mesenteric preparations superfused with platelet-activating factor.[68] In both instances (I/R and PAF superfusion) the ability of CD18 immunoneutralization to prevent emigration is largely a result of the reduction or abolishment of leukocyte adherence, which is a prerequisite for the emigration process.

There is a growing body of evidence which indicates that adhesion molecules expressed on the surface of microvascular endothelium also play an important role in the leukocyte-endothelial cell adhesive interactions associated with acute and chronic inflammatory states. Three of the best characterized endothelial cell adhesion molecules are intercellular adhesion molecule-1 (ICAM-1), endothelial leukocyte adhesion molecule (ELAM-1 or E-selection), and granule membrane protein-140 (GMP-140 or P-selection). ICAM-1 is an inducible cell surface glycoprotein that is constituitively expressed on endothelium. Its surface expression is enhanced during inflammation *in vivo* and on endothelial cell monolayers exposed to cytokines. LFA-1 (CD11a/CD18) appears to act as a ligand for ICAM-1. ELAM-1 is not constituitively expressed on endothelium *in vivo* or *in vitro*, however it is induced by cytokines and endotoxin *in vitro* and in inflamed tissue. The leukocyte receptor for ELAM-1 and its relationship to CD11/CD18 remains unknown. GMP-140 is normally found in Weibel Palade bodies of endothelium, however it is rapidly mobilized to the cell surface when endothelium is exposed to thrombin, histamine, or leukotrienes. Unlike ICAM-1 and ELAM-1, which require >4 h for maximum expression, GMP-140 is expressed within minutes (<20 min) after histamine exposure by a mechanism which is protein synthesis independent.[65,69]

Recently, attempts have been made to determine the relative contributions of both leukocyte and endothelial cell adhesion glycoproteins to the leukocyte adherence elicited by reperfusion (reoxygenation) of ischemic (hypoxic) tissues. In cat mesenteric venules exposed to 1 h of ischemia followed by 1 h of reperfusion, pretreatment with a CD18-specific antibody (MAb IB_4) attenuated the reperfusion-induced increments in both leukocyte adherence and emigration by ~95%, while CD11a- and CD11b-specific antibodies reduced leukocyte adherence by 60 to 65% and emigration by 45 to 50%.[70] An

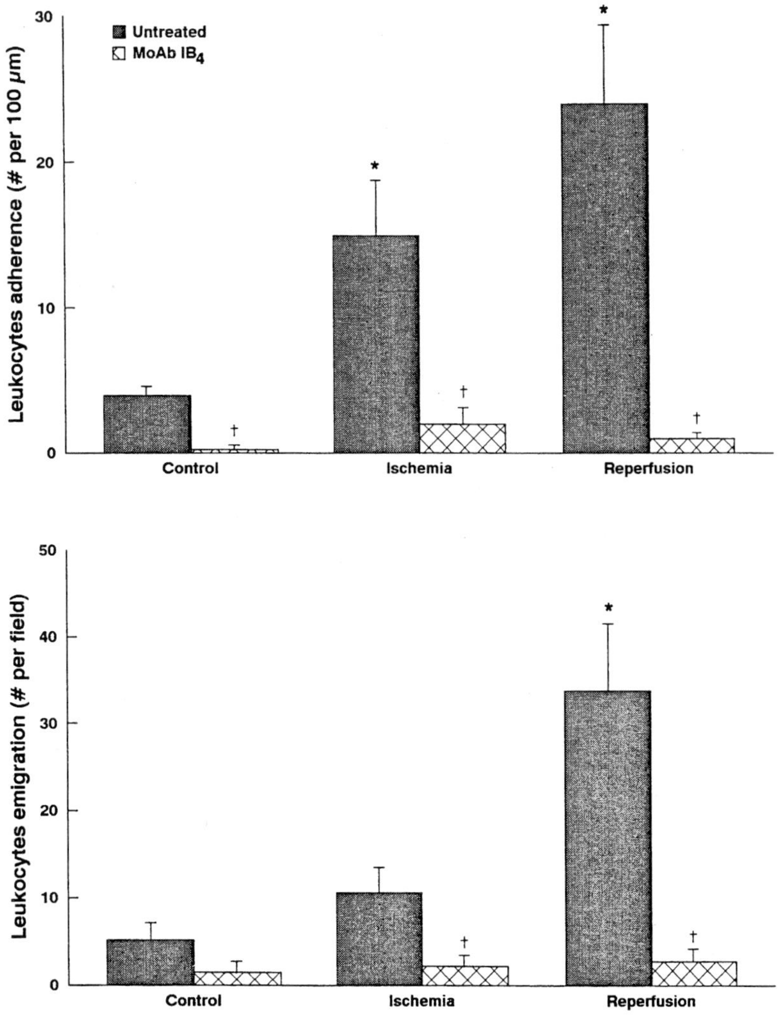

Figure 6-9 Role of CD11/CD18 in I/R-induced leukocyte adherence and emigration in feline mesenteric venules. The small bowel was subjected to 1hr of ischemia followed by 1 h of reperfusion. The CD18-specific antibody (MoAB IB_4) was administered prior to obtaining control measurements. An asterisk denotes significance ($p < 0.05$) compared to the untreated controls, while a dagger indicates significance relative to corresponding value in untreated group. (*Data from Oliver, M. G., Specian, R. D., Perry, M. A., and Granger, D. N., Inflammation, 15, 331, 1991.)*

ICAM-1 specific antibody reduced reperfusion-induced adherence by 40% and emigration by 50%. These results indicate that the leukocyte adherence and emigration observed in postcapillary venules exposed to ischemia/reperfusion are mediated by both CD11/CD18 on neutrophils and ICAM-1 on endothelial cells.

The contribution of different adhesive glycoproteins to ischemia/reperfusion induced leukocyte adhesion has also been addressed in an *in vitro* model that utilizes monolayers of cultured human umbilical vein endothelial cells (HUVEC) and human neutrophils.[71] In this model, the HUVEC monolayers are exposed to sublethal episodes of anoxia and subsequently reoxygenated. Radiolabelled neutrophils are added immediately upon reoxygenation and neutrophil-endothelial cell interactions can be quantitated. Under basal (normoxia) conditions neutrophil adherence to endothelial cell monolayers is inhibited by MAb directed to CD11a and CD18, but not by MAb directed to CD11b. Inhibition is also observed following administration of MAb directed against ICAM-1, but not by MAbs against ELAM-1. Anoxia/reoxygenation leads to a significant increase in neutrophil adherence to the endothelial cell monolayers. The hyperadhesivity of neutrophils on anoxia/reoxygenation-conditioned endothelial cells is inhibited by monoclonal antibodies (MAb) against either CD11a, CD11b, or CD18 (Figure 10). The inhibitory effects of CD11a- and CD11b-specific antibodies were additive when used in combination and this additive effect was equivalent to that of CD18, which completely prevented the hyperadhesivity. The anoxia/reoxygenation-induced increase in neutrophil adherence to endothelial cells was inhibited by MAb directed to ICAM-1, but not by MAb directed to ELAM-1. Enzyme immunoassay studies indicated that ICAM-1 but not ELAM-1 was basally expressed on endothelial cells and that anoxia/reoxygenation did not increase the expression of either of these endothelial cell determinants. Supernatants recovered from endothelial cells exposed to anoxia/reoxygenation increased the expression of CD11b and CD18 on the surface of neutrophils as assessed by flow cytometry. Taken together these findings indicate that endothelial cells exposed to anoxia/reoxygenation release a soluble factor(s) which results in the expression and/or activation of CD11b/CD18 on neutrophils and the increased neutrophil adherence to endothelial cells is a result of interactions between CD11a/CD18 and CD11b/CD18 adherence glycoproteins on neutrophils and ICAM-1 on endothelial cells.

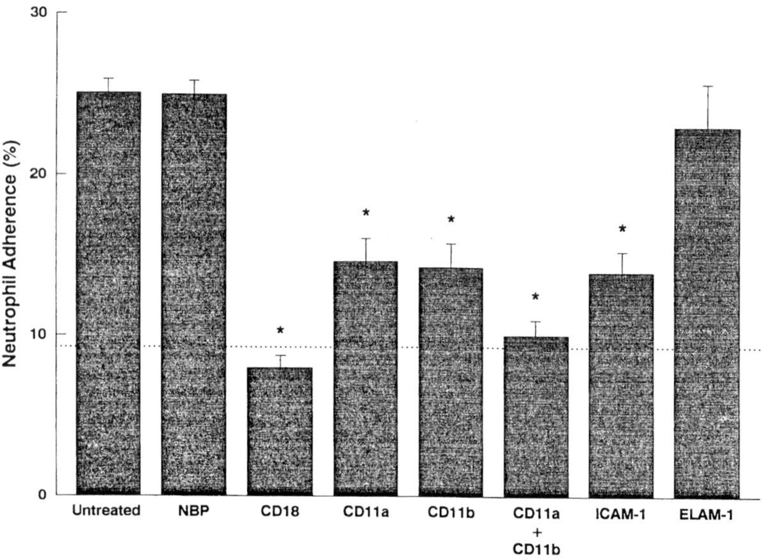

Figure 6-10 Role of neutrophil and endothelial cell adhesion glycoproteins in the hyperadhesivity of neutrophils to endothelial cell monolayers exposed to anoxia-reoxygenation. NBP refers to nonbinding antibody. (*Data from Yoshida, N., Granger, D. N., Anderson, D. C., Rothlein, R., Lane, C., and Kvietys, P. R., Am. J. Physiol., 262, H1891, 1992.*)

2. Reactive Oxygen Metabolites

There is a growing body of evidence which suggests that reactive oxygen metabolites and granule-associated proteins released by activated neutrophils may also play a role in modulating leukocyte-endothelial cell interactions. The possibility that reactive oxygen metabolites may modulate the neutrophil infilitration associated with I/R was first proposed to explain the observation that pretreatment of the cat intestine with either free radical scavenging enzymes (SOD, catalase) or xanthine oxidase inhibitors (allopurinol) significantly reduced the rise in tissue MPO activity normally elicited by I/R.[63,72] These results lead to the hypothesis that xanthine oxidase-derived oxidants play an important role in recruiting neutrophils into postischemic tissues.[10] However, it is also likely that other sources of superoxide and/or H_2O_2 (e.g., granulocytes) may contribute to the process of leukocyte adherence and emigration in postischemic tissues.

There is evidence that implicates both superoxide and H_2O_2 in the neutrophil adherence elicited by I/R. We have recently observed that SOD, but not H_2O_2-inactivated SOD, significantly attenuates the leukocyte adherence and emigration observed in mesenteric venules exposed to I/R, irrespective of whether the active enzyme is administered before or 1 h after reperfusion.[42] Similar antiadhesive effects of SOD have been demonstrated in mesenteric venules exposed to platelet-activating factor.[73] In the latter studies, the SOD-induced reversal of leukocyte adherence was associated with a corresponding reduction in the vascular protein leakage induced by PAF, indicating that the ability of SOD to reduce leukocyte adherence is of importance in maintaining microvascular integrity.

It has also been shown that SOD reduces, in a dose-dependent manner, the neutrophil adherence that occurs when endothelial cell monolayers are exposed to 30 min of hypoxia followed by 60 min of reoxygenation.[42] However, SOD does not interfere with the adherence of activated neutrophils to plastic, suggesting that superoxide-mediated leukocyte adhesion is an endothelium-dependent process. The mechanisms underlying the proadhesive actions of superoxide remain unknown; however, one possibility is that the free radical may interact with an endothelial cell-derived anti-adhesive substance and render it inactive. Nitric oxide is a biologically active compound produced by vascular endothelium and is rapidly inactivated by superoxide. Nitric oxide appears to inhibit neutrophil aggregation *in vitro*, an effect that is potentiated by SOD. Furthermore, we have demonstrated that analogues of L-arginine which inhibit NO production by vascular endothelium greatly increase leukocyte adherence and emigration in postcapillary venules.[74] The proadhesive effects of the L-arginine analogues were largely unrelated to the lower venular wall shear rates associated with NO inhibition, yet were abolished by the CD18-specific MAb IB_4 (Figure 11). These observations, that decreased NO production promotes leukocyte adherence, may explain the ability of SOD to decrease leukocyte adhesion under conditions associated with an increased production of superoxide by either endothelial cells or neutrophils, since the enzyme would prevent superoxide-mediated inactivation of NO.

Relatively little information is available regarding the ability of H_2O_2 to promote leukocyte adherence. We have obtained evidence which indicates that superfusion of cat mesenteric venules with 0.01 to 0.50 mM H_2O_2 results in significant leukocyte adherence to venular endothelium and that the pro-adhesive effect of H_2O_2 can be ameliorated by either CD18-specific antibodies or PAF receptor antagonists.[75] The CD18 dependence of H_2O_2-induced adherence is consistent with the view that H_2O_2 promotes the formation of proinflammatory agents such as PAF and C5a. A role for H_2O_2 in modulating leukocyte adherence is also supported by the observation that active catalase, but not inactivated catalase, exerts a significant anti-adhesive effect in mesenteric venules exposed to I/R.[76] This observation, coupled with published data demonstrating that PAF-receptor antagonists effectively reduce reperfusion-induced leukocyte adherence in postcapillary venules,[77]

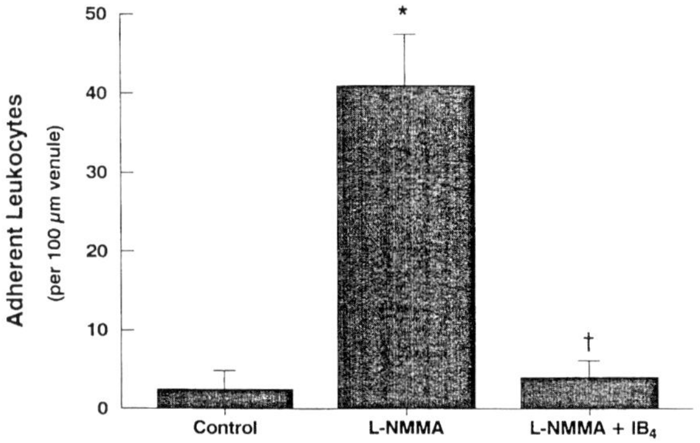

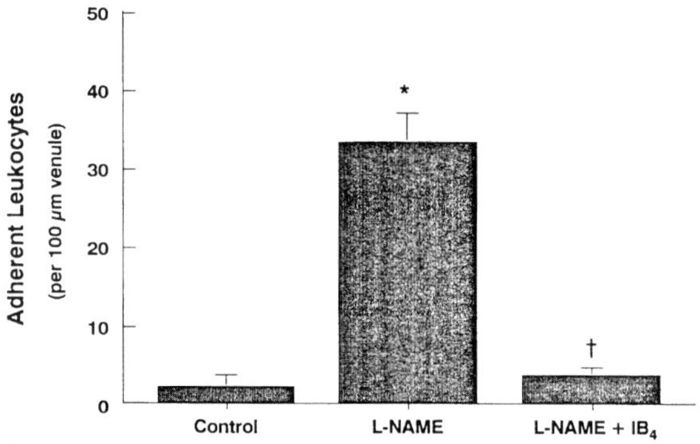

Figure 6-11 Effects of nitric oxide (NO) synthase inhibitors (L-NMMA and L-NAME) on leukocyte adherence in mesenteric venules. The CD18-specific antibody (IB_4) prevented the increased adhesion induced by inhibition of NO synthesis. (*Data from Kubes, P., Suzuki, M., and Granger, D. N., Proc. Natl. Acad. Sci. U.S.A., 88, 465, 1991.*)

supports the view that H_2O_2, generated by either endothelial cells or neutrophils, mediates reperfusion-induced leukocyte adhesion through the production of PAF.

The anti-adhesive action of catalase in experimental models of acute inflammation raises the interesting possibility that neutrophil-derived H_2O_2 may also promote leukocyte adhesion indirectly via the formation of MPO-derived oxidants such as HOCl and monochloramine (NH_2Cl). HOCl and N-chloramines are highly reactive oxidants which may be more or less cytotoxic than H_2O_2, depending on the lipophilicity of the compound. However, intravital microscopic studies of leukocyte adherence in mesenteric venules indicate that NH_2Cl, but not HOCl, exerts a pro-adhesive effect on leukocytes in cat mesenteric venules at concentrations well within the range predicted to occur in inflamed tissue (0.2 to 0.5 m*M*). The pro-adhesive effect of NH_2Cl could be prevented by administration of a CD18-specific antibody but not by PAF receptor antagonists.[75]

3. Neutrophil-Derived Proteins

Proinflammatory agents such as fMLP, LTB_4, and PAF are known to differentially stimulate the exocytosis of primary (azurophilic) and secondary (specific) granules of neutrophils. Elastase, released from activated neutrophils, may play an important role in the emigration of leukocytes across postcapillary venules. Elastase has been shown *in vitro* to degrade several components of vascular basement membrane (collagen, fibronectin, laminin). Thus, one might expect that limited release of elastase by neutrophils during diapedesis could effectively "digest" a route of passage from the vascular compartment into the interstitium. This hypothesis is not supported by the work of Huber and Weiss,[78] which demonstrates that the migration of activated neutrophils across monolayers of cultured endothelial cells with a basement membrane is not altered when neutrophils are pretreated with a serine protease inhibitor. Similar conclusions were drawn from intravital microscopic studies of LTB_4-stimulated leukocyte emigration in hamster cheek pouch. Rosengren and Arfors[79] observed that elastase inhibitors (Eglin C and L658,758) did not alter the LTB_4-induced leukocyte adherence and emigration, and vascular leakage of FITC-dextran. In contrast to the results obtained with LTB_4, I/R-induced leukocyte emigration across cat mesenteric venules is decreased by 90% and leukocyte adherence by 50% in response to pretreatment with a specific elastase inhibitor (L658,758), which does not alter the isoelectric point of the enzyme (Figure 12). This disproportionate effect of elastase inhibition on leukocyte emigration indicates that the enzyme may play an important role in regulating the rate of transendothelial migration following reperfusion of ischemic tissues. The discrep-

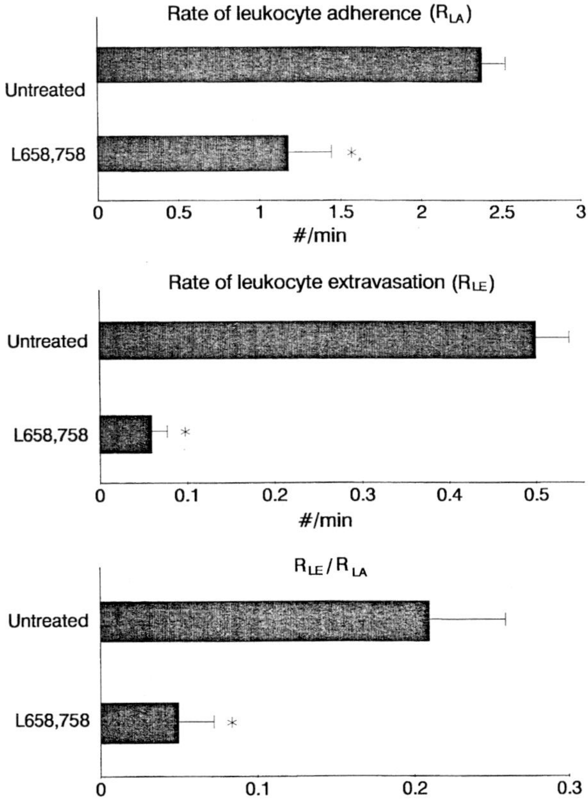

Figure 6-12 Effects of an elastase inhibitor (L658,758) on the rates of leukocyte adherence and emigration, and the proportion of adherent leukocytes that emigrate (R_{LE}/R_{LA}) in mesenteric venules exposed to ischemia and reperfusion. (*Data derived from Zimmerman, B. J. and Granger, D. N., Am. J. Physiol., 259, H390, 1990.)*

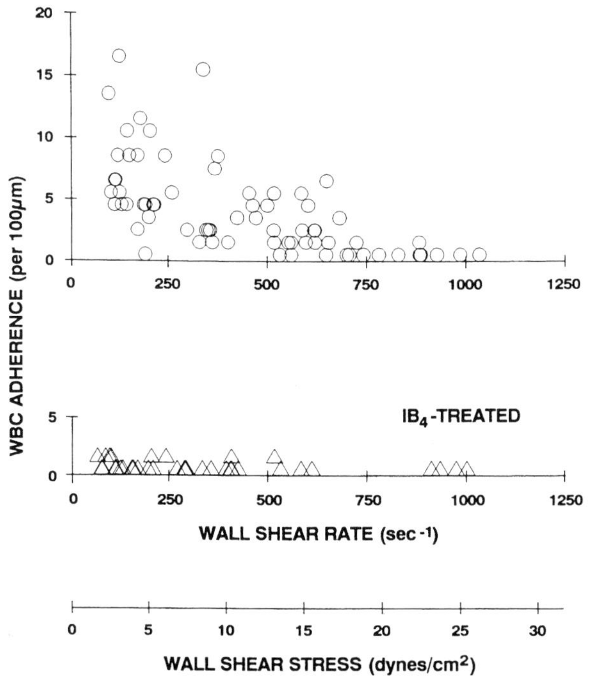

Figure 6-13 Effects of reducing shear rate on leukocyte (WBC) adherence in mesenteric venules both before (untreated) and following administration of a CD18-specific antibody (IB_4). (*Data from Perry, M. A. and Granger, D. N., J. Clin. Invest., 87, 1798, 1991.*)

ancy between the LTB_4 and I/R emigration responses to elastase inhibition may be explained by the relative magnitude of neutrophil degranulation induced by the inflammatory mediator released during I/R vs. LTB_4. However, a potential criticism of the I/R data is that the elastase inhibitor may act by interfering with the production of an elastase-dependent chemoattractant during I/R, rather than by inhibition of elastase-mediated digestion of vessel wall components.

4. Hydrodynamic Dispersal Forces

The shear forces generated by the movement of a viscous fluid (blood) through microvessels also appear to exert a significant influence on leukocyte-endothelial cell adhesive interactions in postcapillary venules. We have recently examined the relationship between leukocyte adhesion and venular wall shear rate in cat mesenteric venules subjected to brief, graded reductions in mesenteric blood flow.[81] Our data indicate that reductions in venular wall shear rate are accompanied by a reversible increase in the number of adherent leukocytes (Figure 13). Based on these data, it can be predicted that 50 to 75% of the leukocyte adherence measured during low flow ischemia results from a reduction in shear forces tending to sweep leukocytes along the blood vessel wall. It has also been reported that shear rate-dependent leukocyte adherence is mediated by the leukocyte adhesion glycoprotein CD11/CD18, since monoclonal antibodies directed against this adhesion glycoprotein abolish the response. Preliminary studies in our laboratory suggest that the increased leukocyte adherence observed in postcapillary venules exposed to low shear rates results in part from an accumulation of leukotriene B_4 in mesenteric tissue. The LTB_4 that accumulates during the low flow state presumably interact with blood neutrophils to upregulate or activate CD11/CD18.

A dependence of leukocyte adhesion on blood flow has also been demonstrated using monolayers of human endothelial cells. Ley et al.[82] have reported that neutrophil adhesion to endothelial cell monolayers averages 36% of the total number of neutrophils added when no shear stress (product of shear rate and fluid viscosity) is applied. However, applying a shear stress of 1.5 dynes/cm^2 reduced adhesion to 21%. Neutrophil adhesion to bovine serum albumin-coated dishes was reduced from 59 to 35% by the same shear stress. Lawrence and co-workers[83] have demonstrated that doubling the wall shear stress from 1 to 2 dynes/cm^2 reduced the number of adherent human neutrophils by more than a factor of four on both control and fMLP-treated endothelial cell monolayers. Doubling the wall shear stress again from 2 to 4 dynes/cm^2 reduced adhesion to virtually zero. These studies support the view that leukocyte adherence to microvascular endothelium is highly dependent on venular blood flow.

A consistent observation in the literature is that leukocyte rolling and adherence is much less common in arterioles than in venules. One explanation that is frequently offered to explain the absence of leukocyte adhesion in arterioles is the much greater shear rate in arterioles compared to venules. However, Perry and Granger[81] demonstrated that the prevalence of leukocyte rolling and adherence in arterioles is much lower than in venules when both vessels are exposed to the same range of shear rates. There are several alternative explanations for the greater adhesive interaction between leukocytes and venular endothelium. One possibility is that there is a lower density of ligand for CD11/CD18 or other leukocyte adhesion molecules on arteriolar endothelium compared to venular endothelium. It is also possible that arterioles may normally produce an anti-adhesive factor (e.g., NO, prostacyclin) that is either not produced or produced to a lower extent in venules. Finally, the greater interaction of leukocytes with venular endothelium could result from the hydrodynamic interaction of leukocytes with red blood cells, which results in a preferential displacement of leukocytes towards the venular wall. The latter phenomenon is thought to occur as vessel diameter increases at the level of postcapillary venules and may enhance the likelihood of leukocyte rolling and adherence.

VI. ROLE OF LEUKOCYTES IN ISCHEMIA/REPERFUSION INJURY

The first quantitative assessment of the contribution of neutrophils to I/R-induced tissue injury was performed in studies of dog myocardium.[84] Depletion of circulating neutrophils resulted in significant reduction of infarct size, a response similar to that observed in animals pretreated with oxy-radical scavengers. Two similar approaches have been used to assess the role of neutrophils in the increased intestinal vascular permeability induced by I/R.[66,85] The I/R-induced increase in vascular permeability is largely prevented in animals that are either rendered neutropenic with polyclonal antiserum or following intravenous administration of monoclonal antibodies (MoAb 60.3 and IB_4) directed against specific leukocyte associated glycoproteins (CD11/CD18) that modulate adherence to vascular endothelium (Figure 14). These results indicate that neutrophils are the major mediators of I/R-induced microvascular injury in the small bowel. The observation that neutrophil depletion and prevention of neutrophil adherence are equally effective in attenuating the microvascular injury suggests that neutrophil adherence to microvascular endothelium is a rate-limiting step in reperfusion-induced, neutrophil-mediated vascular injury. Confirmatory results have been obtained by a number of investigators studying the role of leukocytes in other postischemic tissues.

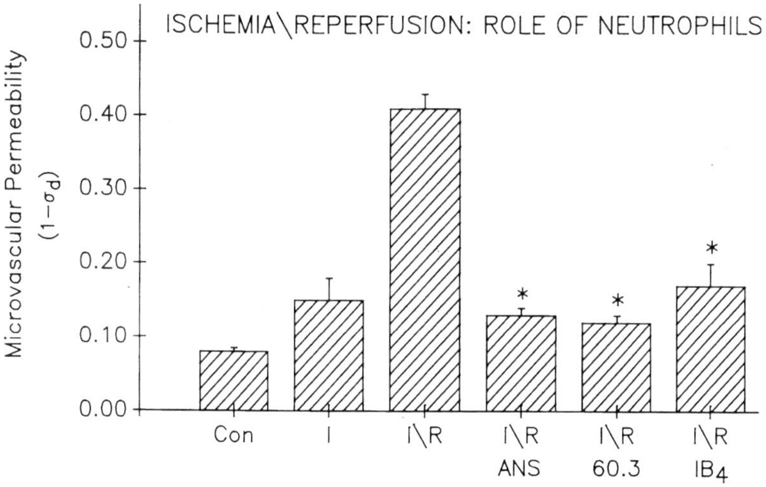

Figure 6-14 Effects of antineutrophil serum (ANS) and monoclonal antibodies against leukocyte adhesion molecules (IB_4 and 60.3) on the increased microvascular permeability associated with I/R.[66,85] (σ) osmotic reflection coefficient of the intestinal microvasculature to total plasma proteins, $^*p < 0.05$ relative to I/R.

A. ROLE OF CHEMOTACTIC AGENTS IN ISCHEMIA/REPERFUSION INJURY

The data discussed above would suggest (1) that neutrophils can adhere to postcapillary venules following I/R and (2) that these white cells mediate much of the vascular injury associated with the reperfusion of ischemic tissue. The mechanism or signal that causes neutrophils to infiltrate postischemic tissue, adhere, and emigrate is presently not well appreciated. Nevertheless, there is data which implicate a number of inflammatory mediators as potential chemotactic molecules involved in the postischemic neutrophil infiltration.

1. Oxidants

It is conceivable that oxygen radicals in combination with some plasmogen mediate reperfusion-induced neutrophil infiltration. The chemotactic potential of feline plasma exposed to an oxy-radical generating system (hypoxanthine and xanthine oxidase) has been examined using both *in vivo* and *in vitro* approaches in our laboratory. The results of these studies indicate that the chemotactic potential of feline extracellular fluid is not enhanced by exposure to oxygen radicals.[63] In contrast, other investigators have reported that human plasma exposed to superoxide becomes potently chemotactic to human neutrophils *in vitro*.[86,87] Intradermal injection of superoxide-treated plasma caused heavy infiltration of neutrophils at the injection site, and SOD inhibited the neutrophil migration.[87] The latter observation would suggest that oxy-radicals react with certain molecules in the extracellular fluid to produce a potent chemoattractant. The discrepancy between feline and human plasma may simply be a species-dependent phenomenon. However, H_2O_2 in the presence of either ferrous iron or hemoglobin did significantly increase the chemotactic activity of cat plasma, suggesting that varying levels of iron, perhaps as a result of hemolysis may be an important factor contributing to the controversial results. Nevertheless, if a plasmogen does exist that in combination with oxidants and iron would promote leukocyte adhesion, its identity remains unknown.

One potential direction to resolving this dilemma may be the observation that peroxide can oxidize phospholipids that will then promote leukocyte adhesion *in vitro*.[88] The leukocyte adhesion is inhibitable by PAF receptor antagonists, suggesting that the oxidized phopholipid although clearly distinct from platelet-activating factor may activate PAF receptors. In fact, Filep et al.[89] reported an increase in PAF-like activity in plasma draining the postischemic intestine, raising the possibility that under certain conditions a substance similar to PAF causes neutrophil infiltration and adhesion to postischemic vessels.

2. Leukotriene B_4

Exposure of cells to oxidants can activate phospholipase A_2, an event known to cause significant alterations in arachidonic acid metabolism as well as the initiation of lipid peroxidation in the postischemic intestine.[46,53] Arachidonic acid metabolism leads to a variety of lipoxygenase products[90,91] including the potent chemoattractant LTB_4, which is frequently implicated as a mediator of reperfusion-induced neutrophil infiltration. Several studies have demonstrated a significant increase in LTB_4 production in tissue[92-94] as well as in plasma[95] following ischemia/reperfusion. Additionally, Zimmerman et al.[96] reported that pretreatment with either a lipoxygenase inhibitor (L663,536) or the LTB_4 antagonist (SC-41930), decreases the magnitude of the reperfusion-induced granulocyte infiltration assessed by MPO activity, providing the first direct evidence that LTB_4 accumulation in the intestinal vasculature is a cause, rather than an effect, of reperfusion-induced granulocyte infiltration.

Recently, in a rabbit model of lower torso I/R, plasma from reperfused animals induced diapedesis into dermabrasion sites in normal rabbits.[97] The plasma contained elevated levels of LTB_4, and neutrophil diapedesis was significantly reduced by the LTB_4 antagonist U 75,302. The authors suggested that LTB_4 may be an important chemoattractant for neutrophils to sites of injury. The investigators observed that the LTB_4 receptor antagonist did not completely inhibit diapedesis of neutrophils into the dermabrasion sites and raised the possibility that a second as yet unidentified chemoattractant may also be released. In another study, this group demonstrated that lipoxygenase inhibition prevents PMN-dependent permeability changes after reperfusion of the ischemic hindlimb.[98] These data would suggest that LTB_4 in postischemic plasma and/or tissue causes PMN adhesion to the vasculature leading to increased microvascular dysfunction. Presently, the source of LTB_4 is not known, however it is conceivable that oxidants may promote the LTB_4 synthesis and release by activating endothelial cells, neutrophils, or some other cell type to cause PMN adhesion in the vasculature. A direct link between oxidants and enhanced LTB_4 production following reperfusion of the ischemic bowel has not been clearly demonstrated.

More recently, Lehr et al.[99] using intravital microscopy have reported that LTB_4 promotes leukocyte adhesion in postischemic vessels of striated muscle, and the hyperadhesivity was essentially abolished by MK-886, an inhibitor of leukotriene biosynthesis. Associated with a reduction in I/R-induced leukocyte adhesion, MK-866 caused a dramatic inhibition of macromolecular leakage from postcapillary venules. To further differentiate the effects of LTB_4 from cysteinyl leukotrienes, the investigators pretreated some animals with the selective LTD_4/LTE_4 receptor antagonist MK-571. The reperfusion-induced macromolecular leakage from postcapillary venules was entirely prevented by pretreatment with MK-571, whereas postischemic leukocyte adhesion was not reduced. These investigators concluded that LTB_4 was responsible for the postischemic leukocyte-endothelial cell interactions while LTD_4/LTE_4 was more important as a mediator of the macromolecular leakage. In keeping with the concept that leukocytes mediate microvascular dysfunction, Lehr et al. proposed that since inhibition of LTD_4/LTE_4 effectively inhibited macromolecular leakage without affecting leukotriene-endothelial cell interactions, the cysteinyl leukotrienes were generated and released by adherent leukocytes and caused the loss of endothelial integrity. This latter hypothesis requires further assessment to determine if indeed leukocytes are the source of LTD_4/LTE_4.

3. Platelet-Activating Factor

There is a growing body of evidence to support a role for platelet-activating factor (PAF) in I/R-induced damage in the vasculture. It has recently been reported that the concentration of PAF increases dramatically after 5 min of reperfusion of the ischemic canine intestine.[89] In that study, pretreatment with the PAF receptor antagonist, BN 52021, prevented the impairment in intestinal function normally induced by ischemia. In another study,[100] increases in lysosomal enzyme release, intestinal permeability, and lipid peroxidation observed following I/R of the rat distal ileum were all significantly reduced with BN 52021. These data suggest that PAF may be a mediator of the microvascular injury that occurs following I/R of the small bowel.

It is well established that PAF promotes leukocyte adhesion, emigration, and activation. Evidence to link PAF to I/R-induced leukocyte adherence and emigration in mesenteric venules has recently been demonstrated using intravital microscopic techniques.[77] In animals pretreated with WEB 2086, a PAF receptor antagonist, reperfusion-induced leukocyte adherence and emigration were reduced by 40 and 85%, respectively. The observation that WEB 2086 reduced leukocyte emigration to a greater degree than leukocyte adherence suggests that the PAF receptor antagonist directly interferes with the emigration process. It is conceivable that platelet-activating factor participates in the emigration process by promoting the limited release of neutrophil proteases and/or oxidants that in turn, facilitate the migration of phagocytic cells across restrictive barriers such as the basement membrane.[101,102]

The signal that activates PAF production following I/R of the intestine remains unclear. In a study by Droy-Lefaix et al.[103] SOD, allopurinol, and PAF antagonists were equally protective against postischemic mucosal damage in rat stomach, suggesting that a link may exist between xanthine oxidase-derived oxidants, PAF formation, and reperfusion injury. This possibility is supported by *in vitro* studies which demonstrate that H_2O_2 can stimulate cultured endothelial cells to produce PAF and consequently promote an adhesive interaction between leukocytes and endothelial cell monolayers.[104] This adhesive interaction could be blocked using different PAF receptor antagonists. Moreover, in the cat mesenteric preparation, it has been demonstrated that H_2O_2 promotes PMN adhesion to postcapillary venules and this adhesion can be attenuated by the PAF receptor antagonist WEB 2086.[75] These data as a whole suggest that a close association exists between oxidants and PAF in the I/R-induced leukocyte adhesion to postcapillary venules.

Although both PAF and LTB_4-receptor antagonists prevent reperfusion-induced PMN accumulation in the small bowel, the role of each inflammatory mediator in this process remains unresolved. LTB_4 appears to play an important role as a chemotactic agent both *in vitro* and *in vivo*. Local intra-arterial infusion of LTB_4 into the small bowel causes leukocyte adhesion in postcapillary venules but interestingly does not promote PMN emigration or increase vascular permeability.[68] Superfusion of tissue with LTB_4 however, has been reported to produce PMN adhesion, emigration, as well as increased vascular permeability.[105,106] Therefore, if during inflammation, levels of LTB_4 are greater in plasma than that in tissue, one would predict based on the aforementioned data that LTB_4 serves more as a chemotactic and pro-adhesive molecule for PMNs. In contrast, PAF has been reported to be a poor chemotactic agent *in vivo*.[107] Indeed, Tagesson et al.[100] have shown that BN52021 (PAF receptor antagonist) has no effect on reperfusion-induced neutrophil infiltration yet it protects the small bowel against reperfusion injury. Our observation that PAF receptor antagonists exert a greater influence on leukocyte emigration than on adherence, coupled to the fact that unlike LTB_4, local intra-arterial infusion of PAF causes a large fraction (>60%) of adherent leukocytes to emigrate out of the vasculature while increasing vascular protein leakage,[68] suggests that the phospholipid may contribute more to reperfusion-induced leukocyte emigration and microvascular dysfunction than does LTB_4.

4. Other Potential Mediators

Numerous vasoactive substances including histamine, prostaglandins, and lysosomal enzymes have been invoked as potential mediators of the tissue injury associated with ischemia. This contention is based on reports that these substances are released into venous blood draining the postischemic small bowel, and increase microvascular permeability when infused into the arterial supply of the nonischemic intestine.[108,109] However, pretreatment of the small bowel with either antihistamines (benadryl + cimetidine), indomethacin, or methylprednisolone does not significantly attenuate the increased microvascular permeability induced by I/R.[1] These data suggest that neither histamine, lysosomal enzymes, nor prostaglandins are involved in the I/R-induced increase in capillary permeability. In contrast, Boros et al.[110] have reported that histamine is released following I/R of the dog ileum in significant amounts. In addition, the increase in histamine levels observed in the dog plasma could be abolished if the animals were pretreated with allopurinol, the xanthine oxidase inhibitor, a superoxide radical scavenger (MTDQ-DA), catalase, or deferroxamine but not with hydroxyl radical scavengers. These data implicate that reactive oxygen metabolites including superoxide and H_2O_2 in the presence of iron are causitive agents in the release of histamine in the postischemic intestine. It should be noted that histamine can cause a brief neutrophil-independent increase in microvascular permeability that may contribute transiently to the reperfusion-induced microvascular dysfunction. There is no evidence to support the latter contention at this time.

Bacterial endotoxin is another possible mediator of reperfusion-induced microvascular dysfunction.[111] However, since lethal doses of *E. coli* endotoxin are required to increase vascular permeability and the magnitude of the increase in permeability produced by the toxin is small relative to I/R, it appears unlikely that endotoxins contribute significantly to the microvascular dysfunction observed at 1 h of reperfusion.[1] Nevertheless, endotoxin has been reported to enhance neutrophil adhesion to hepatic microvasculature via a tumor necrosis factor-mediated event that requires at least 2 to 3 h to occur.[112] Hence, endotoxin and tumor necrosis factor may have a critical role in modulating the long-term effects of I/R injury and possibly animal survival.

VII. CONCLUSIONS

While it has been known for well over a century that severe reductions in tissue blood flow can lead to organ dysfunction and death, only in the past two decades have researchers and clinicians come to appreciate the detrimental consequences of reperfusing an ischemic tissue. Despite the explosion of publications on the topic of reperfusion injury there is not real consensus on the mechanims underlying this paradox. In many tissues there is a large body of compelling evidence which implicates both oxygen-derived free radicals and granulocytes as mediators of reperfusion injury. While these data have led to considerable optimism regarding the potential therapeutic applications of antioxidants and antiadhesion molecules in cardiovascular diseases and organ transplantation, definitive clinical trials are needed to provide the final verdict concerning this issue. There remains, however, many areas of controversy and uncertainty which must be addressed and resolved before major new therapeutic interventions are developed and implemented. A better understanding of reperfusion injury is needed at the cellular, subcellular, and molecular levels. Such information should go a long way in explaining the differential vulnerability of various tissue to both ischemic and postischemic insults, and should provide a basis for understanding regional variations in the mechanisms underlying I/R injury.

REFERENCES

1. **Granger, D. N., Rutili, G., and McCord, J. M.,** Role of superoxide radicals in intestinal ischemia, *Gastroenterology,* 81, 22, 1981.
2. **Granger, D. N., Sennett, M., McElearney P., et al.,** Effect of local arterial hypotension on cat intestinal capillary permeability, *Gastroenterology*, 79, 474, 1980.
3. **Parks, D. A. and Granger, D. N.,** Contributions of ischemia and reperfusion to mucosal lesion formation, *Am. J. Physiol.*, 250, G749, 1986.
4. **Korthuis, R. J., Smith, J. K., and Carden, D. L.,** Hypoxic reperfusion attenuates postischemic microvascular injury, *Am. J. Physiol.*, 256, H315, 1989.
5. **Perry, M. A. and Wadhwa, S. S.,** Gradual reintroduction of oxygen reduces reperfusion injury in cat stomach, *Am. J. Physiol.*, 254, G366, 1988.
6. **Inauen, W., Payne, D. K., Kvietys P. R., and Granger, D. N.,** Hypoxia/reoxygenation increases the permeability of endothelial cell monolayers: role of oxygen radicals, *Free Radical Biol. Med., 9, 219*, 1990.
7. **Nilsson, U. A., Lundgren, O., Haglund U., et al.,** Radical production during intestinal ischemia and reperfusion in vivo in the cat—an ESR study, in *Proc. 4th Int. Cong. Oxygen Radicals,* Simic, M., Ed., 1987, 150.
8. **Morris, J. B., Bulkley, G. B., Haglund, U., et al.,** The direct, real-time demonstration of oxygen free radical generation at reperfusion following ischemia in rat small intestine, *Gastroenterology*, 92, 1541, 1987.
9. **Turrens, J. F., Giulivi, C., Pinus C., et al.,** Low level chemiluminescence from isolated hepatocytes, intact lung and intestine in situ, in *Proc. 4th Int. Cong. Oxygen Radicals,* Simic, M., Ed., 1987, 64.
10. **Granger, D. N.,** Role of xanthine oxidase and granulocytes in ischemia-reperfusion injury, *Am. J. Physiol.*, 255, H1269, 1988.
11. **Del Maestro, R. F.,** An approach to free radicals in medicine and biology, *Acta Physiol. Scand.*, 492 (Suppl.), 153, 1980.
12. **Weiss, S. J.,** Oxygen, ischemia and inflammation, *Acta Physiol. Scand.*, 126, 9, 1986.
13. **Halliwell, B. and Gutteridge, J. M. C.,** Oxygen toxicity, oxygen radicals, transition metals and disease, *Biochem. J.*, 219, 1, 1984.
14. **Grisham, M. B. and McCord, J. M.,** Chemistry and cytotoxicity of reactive oxygen metabolites, in *Physiology of Oxygen Radicals*, Taylor, A. E., Matalon, S., and Ward, P. A., Eds., American Physiological Society, Baltimore, MD, 1986, 1.
15. **Sutton, H. C. and Winterbourn, C. C.,** On the participation of higher oxidation states of iron and copper in Fenten reactions, *Free Radical Biol. Med.*, 6, 53, 1989.
16. **Kooperol, W. H. and Liebman, J. F.,** The oxidizing nature of the hydroxyl radical: a comparison with the ferryl ion (FeO^{+2}), *J. Phys. Chem.*, 88, 99, 1984.
17. **Chance, B., Sies, H., and Boveris, A.,** Hydroperoxide metabolism in mammalian organs, *Physiol. Rev.*, 59, 527, 1979.
18. **Parks, D. A., Bulkley, G. B., and Granger., D. N.,** Role of oxygen-derived free radicals in digestive tract diseases, *Surgery*, 94, 415, 1983.
19. **Korthuis, R. J., and Granger, D. N.,** Ischemia-reperfusion injury: role of oxygen-derived free radicals, in *Physiology of Oxygen Radicals*, Taylor, A. E., Matalon, S., and Ward, P. A., Eds., American Physiological Society, Baltimore, MD, 1986, 217.
20. **Zimmerman, B. J., Parks, D. A., Grisham, M. B., et al.,** Allopurinol does not enhance antioxidant properties of extracellular fluid, *Am. J. Physiol.*, 255, H202, 1988.
21. **Batelli, M. G., Dellacorte, E., and Stirpe, F.,** Xanthine oxidase type D (dehydrogenase) in the intestine and other organs of the rat, *Biochem. J.,* 1263, 747, 1972.
22. **Parks, D. A. and Granger, D. N.,** Xanthine oxidase: biochemistry, distribution and physiology, *Acta Physiol. Scand. Suppl.*, 548, 87, 1986.
23. **Clare, D. A. and Lecce, J. G.,** Copurification of bovine milk xanthine oxidase and immunoglobulin, *Arch. Biochem. Biophys.*, 286, 233, 1991.

24. **Jarasch, E. D., Bruder, G., and Heid, H. W.,** Significance of xanthine oxidase in capillary endothelial cells, *Acta Physiol. Scand. Suppl.*, 548, 39, 1986.
25. **Eddy, L. J., Stewart, J. R., Jones, H. P., Engerson, T. D., McCord, J. M., and Downey, J. M.,** Free radical-producing enzyme, xanthine oxidase, is undetectable in human hearts, *Am. J. Physiol.*, 253, H709, 1987.
26. **Roy, R. S. and McCord, J. M.,** The pathophysiology of superoxide: roles in inflammation and ischemia, *Can. J. Physiol. Pharmacol.*, 60, 1346, 1982.
27. **Parks, D. A., Williams, T. K., and Beckman, J. S.,** Conversion of xanthine dehydrogenase to oxidase in ischemic rat intestine: a re-evaluation, *Am. J. Physiol.*, 254, G768, 1988.
28. **Engerson, T. D., McKelvey, T. G., Rhyne, D. B., et al.,** Conversion of xanthine dehydrogenase to oxidase in ischemic rat tissues, *J. Clin. Invest.*, 79, 1564, 1987.
29. **McKelvey, T. G., Hollwarth, M. E., Granger, D. N., et al.,** Mechanisms of conversion of xanthine dehydrogenase to xanthine oxidase in ischemic rat liver and kidney, *Am. J. Physiol.*, 254, G753, 1988.
30. **Stark, K., Seubert, P., Lynch, G., and Baudry, M.,** Proteolytic conversion of xanthine dehydrogenase to xanthine oxidase: evidence against a role for calcium-activated protease (calpain), *Biochem. Biophys. Res. Comm.*, 165, 858, 1989.
31. **Jarach, E. D., Grund, C., Bruder, G., et al.,** Localization of xanthine oxidase in mammary gland epithelium and capillary endothelium, *Cell*, 25, 67, 1981.
32. **Ratych, R. E., Chuknyiska, R. S., and Bulkley, G. B.,** The primary localization of free radical generation following anoxia/reoxygenation in isolated endothelial cells, *Surgery*, 102, 122, 1987.
33. **Zweijer, J. L., Kuppersamy, P., and Lutty, G. A.,** Measurement of endothelial cell free radical generation: evidence for a central mechanism of free radical injury in postischemic tissues, *Proc. Natl. Acad. Sci.*, 85, 4046, 1988.
34. **Inauen, W., Granger, D. N., Meininger, C. J., Schelling, M. E., Granger, H. J., and Kvietys, P. R.,** An in vitro model of ischemia/reperfusion-induced microvascular injury, *Am. J. Physiol.*, 259, G134, 1990.
35. **Yokoyama, Y., Beckman, J. S., Beckman, T. K., Wheat, J. K., Cash, T. G., Freeman, B. A., and Parks, D. A.,** Circulating xanthine oxidase: potential mediator of ischemic injury, *Am. J. Physiol.*, 258, G564, 1990.
36. **Friedl, H. P., Smith, D. J., Till, G. O., Thomson, P. O., Louis, D. S., and Ward, P. A.,** Ischemia/reperfusion in humans. Appearance of xanthine oxidase activity, *Am. J. Pathol.*, 136, 491, 1990.
37. **Kvietys, P. R., Inauen, W., Bacon, B., and Grisham, M. B.,** Xanthine oxidase-induced injury to endothelium: role of intracellular iron and hydroxyl radical, *Am. J. Physiol.*, 257, H1640, 1989.
38. **Freeman, B. A., Whitfield, K., Gelman, D., and Parks, D. A.,** Heparin-reversible binding of xanthine oxidase to vascular endothelium, *Free Radical Biol. Med.,* 9 (Suppl. 1), 94, 1990.
39. **Hernandez, L. A., Grisham, M. B., and Granger, D. N.,** Effects of Cu-DIPS on ischemia-reperfusion injury, in *Biology of Copper Complexes,* Sorenson, J. R. J., Ed., Humana, Clifton, NJ, 1987, 201.
40. **Parks, D. A., Shah, A. K., and Granger, D. N.,** Oxygen radicals: effects on intestinal vascular permeability, *Am. J. Physiol.,* 247, G167, 1984.
41. **Roldan, E. J. A., Pinus, C. R., Turrens, J. F., and Boveris, A.,** Chemiluminescence of ischaemic and reperfused intestine in vivo, *GUT,* 30, 184, 1989.
42. **Suzuki, M., Inauen, W., Kvietys, P. R., Grisham, M. B., Meininger, C., Schelling, M. E., Granger, H. J., and Granger, D. N.,** Superoxide mediates reperfusion-induced leukocyte-endothelial cell interactions, *Am. J. Physiol.,* 257, H1740, 1989.

43. **Roy, R. S. and McCord, J. M.,** Superoxide and ischemia: conversion of xanthine dehydrogenase to xanthine oxidase, in *Oxy Radicals and Their Scavenger Systems. Volume II: Cellular and Medical Aspects,* Greenwald R. A., and Cohen, G., Eds., Elsevier/North Holland, New York, 1983, 143.
44. **Granger, D. N., Hollwarth, M. E., and Parks, D. A.,** Ischemia-reperfusion injury: role of oxygen-derived free radicals, *Acta Physiol. Scand. Suppl.,* 548, 47, 1986.
45. **Lash, L. H., Hagen, T. M., and Jones, D. P.,** Exogenous glutathione protects intestinal epithelial cells from oxidative injury, *Proc. Natl. Acad. Sci. U.S.A.,* 83, 4641, 1986.
46. **Schoenberg, M. H., Younes, M., Haglund, U., Fredholm, B., Sellin, D., Jung, H., and Schildberg, F. W.,** The participation of the hypoxanthine-xanthine oxidase system in the generation of free radicals after intestinal ischemia, in *Oxygen Radicals in Chemistry and Biology,* Bors, W., Saran, M., and Tait, D., Eds., Walter de Gruyter & Co, Berlin, 1984, 851.
47. **Thomas, C. E., Morehouse, L. A., and Aust, S. D.,** Ferritin and superoxide-dependent lipid peroxidation, *J. Biol. Chem.,* 260, 3275, 1985.
48. **Hernandez, L. A., Grisham, M. B., and Granger, D. N.,** A role for iron in oxidant-mediated ischemic injury to intestinal microvasculature, *Am. J. Physiol.,* 253, G49, 1987.
49. **Buege, J. A. and Aust, S. D.,** Lactoperoxidase-catalyzed lipid peroxidation of microsomal and artificial membranes, *Biochim. Biophys. Acta,* 444, 192, 1976.
50. **Jennings, R. B., Reimer, K. A., Hill, M. L., and Mayer, S. E.,** Total ischemia in dog hearts in vitro, *Circ. Res.,* 49, 892, 1981.
51. **Bielski, B. H. J. and Shiue, G. G.,** Reaction rates of superoxide radicals with the essential amino acids, in *Oxygen Free Radicals and Tissue Damage,* Ciba Foundation, Elsevier, New York, 1979, 43.
52. **Freeman, B. A. and Crapo, J. D.,** Free radicals and tissue injury, *Lab. Invest.,* 47, 412, 1982.
53. **Younes, M., Mohr, A., Schoenberg, M. H., and Schildberg F. W.,** Inhibition of lipid peroxidation by superoxide dismutase following regional intestinal ischemia and reperfusion, *Res. Exp. Med.,* 187, 9, 1987.
54. **Parks, D. A. and Granger, D. N.,** Ischemia-induced vascular changes: role of xanthine oxidase and hydroxyl radicals, *Am. J. Physiol.,* 245, G285, 1983.
55. **Beckman, J. S., Beckman, T. W., Chen, J., Marshall, P. A., and Freeman, B. A.,** Apparent hydroxyl radical production by peroxynitrite implications for endothelial injury from nitric oxide and superoxide, *Proc. Natl. Acad. Sci. U.S.A.,* 87, 1620, 1990.
56. **Lefer, D. J., Ma, X., Johnson, G., III, and Lefer, M. A.,** Endothelium preservation as a major mechanism of cardioprotection by superoxide dismutase in myocardial ischemia reperfusion injury, *Circulation,* 82 (Suppl. 3), 170, 1990.
57. **Aoki, N., Johnson, G., III, and Lefer, A. M.,** Beneficial effects of two forms of NO administration in feline splanchnic artery occlusion shock, *Am. J. Physiol.,* 258, G275, 1990.
58. **Mulligan, M. S., Hevel, J. M., Marletta, M. A., and Ward, P. A.,** Tissue injury caused by deposition of immune complexes is L-arginine dependent, *Proc. Natl. Acad. Sci. U.S.A.,* 88, 6338, 1990.
59. **Antunes, E., Mariano, M., Cirino, G., Levi, S., and deNucci, G.,** Pharmacological characterization of polycation-induced rat hind-paw edema, *Br. J. Pharmacol.,* 101, 986, 1990.
60. **Grisham, M. B. and Granger, D. N.,** Neutrophil-mediated mucosal injury: role of reactive oxygen metabolites, *Dig. Dis. Sci.,* 33, 6S, 1988.
61. **Harlan, J. M.,** Leukocyte-endothelial cell interactions, *Blood,* 65, 513, 1985.
62. **Granger, D. N., Benoit, J. N., Suzuki, M., and Grisham, M. B.,** Leukocyte adherence to venular endothelium during ischemia-reperfusion, *Am. J. Physiol.,* 257, G683, 1989.

63. **Zimmerman, B. J., Grisham, M. B., and Granger, D. N.,** Role of oxidants in ischemia/reperfusion-induced granulocyte infiltration, *Am. J. Physiol.*, 258, G185, 1990.
64. **Oliver, M. G., Specian, R. D., Perry, M. A., and Granger, D. N.,** Morphologic assessment of leukocyte-endothelial cell interactions in mesenteric venules subjected to ischemia and reperfusion, *Inflammation,* 15, 331, 1991.
65. **Tonnesen, M. G.,** Neutrophil-endothelial cell interactions: mechanisms of neutrophil adherence to vascular endothelium, *J. Invest. Dermatol.,* 93, 53s, 1989.
66. **Kubes, P. and Granger, D. N.,** Interaction between circulating granulocytes and xanthine oxidase-derived oxidants in the postischemic intestine, in *Clinical Aspects of O_2 Transport and Tissue Oxygenation,* Reinhart, K. and Eyrich, K., Eds., Springer-Verlag, Berlin, 1989, 133.
67. **Kubes, P., Suzuki, M., and Granger, D. N.,** Platelet activating factor-induced microvascular dysfunction: role of adherent leukocytes, *Am. J. Physiol.*, 258, G158, 1990.
68. **Kubes, P., Grisham, M. B., Barrowman, J. A., Gaginella, T., and Granger D. N.,** Leukocyte-induced vascular protein leakage in cat mesentery, *Am. J. Physiol.*, 261, H1872, 1991.
69. **McEver, R. P.,** Selectins: novel receptors that mediate leukocyte adhesion during inflammation, *Thrombosis Haemostasis,* 65, 223, 1991.
70. **Granger, D. N., Russell, J. M., Arfors, K. E., Rothlein, R., and Anderson, D. C.,** Role of CD11/CD18 and ICAM-1 in ischemia-reperfusion induced leukocyte adherence and emigration in mesenteric venules, *FASEB J.*, 5, A1753, 1991.
71. **Yoshida, N., Granger, D. N., Anderson, D. C., Rothlein, R., Lane, C., and Kvietys, P. R.,** Anoxia/reoxygenation-induced neutrophil adherence to cultured endothelial cells, *Am. J. Physiol.*, 262, H1891, 1992.
72. **Grisham, M. B., Hernandez, L. A., and Granger, D. N.,** Xanthine oxidase and neutrophil infiltration in intestinal ischemia, *Am. J. Physiol.*, 251, G567, 1986.
73. **Kubes, P., Suzuki, M., and Granger, D. N.,** Modulation of PAF-induced leukocyte adherence and increased microvascular permeability, *Am. J. Physiol.*, 259, G859, 1990.
74. **Kubes, P., Suzuki, M., and Granger, D. N.,** Nitric oxide: an endogenous modulator of leukocyte adhesion, *Proc. Natl. Acad. Sci. U.S.A.,* 88, 465, 1991.
75. **Suzuki, M., Asako, H., Kubes, P., Jennings, S., Grisham, M., and Granger, D. N.,** Neutrophil-derived oxidants promote leukocyte adherence in postcapillary venules, *Microvasc. Res.*, 42, 125, 1991.
76. **Suzuki, M., Grisham, M. B., and Granger, D. N.,** Leukocyte-endothelial cell interactions: role of xanthine oxidase-derived oxidants, *J. Leukocyte Biol.*, 50, 488, 1991.
77. **Kubes, P., Ibbotson, G., Russell, J., Wallace, J. L., and Granger, D. N.,** Role of platelet-activating factor in ischemia/reperfusion-induced leukocyte adherence, *Am. J. Physiol.*, 259, G300, 1990.
78. **Huber, A. R. and Weiss, S. J.,** Disruption of the subendothelial cell basement membrane during neutrophil diapedesis in an in vitro contruct of a blood vessel wall, *J. Clin. Invest.*, 83, 1122, 1989.
79. **Rosengren, S. and Arfors, K. E.,** Neutrophil-mediated vascular leakage is not suppressed by leukocyte elastase inhibitors, *Am. J. Physiol.*, in press.
80. **Zimmerman, B. J. and Granger, D. N.,** Reperfusion-induced leukocyte infiltration: role of elastase, *Am. J. Physiol.*, 259, H390, 1990.
81. **Perry, M. A. and Granger, D. N.,** Role of CD11/CD18 in shear rate-dependent leukocyte-endothelial cell interactions in cat mesenteric venules, *J. Clin. Invest.,* 87, 1798, 1991.
82. **Ley, K., Lundgren, E., Berger, E., and Arfors, K. E.,** Shear-dependent inhibition of granulocyte adhesion to cultured endothelium by dextran sulfate, *Blood,* 73, 1324, 1989.
83. **Lawrence, M. B., Smith, C. W., Eskin, S. G., and McIntire, L. V.,** Effect of venous shear stress on CD18-mediated neutrophil adhesion to cultured endothelium, *Blood,*

75, 227, 1990.

84. **Romson, J. L., Hook, B. G., Kunkel, S. L., Abrams, G. D., Schork, A., and Lucchesi, B. R.,** Reduction of the extent of ischemic myocardial injury by neutrophil depletion in the dog, *Circulation,* 67, 1016, 1983.
85. **Hernandez, L. A., Grisham, M. B., Twohig, B., Arfors, K. E., Harlan, J. M., and Granger, D. N.,** Role of neutrophils in ischemia-reperfusion-induced microvascular injury, *Am. J. Physiol.,* 253, H699, 1987.
86. **Petrone, W. F., English, D. K., Wong, K., and McCord, J. M.,** Free radicals and inflammation: superoxide dependent activation of a neutrophil chemotactic factor in plasma, *Proc. Natl. Acad. Sci. U.S.A.,* 77, 1159, 1980.
87. **Perez, H. D., Weksler, B. B., and Goldstein, I. M.,** Generation of chemotactic lipid from arachidonic acid by exposure to a superoxide-generating system, *Inflammation,* 4, 313, 1980.
88. **Smiley, P. L., Stremler, K. E., Prescott, S. M., Zimmerman, G. A., and McIntyre, T. M.,** Oxidatively fragmented phosphatidylcholines activate human neutrophils through the receptor for platelet-activating factor, *J. Biol. Chem.,* 266, 1, 1991.
89. **Filep, J., Herman, F., Braquet, P., and Mozes, T.,** Increased levels of platelet-activating factor in blood following intestinal ischemia in the dog, *Biochem. Biophys. Res. Commun.,* 158, 353, 1989.
90. **Boughton-Smith, N. K., Hawkey, C. J., and Whittle, B. J. R.,** Biosynthesis of lipoxygenase and cyclo-oxygenase products from [14C]-arachidonic acid by human colonic mucosa, *GUT,* 24, 1176, 1983.
91. **Dreyling, K. W., Hoppe, U., Peskar, B. A., Morgenroth, K., Kozuschek, W., and Peskar, B. M.,** Leukotriene synthesis by human gastrointestinal tissues, *Biochim. Biophys. Acta,* 878, 184, 1986.
92. **Mangino, M. J., Anderson, C. B., Murphy, M. K., Brunt, E., and Turk, J.,** Mucosal arachidonate metabolism and intestinal ischemia-reperfusion injury, *Am. J. Physiol.,* 257, G299, 1989.
93. **Lauritsen, K., Laursen, L. S., Bukhave, K., and Rask-Madsen, J.,** In vivo profiles of eicosanoids in ulceratice colitis, Crohn's colitis, and clostridium difficile colitis, *Gastroenterology,* 95, 11, 1988.
94. **Sharon, P. and Stenson, W. F.,** Enhanced synthesis of leukotriene B4 by colonic mucosa in inflammatory bowel disease, *Gastroenterology,* 86, 453, 1984.
95. **Welbourn, R., Goldman, G., Kobzik, L., Paterson, I., Valeri, C. R., Shepro, D., and Hechtman, H. B.,** Neutrophil adherence receptors (CD18) in ischemia, *J. Immunol.,* 145, 1906, 1990.
96. **Zimmerman, B. J., Guillory D. J., Grisham, M. B., Gaginella, T. S., and Granger, D. N.,** Role of Leukotriene B4 in granulocyte infiltration into the postischemic feline intestine, *Gastroenterology,* 99, 1, 1990.
97. **Goldman, G., Welbourn, R., Paterson, I. S., Klausner, J. M., Kobzik, L., Valeri, C. R., Shepro D., and Hechtman, H. B.,** Ischemia induced neutrophil activation and diapedesis are lipoxygenase dependent, *Surgery,* 107, 428, 1990.
98. **Kluasner, J. M., Paterons, I. S., Valeri, C. R., Shepro, D., and Hechtman, H. B.,** Limb ischemia-induced increase in permeability is mediated by leukocytes and leukotrienes, *Ann. Surg.,* 208, 755, 1988.
99. **Lehr, H. A., Guhlmann, A., Nolte, D., Keppler, D., and Messmer, K.,** Leukotrienes as mediators in ischemia/reperfusion injury in a microcirculation model in the hamster, *J. Clin. Invest.,* 87, 2036, 1991.
100. **Tagesson, C., Lindahl, M., and Otamiri, T.,** BN 52021 ameliorates mucosal damage associated with small intestinal ischaemia in rats, in *Ginkgolides: Chemistry, Biology, Pharmacology and Clinical Perspectives,* Braquet, P., Ed., J. R. Prous Science, Barcelona, 1988, 553.
101. **Harlan, J. M., Killen, P. D., Harker, L. A., Striker, G. E., and Wright, D. G.,** Neutrophil-mediated endothelial injury in vitro, *J. Clin. Invest.,* 68, 1394, 1981.

102. **Vercellotti, G. M., Yin, H. Q., Gustafson, K. S., Nelson, R. D., and Jacob, H. S.,** Platelet-activating factor primes neutrophil responses to agonists: role in promoting neutrophil-mediated endothelial damage, *Blood,* 71, 1100, 1988.
103. **Droy-Lefaix, M., Drouet, Y., Geraud, G., and Braquet, P.,** Involvement of platelet activating factor in rat ischemia reperfusion gastric damage, in *Ginkgolides: Chemistry, Biology, Pharmacology and Clinical Perspectives,* Braquet, P., Ed., J. R. Prous, Barcelona, 1988, 563.
104. **Lewis, M. S., Whatley, R. E., Cain, P., McIntyre, T. M., Prescott, S. M., and Zimmerman, G. A.,** Hydrogen peroxide stimulates the synthesis of platelet activating factor by endothelium and induces endothelial cell-dependent neutrophil adhesion, *J. Clin. Invest.,* 82, 2045, 1988.
105. **Bjork, J., Hedqvist, P., and Arfors, K. E.,** Increase in vascular permeability induced by leukotriene B4 and the role of polymorphonuclear leukocytes, *Inflammation,* 6, 189, 1982.
106. **Asako, H., Kubes, P., Baethge, B. A., Wolf, R. E., and Granger, D. N.,** Colchinine and methotrexate reduce leukocyte adherence and emigration in rat mesenteric venules, *Inflammation,* 16, 45, 1992.
107. **Doebber, T. W., Wu, M. S., Robbins, J. C., Choy, B. M., Chang, M. N., and Shen, T. Y.,** Platelet-activating factor (PAF) involvement in endotoxin-induced hypotension in rats. Studies with PAF-receptor antagonist kadsurenone, *Biochem. Biophys. Res. Commun.,* 127, 799, 1985.
108. **Haglund, U., Lundholm, K., Lundgren, O., et al.,** Intestinal lysosomal enzyme activity in regional simulated shock: influence of methylprednisolone and albumin, *Circ. Shock.,* 4, 27, 1977.
109. **Kobold, E. E. and Thal, A. P.,** Quantitation and identification of vasoactive substances liberated during various types of experimental and clinical intestinal ischemia, *Surg. Gynecol. Obstet.,* 117, 315, 1963.
110. **Boros, M., Kaszaki, J., and Nagy, S.,** Oxygen free radical-induced histamine release during intestinal ischemia and reperfusion, *Eur. Surg. Res.,* 21, 297, 1989.
111. **Ballin, H. M. and Meyer, M. W.,** Intestinal lymph flow in dogs after endotoxin, *Proc. Soc. Exp. Biol. Med.,* 103, 93, 1960.
112. **Schlayer, H. J., Laoff, H., Peters, T., Woort-Menker, M., Estler, H. C., Karck, U., Schaefer, H. E., and Decker, K.,** Involvement of tumor necrosis factor in endotoxin-triggered neutrophil adherence to sinusoidal endothelial cells of mouse liver and its modulation in acute phase, *J. Hepatol.,* 7, 239, 1988.

Chapter 7

Diabetic Microangiopathy

Ronald J. Korthuis, Susan P. Fuselier, and Sarah N. Jerome

CONTENTS

I. INTRODUCTION

Vascular disease inflicts a heavy toll on the quality of life and longevity of many patients with diabetes mellitus.[1,2] People with diabetes are at least twice as prone to coronary and cerebrovascular disorders and demonstrate a markedly increased incidence of peripheral vascular disease when compared to nondiabetics. Indeed, diabetes accounts for more than half of all nontraumatic amputations performed each year. Moreover, renovascular disease is at least 17 times more common in diabetic versus nondiabetic subjects and it is now recognized that diabetes is the leading cause of end-stage renal disease in the U.S. Diabetes is also the leading cause of blindness in adults. The most common vascular complications that contribute to visual disability in diabetes include retinopathy, macular edema, and vitreous hemorrhage.

While the mechanisms that contribute to the development of complications late in the course of diabetes remain enigmatic, considerable attention has focused on the role of the microcirculation. This interest stems largely from the remarkable and almost ubiquitous changes that occur within the microvessel wall in diabetes. These alterations include a striking increase in the thickness of capillary basement membranes, a marked impairment in microvascular barrier function, and progressive microvascular occlusion.[1,3-5] Although it generally accepted that these microangiopathic alterations may contribute to the development of diabetic complications by impairing microcirculatory transport function, the mechanisms responsible for these vascular changes remains unclear. However, a growing body of evidence indicates that hyperglycemia may play a critical role in the development of diabetic vascular disease by inducing a number of biochemical changes that act to alter the barrier function of the vasculature and contribute to progressive vascular occlusion. In addition, a number of other changes involving vascular elements contribute to impaired cardiovascular transfer function and include alterations in hemodynamic control and in the function of formed elements within the blood. The overall aim of this chapter is to

0-8493-4547-2/94/$0.00+$.50

provide a comprehensive review of the literature regarding the mechanisms involved in the pathogenesis of diabetic microangiopathy.

II. MECHANISMS INVOLVED IN ENHANCED PROTEIN TRANSFER ACROSS THE VASCULAR WALL IN DIABETES

Diabetic vascular disease is characterized by a marked increase in transvascular protein transfer as evidenced by the presence of albuminuria and the large increment in transcapillary escape rate for macromolecules.[4,5] Although this increase in transcapillary protein flux is commonly attributed solely to enhanced capillary permeability, several other mechanisms also contribute including increased vescicular transport, augmented convective protein transfer secondary to elevated microvascular hydrostatic pressure, as well as biochemical alterations in the permeating macromolecules which allow for easier penetration of the endothelial barrier.

A. ALTERATIONS IN THE VASCULAR WALL — ENDOTHELIUM

The endothelial cell lining of blood vessels and its subjacent basement membrane constitute the principal barriers to transvascular exchange of solutes and water.[6] In diabetes, the barrier function of the vascular wall is impaired such that vascular permeability to macromolecules is increased.[4,5,7-12] Indeed, one of the most important clinical symptoms of developing microvascular disease in diabetes is increased transcapillary protein leak in the kidney with resultant enhanced urinary protein levels. Although the notion that vascular permeability is increased in diabetes is well-accepted, the mechanisms responsible for this reduction in barrier function remain unclear. However, it is likely that hyperglycemia contributes to the pathogenesis of impaired microvascular barrier function in diabetes,[13-16] a notion supported by the observation that the degree to which permeability is increased in diabetes correlates with the quality of metabolic control.[4]

One hypothesis regarding the role of diabetic hyperglycemia in the genesis of increased vascular permeability involves the formation of glycosylated proteins. The level of protein glycosylation increases several-fold in diabetes and is influenced by prevailing glucose concentrations and the half-life of the protein in question.[14,16-19] Protein glycosylation can occur nonenzymatically by a process that involves a condensation reaction between glucose and free amine groups at the N-terminal of proteins or the ε-amino groups of lysine residues within peptide chains.[13,16,17,20-23] The first product to form via this interaction is an aldimine (Schiff base) which then undergoes an internal rearrangement (Amadori rearrangement) of the double bond to form a stable ketoamine. The aldimine products may also undergo further reactions in the presence of prolonged hyperglycemia to form advanced glycosylation end-products (AGEs) which accumulate on long-lived matrix proteins. As a consequence of glycosylation, the structure and three-dimensional organization of the endothelial cell glycocalyx in the interendothelial cleft may be altered so that the restrictive properties of this fibrous matrix are reduced (Figure 1).

Another important repercussion of glycosylation relates to the ability of AGEs to quench nitric oxide,[24] an endothelial-derived vasorelaxant. Based on this observation, it has been suggested that inactivation of nitric oxide by AGEs may contribute to the development of hypertension in diabetes.[24] This may also represent a causative factor for impotence in diabetic men.[25] Since nitric oxide is also known to promote the barrier function of the microvasculature,[26] nitric oxide quenching by AGEs may contribute to the increase in vascular permeability associated with diabetes mellitus.

In addition to alterations in the three-dimensional array of the endothelial glycocalyx, it also appears that the charge characteristics of the endothelium (and basement mem-

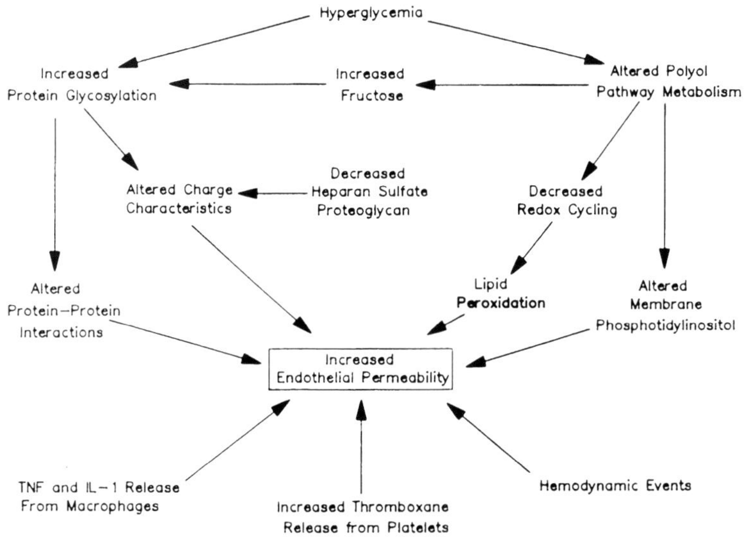

Figure 7-1 Mechanisms involved in the genesis of microvascular barrier disruption in diabetes mellitus.

brane — see below) may be altered in diabetes. This notion is based on the observation that diabetes is associated with a decrease in the synthesis of the heparan sulfate, a proteoglycan that contains a high number of anionic sites.[5,27-29] The reduction in negative charge on the endothelial cell surface reduces the electrostatic repulsion between anionic solutes such as albumin and the endothelial cell glycocalyx.[6] As a consequence of this reduction in the charge characteristics exhibited by endothelium, the permeation of negatively charged solutes is increased (Figure 1).

Hyperglycemia may also play a role in the develoment of increased microvascular permeability by inducing alterations in cellular glucose metabolism.[30-32] Normally, glucose is preferentially converted to glucose-6-phosphate by hexokinase in the glycolytic pathway (Figure 2). However, hexokinase becomes saturated in the presence of the high intracellular glucose concentrations. Thus, hyperglycemia is associated with substantial conversion of glucose to sorbitol by the enzyme aldose reductase. Although sorbitol can then be oxidized to D-fructose by NAD^+-dependent polyol (sorbitol) dehydrogenase (Figure 2), the rate of this reaction is slow relative to the rate of sorbitol formation. This, coupled with the fact that sorbitol does not readily penetrate cell membranes due to its polarity, results in an accumulation of this sugar alcohol in cells. Sorbitol accumulation, in turn, results in increased cellular osmolarity and fluid influx.

Aldose reductase has been shown to exist in many tissues including those prone to diabetic complications such as the retina and lens, peripheral nerves, and renal glomerulus.[30,33] Since glucose transport is independent of insulin in these tissues, intracellular glucose equilibrates with blood glucose.[30,33] Therefore, sorbitol accumulation is especially pronounced in these tissues during periods of hyperglycemia and suggests a possible link between hyperglycemia, aldose reductase, and the development of diabetic complications.

Aldose reductase is also capable of reducing other sugars in addition to glucose.[30,34] This broad specificity has been exploited to examine the role of aldose reductase in the the genesis of diabetic microangiopathy. For example, galactose is more rapidly reduced

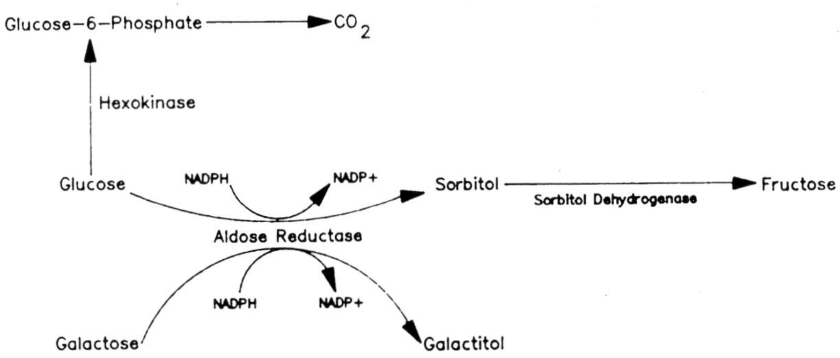

Figure 7-2 Metabolism of glucose and galactose in the polyol pathway.

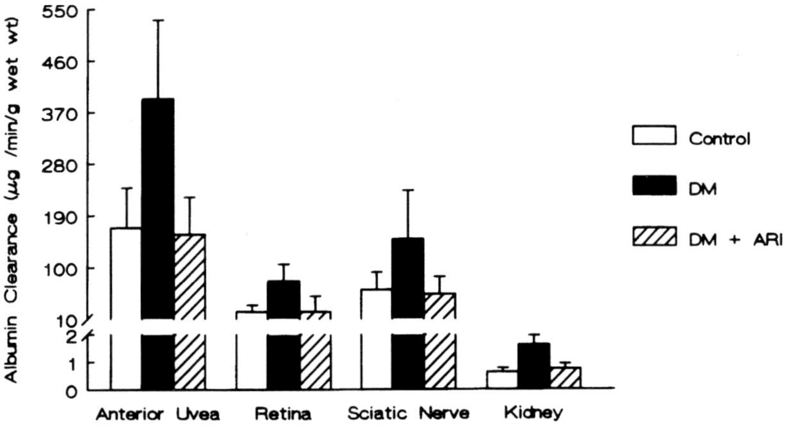

Figure 7-3 Diabetes mellitus (DM)-induced increase in albumin clearance across microvessels in the anterior uvea, retina, peripheral nerves, and kidneys is attenuated by aldose reductase inhibition (ARI). *(Modified from Pugliese, G., Tilton, R. G., and Williamson, J. R., Diabetes Metab., 7, 35, 1991.)*

by aldose reductase than glucose and thus accumulates more rapidly within the cell (Figure 2).[34] Since the product of this reaction, galactitol, is not metabolized by sorbitol dehydrogenase, galactitol levels remain elevated for longer periods of time within the cell. Animals fed galactose-rich diets develop retinal and renal complications that are very similar to that noted in diabetes mellitus.[29,34] In addition, these animals also demonstrate increased albumin permeation and blood flow in the retina, kidneys, and peripheral nerves,[29] tissues which contain particularly high levels of aldose reductase.[30] When coupled with the observation that aldose reductase inhibition effectively prevented microvascular barrier disruption in both diabetic rats and animals fed a galactose-enriched diet (Figure 3), these studies strongly support the notion that the polyol pathway plays an important role in the development of an impaired microvascular barrier in diabetes.[29,33] Similarly, use of aldose reductase inhibitors in galactose-fed dogs produced a dose-dependent reduction in the destruction of retinal pericytes (the hallmark of diabetic retinopathy) and subsequent microaneurysm formation,[30,32,34] indicating that these agents may be quite useful in the treatment of diabetic complications.

Several mechanisms have been proposed to explain how an increase in polyol activity and the resultant sorbitol accumulation may be involved in the pathogenesis of diabetic microangiopathy. One of the first relates to the increase in cell osmolarity induced by accumulation of sorbitol.[30,32] This produces an influx of fluid into cells and results in loss of cellular integrity. Support for this hypothesis has come mainly from studies regarding the formation of cataracts in rat lens. That is, as cellular sorbitol levels increase, lens fibers swell due to the osmotic effects of the accumulated sorbitol. Water influx continues to cause further swelling until the lens fibers rupture to cause lens opacification.[30-34] According to this scenario, cataract formation is not caused by the presence of sorbitol per se but rather by the influx of water produced by the osmotic gradient.[33,34] Strong support for the involvement of aldose reductase in diabetic cataractogenesis is derived from studies in which inhibition of the enzyme has been shown to prevent lens opacification in diabetic rats and animals fed galactose-enriched diets.[34] Although the osmotic theory appears to explain the pathologic events associated with diabetic cataract formation, many believe that this mechanism does not account for complications in other organs.

Since NADPH is consumed during the conversion of glucose to sorbitol, the ability of susceptible tissues to resist an oxidative stress may be impaired.[35] This concept is based on the fact that NADPH is required for redox cycling of oxidized free radical scavengers to the reduced form. For example, the increase in NADPH utilization associated with enhanced polyol metabolism can result in depletion of reduced glutathione (GSH), an important component of the cell's defense against oxidative damage.[32,35] In addition, diabetic patients exhibit lower levels of several other biologically important antioxidants including vitamins C and E.[37-40] Reports of increased lipid peroxidation in diabetes[41-44] and the fact that glycated proteins can interact with oxygen to form oxidants[36] are consistent with the aforementioned observations. Enhanced susceptibilty to oxidative damage may play an important role in the impairment in microvascular barrier function induced by diabetes since it is well-known that oxidants are directly cytotoxic to the endothelial cells (Figure 1).

The increase in cellular fructose levels associated with enhanced polyol pathway metabolism may also play a role in the genesis of increased microvascular permeability in diabetes. This notion is based on the fact that fructose is a preferred substrate for the nonenzymatic glycoslyation of proteins (Figure 1).[46] Thus, fructose accumulation may facilitate the protein glycoslyation in the endothelial cell glycocalyx. As outlined above, protein glycosylation has the potential to markedly alter the permeability characteristics of the endothelial fiber matrix. Increased fructose levels may also result in enhanced tissue lactate levels due to its ability to be phosphorylated to fructose-6-phosphate and fructose-1-phosphate and enter the glycolytic pathway.[33] As a consequence, local pH changes may ensue which could conceivably alter the architectural characteristics of the microvascular barrier.

Other potential mechanisms whereby altered polyol metabolism may contribute to increased microvascular permeability in diabetes include depletion of cellular myoinositol levels and accumulation of amphipathic lipids such as diacylglycerol.[32] Myoinositol depletion may interfere with membrane phosphoinositide turnover. Although it is clear that such alterations reduce Na^+/K^+ ATPase activity,[32] the effect of such changes in the endothelium are unknown. However, the accumulation of diacylglycerol may increase endothelial protein kinase C activity, thereby promoting increased vascular permeability.[32]

B. ALTERATIONS IN THE VASCULAR WALL — BASEMENT MEMBRANE

Thickening of the capillary basement membrane is widely recognized as the ultrastructural hallmark of microvascular damage in diabetes mellitus.[28,29,32] Although initially and most often seen in the retina and renal glomerulus, capillary basement membrane thickening appears to be ubiquitous, occurring in nearly every organ examined.[34] This manifestation of diabetic microangiopathy appears to be due, at least in part, to substantial alterations in the production and distribution of its functional components. For example, type IV collagen levels are increased by approximately 1.5- to 3-fold in glomerular basement membranes of diabetic humans and animals.[3,28,29] There is also an increase in the proportion of hydroxylysine and its glycosidically linked dissacharide units in diabetic basement membranes, an effect that may be related to an increase in the activity of lysine hydroxylase, galactose transferase, and glucosyltransferase.[1,29] Basement membranes of diabetics also contain large amounts of albumin, fibronectin, IgG, and complement relative to that seen in normal individuals.[29] On the other hand, heparan sulfate proteoglycans are reduced by almost 70%, while laminin levels have been reported to increase or decrease.[3,27-29] Excessive nonenzymatic glycosylation of matrix components is also a prominent feature of the diabetic basement membrane.[28,29]

The cellular mechanisms responsible for hyperglycemia-induced alterations in basement membrane structure are not clear. However, the fact that glucose enhances the biosynthesis of basement membrane components by endothelial cell monolayers suggests that hyperglycemia may play an important role.[47] Since these changes are associated with increased glucose metabolism via the polyol pathway, it has been suggested that capillary basement membrane thickening is related to the accumulation of sorbitol.[29,32] This notion is strongly supported by the observation that aldose reductase inhibitors prevent retinal and renal capillary basement membrane thickening induced by galactosemia.[29,32]

Nonenzymatic glycosylation of proteins and other biomolecules is also thought to contribute to capillary basement membrane thickening. For example, DNA glycation is thought to result in increased synthesis of mRNAs for specific extracellular matrix components, thereby promoting increased thickness of capillary basement membranes.[47] Excessive glycosylation of basement membrane components may increase the resistance of collagen to degradation by collagenase, result in reduced cross-linking, alter the binding of fibronectin to basement membrane components, and covalently trap low-density lipoproteins within the matrix.[48-54] As a consequence, the orderly arrangement of the extracellular matrix components in the basement membrane may be compromised leading to increased thickness and a reduction in the restrictive properties of this component of the barrier to transcapillary solute exchange (Figure 1).[28,55,56] Such changes in extracellular matrix proteins in renal podocytes may contribute to increased glomerular protein clearance noted in diabetes.

It has also been suggested that diabetes induces proliferative responses in endothelial cells that contribute to basement membrane thickening.[57,58] As a result of increased cell turnover, basal laminae accumulate and thicken in diabetes. Although the mechanism involved in increased turnover of endothelial cells in diabetes is unclear, it has been suggested that endothelial cell injury and/or elevated capillary pressure or shear rate may contribute to this proliferative response (Figure 1).[3] This notion is based on the observation that blood flow (and presumably shear rate) and capillary pressure are elevated early in the course of the disease in the kidney, retina, intestine, and periphery (nailfold).[3,4,10,11,29] If these hemodynamic events are prevented from occurring, microangiopathy is reduced.[10,59,60] The influence of capillary pressure on the accumulation of excess basement membrane may also explain why basement membranes are thicker in capillaries of the distal lower limb relative to the thigh.[10,29] In any event, these observations suggest that while hyperglycemia induces a number of important biochemical changes that ultimately result in basement membrane thickening, the extent and nature of these changes may be modified by hemodynamic events.[3,10,11,29]

In addition to alterations in the three-dimensional array of extracellular matrix components in diabetes, it also appears that the charge characteristics of the basement membrane may be altered. As noted above, basement membranes obtained from diabetic animals exhibit a 70% reduction in heparan sulfate proteoglycan content,[5,27-29] an effect that may be related to alterations in the activity of N-acetylase, the key enzyme involved in sulfation of heparan.[5] As a consequence, the number of anionic sites within diabetic basement membranes is reduced, thereby diminishing the effectiveness of the basement membrane as a barrier to the movement of negatively charged macromolecules (Figure 1).[5,61,62] The decreased orderliness of the extracellular matrix array and reduced charge barrier may explain the apparent paradox of increased permeability in the face of a thickened basement membrane.[5,45,63]

Alterations in the selectivity of basement membranes for macromolecules would most likely be manifest in capillaries lined by discontinuous or fenestrated endothelium since the extracellular matrix of this structure is an important component of the serial barrier to transmicrovascular exchange in these types of capillaries.[6] However, the sieving characteristics of the basement membrane assumes critical importance in restricting macromolecule exchange in continuous capillaries when the endothelial permeability is increased. On the other hand, the interdigitating podocytes represent the most important structural barrier to fluid and solute transfer in the renal glomerulus. Although it is not clear to what extent the proteinuria associated with diabetes can be attributed to changes in the glomerular basement membrane versus podocytes, it is clear that altered charge characteristics of these structures contribute to enhanced transglomerular macromolecule permeation.[5,45]

Since basement membranes provide the physical support required for attachment of endothelial cells to the underlying connective tissue,[28,29] it is possible that disruption in their normal organization may contribute capillary acellularity that is occasionally encountered. A similar argument can be made for podocytes in the glomerulus. Given that the endothelium (in general) and podocytes (in glomeruli) regulate solute penetration into the interstitium or renal tubule, respectively, adherence of these cells to basement membranes may play an important role in the maintenance of a normal microvascular barrier. Indeed, focal separation of podocytes from basement membrane may contribute to enhanced renal protein loss in severely proteinuric diabetics.[45]

C. ALTERATIONS IN THE PERMEATING SOLUTES

Glycosylation of proteins in diabetes is not limited only to peptides associated within the extracellular matrix. Indeed, plasma proteins can also be covalently modified by nonenzymatic attachment of glucose. In normal individuals and diabetics with good metabolic control, only 2 to 5% of plasma albumin is glycosylated. However, this can increase to as high as 30% in poorly controlled diabetics.[17,21-23] Since glycosylation alters the conformation and decreases the pH of albumin, one would predict that its transport across the microvascular barrier may be modified, a postulate supported by several studies in the literature.[9,11,64-68] For example, glycosylation of albumin appears to enhance the vesicular transport of this protein across the endothelium relative to unmodified albumin.[65-67] These changes may explain why diabetes is associated with an increase in albumin permeation that is much greater than that for other macromolecules.[68] However, the effect of covalent modification of proteins by nonenzymatic attachment of glucose is not limited exclusively to albumin since glycosylation of myoglobin and ovalbumin enhances the vesicular transport of these macromolecules as well.[67]

III. MECHANISMS INVOLVED IN THE DEVELOPMENT OF CAPILLARY SCLEROSIS IN DIABETES

A. ROLE OF ADVANCED GLYCOSYLATION END-PRODUCTS

The accumulation of proteins cross-linked by glucose-derived AGEs alters the three-dimensional array of basement membrane constituents and is thought to contribute to narrowing of the blood vessel wall (Figure 4).[69] However, AGEs contribute to diabetic

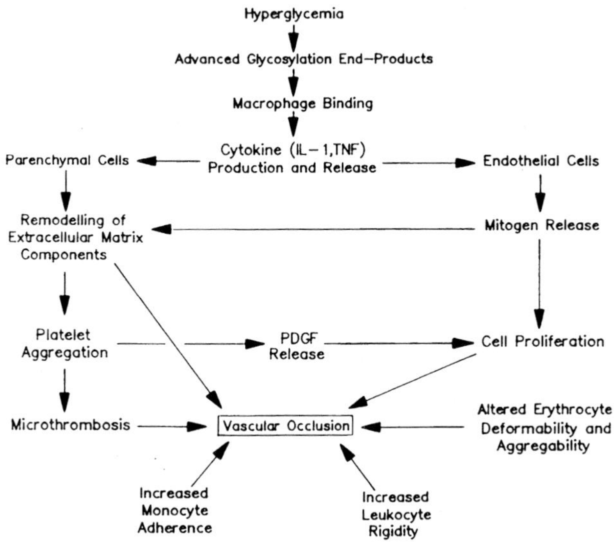

Figure 7-4 Mechanisms involved in the genesis of vascular occlusion in diabetes mellitus.

vascular occlusion through other mechanisms in addition to the structural abnormalities induced by protein cross-linking. One of the most important relates to the ability of AGE-modified proteins to induce proliferation of smooth muscle, mesangial, and endothelial cells via macrophage activation.[69] Macrophages express receptors that specifically recognize and bind to AGE-modified proteins.[69-74] The AGE-dependent macrophage activation in down-regulated by insulin.[69] These receptors do not bind to proteins that are recognized by the macrophage scavenger or glycoprotein receptors nor do they recognize proteins that have been modified by attachment of early glycosylation products.[72] Once bound to AGE-modified protein receptors, macrophages synthesize and secrete a variety of multifunctional cytokines, including tumor necrosis factor and interleukin-1 (Figure 4).[69,74] These cytokines bind to various cellular elements in the vascular wall and also to parenchymal cells where they initiate a combination of proliferative and degradative processes that ultimately contribute to vascular occlusion.[69] For example, cytokine-activated mesenchymal cells secrete a variety of proteases, including collagenase, which contribute to remodelling of extracellular matrix components (Figure 4). TNF also induces proliferative responses within the vascular wall by inducing the release of platelet-derived growth factor-like activity. In addition, these cytokines promote the proliferation of fibroblasts and contribute to impaired microvascular barrier function through their ability to increase microvascular permeability (Figure 1).

Strong support for the notion the AGEs contribute to structural and functional alterations in the diabetic extracellular matrix are provided by studies utilizing aminoguanidine, a nucleophilic hydrazine compound which has been shown to inhibit cross-linking between collagen fibers and plasma proteins and collagen.[69] In addition, this agent attenuates the defects in heparin and heparan sulfate binding to collagen/fibronectin substrate and basement membranes, respectively, induced by cross-linking. More importantly, aminoguanidine has been shown to reduce AGE content and cross-linking in glomerular basement membrane and aortic connective tissue in diabetic animals. As a consequence, the thickening of the glomerular basement membrane is prevented in long-term diabetic animals suggesting that this agent may be useful in the treatment of diabetic renovascular disease.

B. MICROVASCULAR OBSTRUCTION AND FORMED ELEMENTS

Capillary obstruction by activated leukocytes may also contribute to microvascular occlusion in diabetes. This notion is based on the observation that leukocytes obtained from diabetic patients are more rigid that those obtained from healthy individuals.[75,76] In addition, monocytes express receptors for nonenzymatic glycation adducts which may explain why these cells, when isolated from diabetic patients, demonstrate increased adhesion to fibronectin.[76] Because the granulocyte and monocyte diameters exceed the luminal dimensions of capillaries, these observations suggest that leukocytes are likely to become entrapped in the microcirculation, an event that can result in microvascular occlusion (Figure 4).[75] The likelihood of such an event occuring is further enhanced by the fact that diabetes is often associated with endothelial cell swelling which reduces luminal diameter.[75] Furthermore, granulocytes and monocytes can cause endothelial cell dysfunction through the stimulated release of cytotoxic oxidants and hydrolytic enzymes. Indeed, diabetes is associated with vacuolization and swelling of endothelial cells in retinal capillaries, manifestations of diabetic retinopathy that occur predominately in regions where leukocyte infiltration is most pronounced.[75] Finally, leukocyte adherence to arteriolar endothelium occurs only rarely in normal animals has been noted in diabetes.[77,78] This may be related to the ability of AGEs to quench nitric oxide, a potent endogenous anti-adhesive agent.[79] It is also possible that oxidized low-density lipoproteins contribute to the adhesive interactions between arteriolar endothelium and leukocytes in diabetes.[80,81]

Since capillary nonperfusion is strongly correlated with the development of microaneurysms and neovascularization, it has been suggested that ischemia may induce the production of angiogenic factors.[82,83] Recent observations in alloxan diabetic rats indicate that capillary sclerosis and neovascularization are always associated with monocyte and macrophage infiltration.[75] Since these cells are also capable of producing angiogenic factors, monocytes and macrophages may play a critical role in the development of diabetic retinopathy by inducing capillary sclerosis.[75]

Platelets may also play a role in the development of microvascular sclerosis in diabetes (Figure 4).[84,85] When isolated from diabetic animals and patients, platelets exhibit increased aggregation and mediator release when exposed to agonists such as ADP, epinephrine, arachidonate, thrombin, and collagen.[85-87] These alterations in platelet function occur early in the course of the disease and thus precede the development of microangiopathy. Increased release of thromboxane and other mediators may contribute to the increase in endothelial permeability exhibited by diabetic microvessels (Figure 1) while platelet aggregation may result in microthrombosis, tissue ischemia, and ultimately, capillary sclerosis (Figure 4).[85] Platelets also secrete a mitogen (e.g., platelet-derived growth factor) that induces proliferation of vascular smooth muscle which may contribute to vascular occlusion in diabetes (Figure 4).[85] This notion is supported by the observation that supernatant obtained after activation of diabetic platelets promotes growth in cultured smooth muscle cells and fibroblasts obtained from nondiabetic patients, an effect that was reversed by insulin therapy.[85] However, this effect was not noted when platelets were obtained from spontaneously diabetic or streptozotocin-treated rats.[85]

The potency of basement membrane and extracellular matrix components as stimuli for platelet activation may increase dramatically as a consequence of glycosylation.[85] Indeed, greater platelet deposition occurs in vessels damaged by indwelling catheters in diabetic versus normal rats. This response is probably due to the altered extracellular matrix array since platelets obtained from diabetic rats respond to collagen in a fashion similar to normal platelets while platelets have been observed to aggregate more readily when exposed to glycosylated vs. nonglycosylated collagen. The fact that platelet microthrombi are more common in retinal and endoneural vessels of diabetic patients and animals suggests that there may be an association between diabetes and the propensity for thrombosis. This notion is further supported by the observation that diabetic blood induces platelet aggregation *in vitro* and facilitates thrombus formation *in vivo*.

Another hemorheologic factor that may contribute to diabetic microangiopathy relates to altered red cell deformability and aggregability in diabetes (Figure 4).[3,88,89] This notion appears to stem largely from the observation that red cell aggregates are capable of disrupting flow in the conjuctiva of both diabetic and nondiabetic subjects.[88] If erthrocyte deformability was reduced or the propensity for red cell aggregation was increased in diabetes, these hemorheologic alterations could contribute to transient or sustained ischemia in affected organs. There is some support for this concept in that red cells obtained from animals and patients with long-standing diabetes demonstrate a reduced filterability through polycarbonate filters.[88,90] This effect appears to be related to the degree to which plasma glucose is regulated. Moreover, diabetics with long-standing disease who are free from complications exhibit a lesser disturbance in rheological behavior.[88]

Although the mechanisms involved in altered erythrocyte deformability are uncertain, this alteration in rheologic behavior may be due to changes in cholesteral/lipid ratios in the diabetic red cell membrane.[3,88,91] In addition, changes in phosphorylated membrane lipid components may contribute to altered erythrocyte deformability.[88] For example, diabetic red cell membranes contain less phosphatidic acid and phosphoinositol diphosphate levels. As a consequence, the negative charge exhibited by the erythrocyte membrane is reduced which may alter the interaction between the cell membrane and underlying spectrin network and reduce deformability. Glycosylation of cytoskeletal proteins in the erythrocyte may also contribute to this phenomenon in diabetic red cells.

Diabetic erythrocytes also exhibit a greater tendency for Rouleaux formation.[88] The tendency for diabetic red cells to aggregate appears to be largely due to elevations in plasma fibrinogen and haptoglobin, acute phase proteins that increase in diabetes. The reduction in negative charge on the red cell surface may also act to promote red cell aggregation by reducing the electrostatic repulsion between erythrocytes. The aforementioned alterations in the hemorheologic behavior of diabetic red erythrocytes increase blood viscosity, especially at low shear rates. Since an increase in viscosity tends to elevate the resistance to blood flow, local changes in these hemorheologic behaviors may contribute to tissue ischemia and ultimately, capillary sclerosis (Figure 4).[88]

IV. HEMODYNAMIC HYPOTHESIS OF DIABETIC MICROANGIOPATHY

There is a large body of circumstantial evidence which implicates microvascular hemodynamic abnormalities in the genesis of increased microvascular permeability and sclerosis in diabetes.[3,4,10,11] According to this hemodynamic hypothesis, widespread vasodilation early in the course of the disease may be an important initiating event in the development of diabetic microangiopathy. Indeed, the results of several studies indicate that blood flow is elevated in many organs (e.g., stomach, small bowel, colon, liver, fat, skeletal muscle, retina, and skin) early in the course of the disease.[92-107] As a consequence of this widespread vasodilation, blood flow and capillary pressure are increased and it is thought that these hemodynamic events directly promote increased vascular wall proliferation and permeability, capillary basement membrane thickening, and luminal narrowing with eventual sclerosis.[3,4,10,11,29,98,101] Strong support for this notion is provided by the observation that renal artery stenosis prevents thickening of the glomerular basement membrane while unilateral carotid artery stenosis limits retinopathy on that side in diabetic animals.[59,60] Similarly, diabetic glomerulopathy is attenuated by pharmacologic reductions in glomerular capillary pressure.[10] These considerations have led to the development of the concept that while hyperglycemia induces a number of important biochemical changes that ultimately result in microangiopathy, the extent and nature of these changes may be modified by hemodynamic events.[3,10,11,29]

While it is clear that there is an increase in blood flow in many organs during early diabetes, the mechanisms involved in the genesis of this hyperemic response are unclear. However, there is evidence implicating atrial natriuretic peptide, growth hormone, and elevated intermediary metabolite levels in the genesis of increased renal plasma flow and glomerular filtration rate.[102-104] In addition, the diabetic kidney appears to produce greater quantities of vasodilator prostaglandins.[105] On the other hand, the vasoconstrictor response to angiotensin II is reduced in diabetes.[105]

Retinal and cutaneous blood flow are also elevated early in the development of diabetes. Although the mechanisms responsible for the increased blood flow in these organs are unclear, it has been suggested that hypoxemia may play a role in the retinal hyperemia,[106] whereas diabetes-induced elevations in metabolic rate may produce vasodilation in the skin as a means to promote thermoregulation.[107] The finding that aldose reductase inhibition reduces the diabetes-induced hyperemia in the anterior and posterior uvea, kidney, and skin granulation tissue suggests that alterations in polyol metabolism may play an important role in vasoregulation in these tissues (Figure 5).[32]

Cross-perfusion experiments indicate that the pronounced intestinal hyperemia that occurs in diabetic animals is related to an increase in circulating humoral factors (Figure 6).[97] Hyperglucagonemia appears to play an important role in mediating the intestinal hyperemia induced by diabetes since immunoneutralization of this hormone attenuates the increase in blood flow to the proximal small bowel (Figure 7).[101] Another mechanism which may explain the hyperemia associated with diabetes is impaired sympathetic vascular regulation (Figure 8).[97] While the mechanism responsible for the reduction in vascular sensitivity to norepinephrine is uncertain, it may be related to the hyperglucagonemia induced by diabetes mellitus.[97]

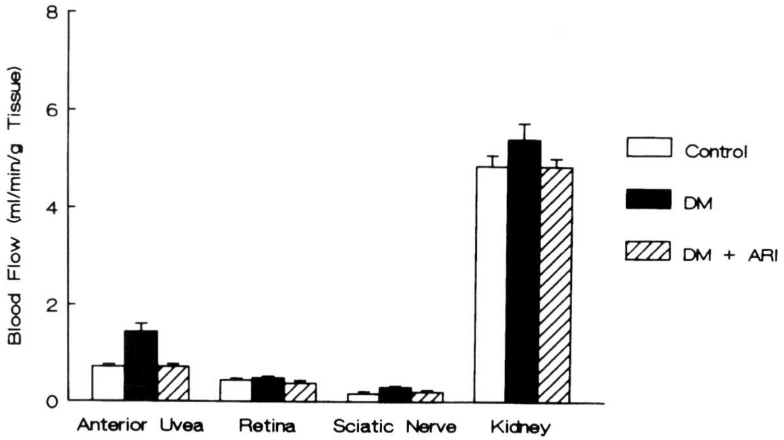

Figure 7-5 Aldose reductase inhibition (ARI) reduces the hyperemia induced by diabetes mellitus (DM) in the anterior uvea, retina, sciatic nerve, and kidney.

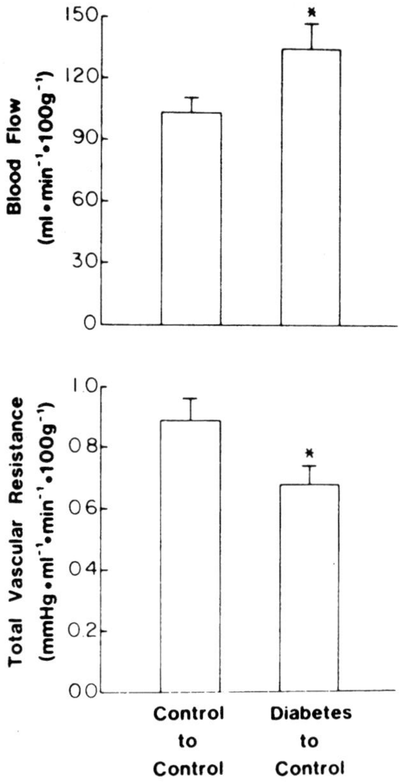

Figure 7-6 Cross-perfusion of the small intestine of normal rats with blood obtained from diabetic animals increases intestinal blood flow. This result suggests that humoral factors contribute to the intestinal hyperemia noted in experimental diabetes mellitus. *(Data from Korthuis, R. J., Benoit, J. N., Kvietys, P. R., Laughlin, M. H., Taylor, A. E., and Granger, D. N., Am. J. Physiol., 253, G26, 1987.)*

V. SUMMARY

Almost 12 million people (almost 1 in 20) in the U.S. currently have diabetes.[2] A more ominous fact is that almost 20% of the American population may develop the disease by age 65 to 74.[2] Given the incidence of diabetes and the severity of its complications, it is not surprising that diabetes ranks as the third largest cause of death by disease in the U.S. The prognosis for diabetics afflicted with the disease prior to age 31 is particularly distressing, with only 30 to 50% of these patients surviving to the age of 50. The major factor contributing to the high incidence of morbidity and mortality is end-organ dysfunction that arises secondary to diabetic microangiopathy.[2] Thus, it should not be surprising that elucidation of the mechanisms involved in the development of microangiopathy has become a central focus of research aimed at reducing end-organ complications in diabetes.

Despite this concerted research effort, the pathogenetic mechanisms underlying the development of diabetic microangiopathy remain enigmatic. However, evidence is accumulating which suggests that a variety of different mechanisms appear to contribute to the pathogenesis of diabetic microangiopathy. These include alterations in the vascular wall, hemodynamics, and circulating formed elements that contribute to the development of

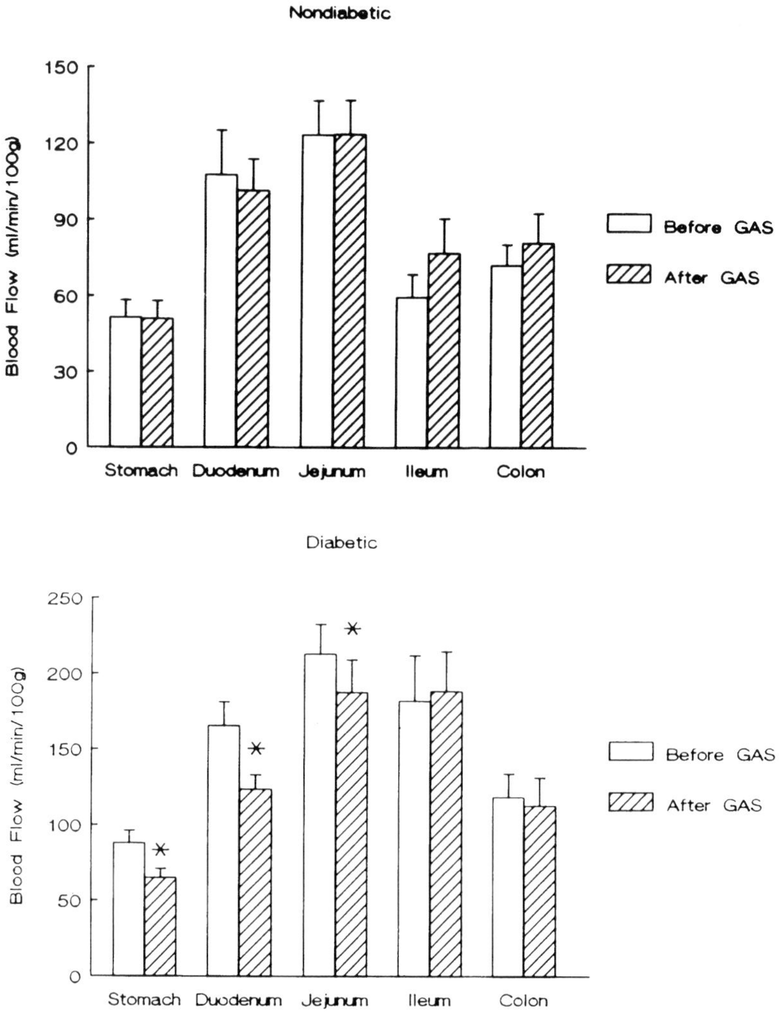

Figure 7-7 Diabetes is associated with a hyperemia in the small intestine (compare values in upper and lower panels) of fasted animals that was partially attenuated by glucagon antiserum (GAS) (Lower Panel). Note that the antiserum was without effect in normal animals (Upper Panel). *(Modified from Yrle, L. F., Smith, J. K., Benoit, J. N., Granger, D. N., and Korthuis, R. J., Am. J. Physiol., 253, G542, 1988.)*

increased vascular permeability and capillary sclerosis. Increased permeability may facilitate the accumulation of plasma proteins in vessel walls where they act to accelerate the rate of microvascular occlusion by inducing abnormal matrix thickening and fibrin deposition. Capillary sclerosis results in impaired blood flow in small regions of the affected organ with compensatory hyperperfusion in other areas. Local hypoperfusion may induce the secretion of growth factors which, in turn, may contribute to proliferative changes noted in the vascular wall. On the other hand, the compensatory hyperperfusion accentuates the deposition of proteins in the vascular wall (as a result of increased convective solute flux), thereby perpetuating the cycle of vascular and tissue damage. The recognition of these abnormalities as potential contributors to the pathogenesis of diabetic

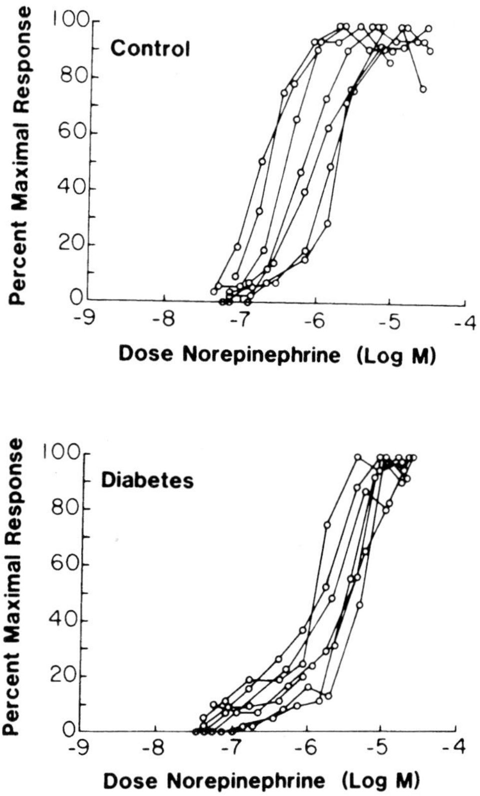

Figure 7-8 Vascular responsiveness to norepinephrine is reduced in diabetes mellitus. *(Data from Korthuis, R. J., Benoit, J. N., Kvietys, P. R., Laughlin, M. H., Taylor, A. E., and Granger, D. N., Am. J. Physiol., 253, G26, 1987.)*

microangiopathy may lead to the development of several new therapeutic approaches which may prove useful in the treatment of diabetic complications.

ACKNOWLEDGMENTS

This work was supported by a grant from the National Heart, Lung, and Blood Institute (HL-36069). R. J. Korthuis is the recipient of an Established Investigatorship from the American Heart Association.

REFERENCES

1. **Skyler, J. S.,** Strategies in diabetes mellitus, *Postgrad. Med.,* 89, 45, 1991.
2. **Siperstein, M. D.,** Diabetic microangiopathy, genetics, environment, and treatment, *Am. J. Med.,* 85 (Suppl. 5a), 119, 1988.
3. **Tooke, J. E.,** Microcirculation and diabetes, *Br. Med. Bull.,* 45, 206, 1989.
4. **Parving, H.-H.,** Impact of blood pressure and antihypertensive treatment on incipient and overt nephropathy, retinopathy, and endothelial permeability in diabetes mellitus, *Diab. Care,* 14, 1991.

5. **Deckert, T., Feldt-Rasmussen, B., Borch-Johnson, K., and Kofoed-Enevoldsen, A.,** Albuminuria reflects widespread vascular damage: the Steno hypothesis, *Diabetologia*, 32, 219, 1989.
6. **Taylor, A. E. and Granger, D. N.,** Exchange of macromolecules across the circulation, in *Handbook of Physiology — The Cardiovascular System, Microcirculation, Part 1,* Vol. 4, Renkin, E. M. and Michel, C. C., Eds., American Physiological Society, Bethesda, MD, 1984, chap. 11.
7. **Stauber, W. T., Ong, S.-H., and McCuskey, R. S.,** Selective extravascular escape of albumin into cerebral cortex of the diabetic rat, *Diabetes,* 30, 500, 1981.
8. **O'Hare, J. A., Ferriss, J. B., Twomey, B., and O'Sullivan, D. J.,** Poor metabolic control, hypertension, microangiopathy independently increase the transcapillary escape rate of albumin in diabetes, *Diabetologia,* 25, 260, 1983.
9. **Kilzer, P., Chang, K., Marvel, J., Rowlod, E., Jaudes, P., Ullensvang, S., Kilo, C., and Williamson, J. R.,** Albumin permeation of new vessels is increased in diabetic rats, *Diabetes*, 34, 333, 1985.
10. **Zatz, R. and Brenner, B. M.,** Pathogenesis of diabetic microangiopathy: the hemodynamic view, *Am. J. Med.,* 80, 443, 1986.
11. **Parving, H.-H., Viberti, G. C., Keen, H., Christiansen, J. S., and Lassen, N. A.,** Hemodynamic factors in the genesis of diabetic microangiopathy, *Metabolism,* 9, 943, 1983.
12. **Bent-Hansen, L., Feld-Rasmussen, B., Kverneland, A., and Deckert, T.,** Transcapillary escape rate and relative metabolic clearance of glycated and nonglycated albumin in Type 1 (insulin-dependent) diabetes mellitus, *Diabetologia,* 30, 2, 1987.
13. **Brownlee, M. and Cerami, A.,** The biochemistry of the complications of diabetes mellitus, *Ann. Rev. Biochem.,* 50, 385, 1981.
14. **Kennedy, L. and Baynes, J. W.,** Nonenzymatic glycosylation and the chronic complications of diabetes: an overview, *Diabetologia*, 26, 93, 1984.
15. **McMillen, D. E.,** The microcirculation in diabetes, *Microcirc. Endo. Lymph.,* 1, 3, 1984.
16. **Vlassera, H., Brownlee, M., and Cerami, A.,** Nonenzymatic glycosylation: role in pathogenesis of diabetic complications, *Clin. Chem.,* 32, B37, 1986.
17. **Iberg, N. and Fluckinger, R.,** Nonenzymatic glycosylation of albumin in vivo: identification of multiple glycosylation sites, *J. Biol. Chem.,* 261, 13542, 1986.
18. **Dolhofer, R. and Wieland, O. A.,** Increased glycosylation of serum albumin in diabetes mellitus, *Diabetes,* 29, 417, 1980.
19. **Murtiashaw, M. H. and Winterhalter, K. H.,** Non-enzymatic glycation of human albumin does not alter its palmitate binding, *Diabetologia,* 29, 366, 1987.
20. **Garlick, R. L. and Mazer, J. S.,** The principle site of nonenzymatic glycosylation of human serum albumin in vivo, *J. Biol. Chem.,* 258, 6142, 1983.
21. **Day, J. F., Thorp, S. R., and Baynes, J. W.,** Nonenzymatic glucosylation. In vitro preparation and isolation from normal human serum, *J. Biol. Chem.,* 254, 595, 1979.
22. **Shalkai, N., Garlick, R. L., and Bunn, H. F.,** Nonenzymatic glycosylation of human serum albumin alters its conformation and function, *J. Biol. Chem.,* 259, 3812, 1984.
23. **Baynes, J. W., Thorpe, S. R., and Murtiashaw, H. M.,** Nonenzymatic glucosylation of lysine residues in albumin, *Meth. Enzymol.,* 106, 88, 1984.
24. **Buccala, R., Tracey, K. J., and Cerami, A.,** Advanced glycosylation products quench nitric oxide and mediate defective endothelium-dependent vasodilation in experimental diabetes, *J. Clin. Invest.,* 87P, 432, 1991.
25. **de Tejaden, I. S., Goldstein, I., Azadzoi, K., Krane, R. J., and Cohen, R. A.,** Impaired neurogenic and endothelium mediated relaxation of penile smooth muscle from diabetic men with impotence, *N. Engl. J. Med.,* 320, 1025, 1989.

26. **Kubes, P. and Granger, D. N.,** Nitric oxide modulate microvascular permeability, *Am. J. Physiol.,* 262, H611, 1992.
27. **Shimomura, H. and Spiro, R. G.,** Studies on macromolecular components of human glomerular basement membrane and alterations in diabetes: decreased levels of heparan sulfate proteoglycan and laminin, *Diabetes,* 36, 374, 1987.
28. **Boyd, R. B., Burke, J. P., Atkin, J., Thompson, V. W., and Nugent, J. F.,** Significance of capillary basement membrane changes in diabetes mellitus, *J. Am. Pod. Med. Assoc.,* 6, 307, 1990.
29. **Williamson, J. R. and Kilo, C.,** Basement membrane thickening in diabetes mellitus, in *Complications of Diabetes Mellitus,* Vol. 3, Draznin, B., Melmed, S., and LeRoith, D., Eds., Alan R. Liss, New York, chap. 3.
30. **Collier, A. and Small, M.,** The role of the polyol pathway in diabetes mellitus, *Br. J. Hosp. Med.,* 45, 38, 1991.
31. **Zenon, G. J., Abobo, C. V., Carter, B. L., and Ball, D. W.,** Potential use of aldose reductase inhibitors to prevent diabetic complications, *Clin. Pharm.,* 9, 446, 1990.
32. **Pugliese, G., Tilton, R. G., and Williamson, J. R.,** Glucose-induced metabolic imbalances in the pathogenesis of diabetic vascular disease, *Diabetes Metab. Rev.,* 7, 35, 1991.
33. **Harrison, H. E., Stribling, D., Armstrong, F. M., and Perkins, C. M.,** Aldose reductase in the etiology of diabetic compliations. I. Introduction, *J. Diabetes Complic.,* 3, 6, 1989.
34. **Kador, P. F.,** The role of aldose reductase in the development of ocular diabetic complications, in *Complications of Diabetes Mellitus,* Vol. 3, Draznin, B., Melmed, S., and LeRoith, D., Eds., Alan R. Liss, New York, chap. 12.
35. **Barnett, P. A., Gonzalez, R. G., Chylack, L. T., and Chen, H.-M.,** The effect oxidation on sorbitol pathway kinetics, *Diabetes,* 35, 426, 1986.
36. **Gillery, P., Monboisse, J.-C., Maquart, F.-X., and Borel, J.-P.,** Does oxygen free radical increased formation explain long term complications of diabetes mellitus, *Med. Hypoth.,* 29, 47, 1989.
37. **Chari, S. W., Nath, H., and Rathi, A. B.,** Glutathione and its redox system in diabetic polymorphonuclear leukocytes, *Am. J. Med. Sci.,* 287, 1984.
38. **Stankova, L., Riddle, M., and Larned, J.,** Plasma ascorbate concentrations and blood cell dehydro-ascorbate transport in patients with diabetes mellitus, *Metabolism,* 33, 347, 1984.
39. **Jennings, P. E., Chirico, S., Jones, A. F., Lunec, J., and Barnett, A. H.,** Vitamin C metabolites and microangiopathy in diabetes mellitus, *Diabetes Res.,* 6, 151, 1987.
40. **Karpen, C. W., Cataland, S., O'Dorisio, T. M., and Pangamamal, R. V.,** Production of 12 HETE and vitamin E status of platelets from type 1 diabetic subjects, *Diabetes,* 34, 526, 1985.
41. **Nishigaki, I., Hagihara, M., Tsunekawa, H., Maseki, M., and Yagi, K.,** Lipid peroxide levels of serum lipoprotein fractions of diabetic patients, *Biochem. Med.,* 25, 373, 1981.
42. **Kaji, H., Kurasaki, M., and Ito, K.,** Increased lipoperoxide value and glutathione peroxidase activity in blood plasma of type II (non-insulin dependent) diabetic women, *Klin. Wochenschr.,* 63, 765, 1985.
43. **Sato, Y., Hotta, N., Sakamoto, N., Matsuoka, S., Ohishi, N., and Yagi, K.,** Lipid peroxide levels in plasma of diabetic patients, *Biochem. Med.,* 21, 104, 1979.
44. **Morel, D. W. and Chisolm, G. M.,** Vitamin E treatment decreases in vivo oxidation and in vitro cytotoxicity of lipoproteins from rats in experimental diabetes, *Fed. Proc.,* 46, 416, 1987.

45. **Barnett, A. H.,** Pathogenesis of diabetic microangiopathy: an overview, *Am. J. Med.,* 90 (Suppl. 6a), 6A-67S, 1991.
46. **Steven, V. J., Vlassara, H., Abati, A., and Cerami, A.,** Nonenzymatic glycosylation of hemoglobin, *J. Biol. Chem.,* 252, 2998, 1977.
47. **Cagliero, E., Maiello, M., Boeri, D., Roy, S., and Lorenzi, M.,** Increased expression of basement membrane components in human endothelial cells cultured in high glucose, *J. Clin. Invest.,* 82, 735, 1988.
48. **Schneider, S. K. and Kohn, R. R.,** Effects of age and diabetes mellitus on the solubility and nonenzymatic glycosylation of human skin collagen, *J. Clin. Invest.,* 67: 1630, 1985.
49. **LePape, A., Guitten, J. D., and Muh, J. P.,** Modification of glomerular basement membrane cross-links in experimental diabetic rats, *Biochem. Biophys. Res. Commun.,* 100, 1214, 1981.
50. **Lein, Y.-H, Stern, R., and Fu, J. C. C.,** Inhibition of collagen fibril formation in vitro and subsequent cross-linking by glucose, *Science,* 225, 1489, 1984.
51. **Pongor, S., Ulrich, P. C., and Bencsath, F. A.,** Aging of proteins: isolation and identification of fluorescent chromophore from the reaction of polypeptides with glucose, *Proc. Natl. Acad. Sci. U.S.A.,* 81, 2684, 1984.
52. **Brownlee, M., Vlassara, H., and Cerami, A.,** Nonenzymatic glycosylation products on collagen covalently trap low-density lipoproteins, *Diabetes,* 34, 938, 1985.
53. **Cohen, M. P. and Ku, L.,** Inhibition of fibronectin binding of matrix components by nonenzymatic glycosylation, *Diabetes,* 33, 970, 1984.
54. **Tarsio, J. F., Wigness, B., and Rhode, T. D.,** Nonezymatic glycation of fibronectin and alterations in the molecular association of cell matrix and basement membrane components in diabetes mellitus, *Diabetes,* 34, 477, 1985.
55. **Beisswenger, P. J. and Spiro, R. G.,** Studies on the human glomerular basement membrane: composition, nature of carbohydrate units and chemical changes in diabetes mellitus, *Diabetes,* 22, 180, 1973.
56. **Siperstein, M. D.,** Diabetic microangiopathy, *West. J. Med.,* 212, 404, 1974.
57. **Vracko, R.,** A comparison of the microvascular lesions in diabetes mellitus with those in normal aging, *J. Am. Geriatr. Soc.,* 30, 201, 1985
58. **Porta, M., La Selva, M., Molinatti, P., and Molinatti, G. M.,** Endothelial cell function in diabetic microangiopathy, *Diabetologia,* 30, 601, 1987.
59. **Berkman, J. and Rifkin, H.,** Unilateral nodular diabetic glomerulosclerosis (Kimmelstiel-Wilson). Report of a case, *Metab. Clin. Exp.,* 22, 715, 1973.
60. **Behrendt, T. and Duane, T. D.,** Unilateral complications in diabetic retinopathy, *Trans. Am. Acad. Opthamol. Otol.,* 74, 28, 1970.
61. **Nakamura, Y. and Myers, B. D.,** Charge selectivity of proteinuria in diabetic glomerulopathy, *Diabetes,* 37, 1202, 1988.
62. **Houhala, I. A. and Pasternak, A.,** Fractional dextran and protein clearances in glomerulonephritis and in diabetic nephropathy, *Clin. Sci.,* 72, 289, 1989.
63. **Sternberg, M., Cohen-Forterre, L., and Peyroux, J.,** Connective tissue in diabetes mellitus: biochemical alterations of the intracellular matrix with special reference to proteoglycan, collagens, and basement membrane, *Diabetes Metab.,* 11, 27, 1985.
64. **Sampietro, T., Colantuoni, A., Lenzi. S., Bertuglia, S., Bionda, A., and Donato, L.,** Increased permeability of hamster microcirculation to glycosylated albumin, *Lancet,* 994, 1988.
65. **Wagner, R. C., Williams, S. K., Mathews, M. A., and Andrews, B. S.,** Exclusion of albumin from vesicular ingestion by isolated microvessels, *Microvasc. Res.,* 19, 127, 1980.

66. **Williams, S. K.,** Vesicular transport of proteins by capillary endothelium, *Ann. N.Y. Acad. Sci.,* 416, 457, 1983.
67. **Williams, S. K. and Solenski, N. J.,** Enhanced vesicular ingestion of nonenzymatically glucosylated proteins by capillary endothelium, *Microvasc. Res.,* 28, 311, 1984.
68. **Poduslo, J. F., Curran, G. L., and Dyke, P. J.,** Increase in albumin, IgG, and IgM blood-nervé indices in human diabetic neuropathy, *Proc. Natl. Acad. Sci. U.S.A.,* 85, 4879, 1988.
69. **Brownlee, M.,** The role of nonenzymatic glycosylation in the pathogenesis of diabetic angiopathy, in *Complications of Diabetes Mellitus,* Vol. 3, Draznin, B., Melmed, S., and LeRoith, D., Eds., Alan R. Liss, New York, chap. 2.
70. **Radoff, S., Vlassara, H., and Cerami, A.,** Isolation of a macrophage receptor for proteins modified by advanced glycosylation endproducts (AGE), *Fed. Proc. Exp. Biol.,* 46, 2116, 1987.
71. **Vlassara, H., Brownlee, M., and Cerami, A.,** Novel macrophage receptor for glucose-modified proteins is distinct from previously describe scavenger receptors, *J. Exp. Med.,* 164, 1301, 1986.
72. **Vlassara, H., Brownlee, M., and Cerami, A.,** High-affinity-receptor-mediated uptake and degradation of glucose-modified proteins: a potential mechanism for the removal of senescent macromolecules, *Proc. Natl. Acad. Sci. U.S.A.,* 82, 5588, 1985.
73. **Vlassara, H., Brownlee, M., and Cerami, A.,** Specific macrophage receptor activity for advanced glycosylation endproducts inversely correlates with insulin levels in vivo, *Diabetes,* 37, 456, 1988.
74. **Vlassara, H., Brownlee, M., and Cerami, A.,** Advanced glycosylation endproduct (AGE) binding to its macrophage receptor stimulates secretion of a multifunctional growth-promoting monokine, *Science,* 240, 1546, 1988.
75. **Schroder, S., Palinski, W., and Schmid-Schonbein, G. W.,** Activated monocytes and granulocytes, capillary nonperfusion, and neovascularization in diabetic retinopathy, *Am. J. Pathol.,* 139, 81, 1991.
76. **Setiadi, H., Wautier, J. L., Courillon-Mallet, A., Passa, P., and Caen, J.,** Increased adhesion to fibronectin and MO-1 expression by diabetic monocytes, *J. Immunol.,* 138, 3230, 1987.
77. **Bohlen, H. G. and Niggl, B. A.,** Early arteriolar disturbances following streptozotocin-induced diabetes mellitus in adult mice, *Microvasc. Res.,* 20, 19, 1980.
78. **Lash, J. and Bohlen, H. G.,** Structural and functional origins of suppressed acetylcholine vasodilation in diabetic rat intestinal arterioles, *Circ. Res.,* 69, 1259, 1991.
79. **Kubes, P., Suzuki, M., and Granger, D. N.,** Nitric oxide: an endogenous modulator of leukocyte adhesion, *Proc. Natl. Acad. Sci. U.S.A.,* 88, 4651, 1991.
80. **Lehr, H.-A., Hubner, C., Nolte, D., Finckh, B., Beisiegel, U., Kohlschutter, A., and Messmer, K.,** Oxidatively modified human low density lipoprotein stimulates leukocyte adherence to the microvascular endothelium in vivo, *Res. Exp. Med.,* 191, 85, 1991.
81. **Lehr, H.-A., Hubner, C., Finckh, B., Angersmuller, S., Nolte, D., Kohlschutter, A., Beisiegel, U., and Messmer, K.,** Role of leukotrienes in leukocyte adhesion following systemic administration of oxidatively modified human low density lipoprotein in hamsters, *J. Clin. Invest.,* 88, 9, 1991.
82. **Wise, G. N.,** Retinal neovascularization, *Trans. Am. Opthamol. Soc.,* 54, 729, 1956.
83. **Davis, M. D., Myers, F. L., Engerman, R. L., De Venecia, G., and Magli, Y. L.,** Clinical observations concerning the pathogenesis of diabetic retinopathy, in *Symposium on the Treatment of Diabetic Retinopathy,* Goldberg, M. F. and Fine, S. L., Eds., U.S. Government Printing Office, Washington, D.C., 1969, 47.
84. **Colwell, J. A., Winocour, P. D., and Halushka, P. V.,** Do platelets have anything to do with diabetic microvascular disease, *Diabetes,* 32, 14, 1983.

85. **Winocour, P. D.,** The role of platelets in the pathogenesis of diabetic vascular disease, in *Complications of Diabetes Mellitus,* Vol. 3, Draznin, B., Melmed, S., and LeRoith, D., Eds., Alan R. Liss, New York, chap. 5.
86. **Winocour, P. D., Kinlough-Rathbone, R. L., and Mustard, J. F.,** Pathways responsible for platelet hypersensitivity in rats with diabetes. I. Streptozotocin-induced diabetes, *J. Lab. Clin. Med.,* 107, 148, 1986.
87. **Winocour, P. D., Kinlough-Rathbone, R. L., and Mustard, J. F.,** Pathways responsible for platelet hypersensitivity in rats with diabetes. I. Spontaneous diabetes in BB Wistar rats, *J. Lab. Clin. Med.,* 107, 154, 1986.
88. **McMillan, D. E.,** The role of the diabetic erythrocyte in the development of microvascular disease, in *Complications of Diabetes Mellitus,* Vol. 3, Draznin, B., Melmed, S., and LeRoith, D., Eds., Alan R. Liss, New York, chap. 6.
89. **Stuart, J. and Juhan-Vague, I.,** Erythrocyte rheology in diabetes mellitus, *Clin. Hemorheol.,* 7, 239, 1987.
90. **McMillan, D. E., Utterback, N. G., and Mitchell, T. P.,** Reduced erythrocyte deformability in diabetes, *Diabetes,* 27, 895, 1978.
91. **Juhan-Vague, I., Driss, F., and Roul, C.,** Abnormalities of erythrocyte membrane lipids in insulin-dependent diabetics are improved by short term strict control of diabetics, *Clin. Hemorheol.,* 4, 455, 1984.
92. **Bohlen, H. G. and Hankins, K. D.,** Early arteriolar and capillary changes in streptozotocin-induced diabetic rats and intraperitoneal hyperglycaemic rats, *Diabetologia,* 22, 344, 1982.
93. **Gunderson, H. J. G.,** Peripheral blood flow and metabolic control in juvenile diabetics, *Diabetologia,* 10, 225, 1974.
94. **Haggendale, E., Steen, B., and Svanborg, A.,** Blood flow in subcutaneous fat tissue in patients with diabetes mellitus, *Acta Med. Scand.,* 187, 49, 1970.
95. **Hill, M. A. and Larkins, R. G.,** Functional microvascular alterations in early experimental diabetes mellitus, in *Microcirculation — An Update,* Vol. 2, Tsuchiya, M., Ed., Elsevier, New York, 1987, 619.
96. **Kohner, E. M., Hamilton, A. M., Saunders, S. J., Sutcliffe, B. A., and Bulpitt, C. J.,** The retinal blood flow in diabetes mellitus, *Diabetologia,* 11, 27, 1975.
97. **Korthuis, R. J., Benoit, J. N., Kvietys, P. R., Laughlin, M. H., Taylor, A. E., and Granger, D. N.,** Intestinal hyperemia in experimental diabetes mellitus, *Am. J. Physiol.,* 253, G26, 1987.
98. **Korthuis, R. J., Pitts, V. H., and Granger, D. N.,** Intestinal capillary filtration in experimental diabetes mellitus, *Am. J. Physiol.,* 253, G20, 1987.
99. **Lucas, P. D. and Foy, J. M.,** Effects of experimental diabetes and genetic obesity on regional blood flow in the rat, *Diabetes,* 26, 786, 1977.
100. **Rosenblum, W. I., Bryan, D., and Choi, S. C.,** Effect of diabetes on microvascular responses in mouse mesentery, *Microcirc. Endothelium Lymph.,* 2, 195, 1985.
101. **Yrle, L. F., Smith, J. K., Benoit, J. N., Granger, D. N., and Korthuis, R. J.,** Role of glucagon in intestinal hyperemia associated with early experimental diabetes mellitus, *Am. J. Physiol.,* 253, G542, 1988.
102. **Trevisan, R., Nosadini, R., Fioretto, P., and Velussi, M.,** Metabolic control of kidney haemodynamics in normal and insulin-dependent diabetic subjects, *Diabetes,* 36, 1073, 1987.
103. **Ortola, F. V., Ballerman, B. J., Anderson, S., and Mendez, R. E.,** Elevated plasma atrial natriuretic peptide levels in diabetic rats, potential mediator of hyperfiltration, *J. Clin. Invest.,* 80, 670, 1987.
104. **Sandahl-Christiensen, J., Gammelgaard, J., and Frandsen, M.,** Kidney function and size in type I (insulin-dependent) diabetic patients before and during growth hormone administration for one week, *Diabetologia,* 22, 333, 1982.

105. **Kreisberg, J. I. and Patel, P. Y.,** The effects of insulin, glucose, and diabetes on prostaglandin production by rat kidney glomeruli and cultured mesangial cells, *Prostaglandins Leukotrienes Med.,* 11, 431, 1983.
106. **Stefansson, E., Landers, M. B., and Wolbarsht, M. L.,** Oxygenation and vasodilation in relationship to diabetic and other proliferative retinopathy, *Opthalmic Surg.,* 14, 209, 1983.
107. **Leslie, P., Jung, R. T., and Isles, T. E.,** Effect of optimal glacemic control with subcutaneous insulin infusion on energy expenditure in type I diabetes mellitus, *Br. Med. J.,* 293, 1121, 1986.

Chapter 8

Immunologic Injury

David J. Dzielak, Robert L. Hester, and Joey P. Granger

CONTENTS

I. INTRODUCTION

Endothelial cells, positioned between the interface of blood and extravascular tissue, play an important role in the pathogenesis of permeability changes and leukocyte infiltration characteristic of inflammatory and immune reactions. Although investigators once believed that the vascular endothelium was a passive bystander in these reactions, this view has changed considerably over the past decade. Vascular endothelial cells are now recognized as having an active role in both inflammatory and immune reactions.

Endothelial cells can express leukocyte specific adhesion molecules as well as both Class I and Class II Major Histocompatibility Complex (MHC) antigens. Endothelial cells are now known to respond to and produce a variety of cytokines. These functions allow vascular endothelial cells to participate not only in the normal protective response to a foreign antigen, but also in potentially harmful autoreactive processes that are characteristic of some immunologic diseases. This chapter will focus on the role of the endothelium in inflammatory and immunologic injury to the microvasculature.

II. ENDOTHELIAL RESPONSE TO CYTOKINES

Antigen-stimulated leukocytes secrete protein mediators that can activate and recruit cells that take part in the inflammatory response. Originally these mediators were thought to be derived only from cells that traditionally were considered to be part of the immune system. Therefore, they were identified as lymphokines, monokines, and interleukins. Subsequently, it has been discovered that other cell types can secrete similar mediators, now collectively called cytokines.[1] A major target of cytokine action is the microvascular endothelium. Interleukin-I (IL-1), tumor necrosis factor (TNF), lymphotoxin (LT), and interferon-gamma (IFN-γ), and their effects on endothelial cells are the focus of the following discussion.

0-8493-4547-2/94/$0.00+$.50

A. INTERLEUKIN-1

Early in the course of an inflammatory response, leukocytes are activated and recruited to the site of the initiating disturbance (i.e., foreign antigen). One of the initial steps in this process is the adhesion of leukocytes to the endothelium of the postcapillary venules. IL-1 is believed to be involved in this process by inducing adhesiveness of the endothelium for neutrophils, eosinophils, basophils, and monocytes.[2-8]

Under basal conditions cultured endothelial cells are poorly adhesive for leukocytes.[9] However, when exposed to IL-1, endothelial cells avidly bind leukocytes as a result of the induction of leukocyte adhesion receptors on the surface of endothelial cells by IL-1. IL-1 induces the synthesis and cell surface expression of a 115 kD glycoprotein called endothelial-leukocyte adhesion molecule 1 (ELAM-1),[10] which binds neutrophils to endothelial cells. The receptor for ELAM-1 on the surface of neutrophils has not been identified, but is not believed to be part of the CD11/18 complex of adhesion molecules.[11] The expression of ELAM-1 peaks at 4 to 6 h after exposure to IL-1 and appears to be specific for endothelial cells. Other cell types (e.g., fibroblasts, smooth muscle cells) do not express ELAM-1 when exposed to IL-1 or other cytokines. In addition to the induction of ELAM-1, IL-1 also increases the expression of ICAM-1 (intercellular adhesion molecule 1) by endothelial cells. ICAM-1 is a 90-kD glycoprotein that is expressed basally by endothelial cells.[12,13] Peak expression of ICAM-1 occurs 24 h after exposure to IL-1. ICAM-1 expression remains stable as long as IL-1 is present in the media.[14,15] ICAM-1 appears to be the endothelial cell ligand for lymphocytes, macrophages, and neutrophils.[12] The temporal role of these endothelial adhesion molecules is not known. Maximal ICAM-1 expression occurs well past that for ELAM-1, suggesting a role for ICAM-1 during the latter phase of the inflammatory response. IL-1 can also induce the expression of both ELAM-1 and ICAM-1 on postcapillary endothelial cells *in situ*.[9]

In addition to the effect of enhancing the expression of adhesion molecules, IL-1 can also promote the production of leukocyte-activating factors. It has been reported that IL-1 stimulates endothelial cells to synthesize platelet-activating factor (PAF),[15] which promotes leukocyte aggregation, microcirculatory sludge, diapedesis, plasma extravasation, and intercellular edema.[16] PAF can also induce the release of IL-1 from macrophages and increase the expression of surface adhesion molecules on neutrophils. PAF has been implicated in the generation of positive feedback cycles that may play a significant role in pathophysiological processes.[16]

IL-1 can stimulate endothelial cells to synthesize and express membrane IL-1.[17] In addition, IL-1 can induce a secretion of IL-1 itself, suggesting a potential for a positive feedback cycle.[18] IL-1 also stimulates endothelial cells to synthesize granulocyte-macrophage-colony stimulating factor (GM-CSF) and granulocyte-colony stimulating factor (G-CSF).[19,20]

IL-1 has multiple effects on endothelial cells that serve to promote the inflammatory response. IL-1 has not been shown to be directly toxic to endothelial cells. However, IL-1 pretreatment has been reported to enhance the destruction of endothelial cells by activated neutrophils.[21] Thus, IL-1 may predispose endothelial cells to immunologic injury under certain pathophysiological conditions.

B. TUMOR NECROSIS FACTOR AND LYMPHOTOXIN

Tumor necrosis factor (TNF) is a product of endotoxin-stimulated mononuclear phagocytes.[22] LT is a product of antigen-activated T-cells.[23,24] While antigen-activated T-cells are capable of producing both LT and TNF, the major source of TNF is mononuclear phagocytes.[25,26] Both cytokines are strikingly similar to IL-1 with respect to their actions on endothelial cells. However, it requires approximately one-hundred-fold greater concentrations of both TNF and LT to produce the same biological effects on endothelium as IL-1.

TNF and LT mimic every known action of IL-1 on cultured endothelial cells.[9,27] Both cytokines induce ELAM-1 expression;[10,28] augment ICAM-1 expression;[28] increase adhesiveness of endothelial cells for granulocytes and lymphocytes;[2,4,6,7,29,30] induce membrane expression of IL-1[17] and cause secretion of IL-1[31-33] and GM-CSF;[34-36] and stimulate PAF synthesis.[37] TNF and LT also act on postcapillary venules *in situ* to induce ELAM-1 expression[38] and to augment ICAM-1 expression.[39]

There are two major differences in the actions of either TNF or LT and IL-1. Both TNF and LT cause an increase in the expression of Class I MHC antigens whereas IL-1 does not.[40] In addition, TNF and LT activate neutrophils and increase adhesion of the endothelium for lymphocytes.[31,41]

The multiple actions of TNF and LT on endothelial cells serve to promote the inflammatory response. Through their effects on MHC antigen expression, both TNF and LT promote lymphocyte-dependent inflammation, an action that distinguishes these cytokines from IL-1, which does not affect MHC expression.

C. INTERFERON-γ

Interferons are a class of cytokines that interfere with viral replication in host cells. Interferons are produced in response to viral infection and are thought to perform an altruistic function in protecting neighboring cells from viral pathogens by inducing self-destruction. Interferon brings on self-destruction by activating natural killer cells and by enhancing susceptibility of the virus-infected cells to cytotoxic T-lymphocytes. IFN-γ is secreted by T-cells in response to antigen. IFN-γ induces maturation of B and cytotoxic T-lymphocytes and is a potent macrophage-activating factor.[42]

IFN-γ has numerous effects on endothelial cells. It induces the synthesis of IP-10 (a putative cytokine of unknown function) and the proteins of the alternative complement pathway.[43-45] IFN-γ enhances the expression of ICAM-1 and Class I MHC antigens.[13] A unique characteristic of IFN-γ is its ability to induce the expression of Class II MHC antigens by its action on endothelial cells.[46-50] The expression of Class II MHC antigens allows the endothelial cells to present antigen to $CD4^+$ T-cells (helper cells). This action of IFN-γ on endothelial cells allows them to act as antigen-presenting cells and to perform accessory cell function.

IFN-γ selectively increases endothelial adhesion for lymphocytes without increasing adhesion for other white cell populations.[30,51] Some experimental evidence suggests that IFN-γ increases endothelial adhesiveness only for the $CD4^+$ T-cell subpopulation.[48,52] These actions of IFN-γ on endothelial cells also have been observed *in vivo* during cell-mediated responses to foreign antigens.[39,53]

The endothelial effects of IFN-γ can be modulated by TNF and LT. IFN-γ acts synergistically with TNF and LT to increase ICAM-1 and Class I MHC antigen expression.[9,40] This interaction may be important *in situ* because these cytokines are often released concomitantly by antigen-activated T-cells. The fact that IFN-γ enhances Class I MHC expression and induces Class II MHC expression on endothelial cells is an important feature that allows the endothelium to participate in lymphocyte-mediated inflammation. Class I MHC antigens are important in the recognition of foreign antigen by cytolytic T-lymphocytes. Class II MHC antigens are required for the presentation of antigen to helper T-cells. The expression of Class II MHC by IFN-γ allows allogeneic endothelial cells to activate T-lymphocytes.

Cytokines are important modulators of endothelial cell phenotype. IL-1, TNF, and LT influence endothelial cells' surface leukocyte adhesiveness and promote other pro-inflammatory actions. IFN-γ enhances Class I MHC antigen expression and induces *de novo* expression of Class II MHC antigens. The modifications induced by these cytokines allow the vascular endothelium to be an active participant in the inflammatory process.

III. THE ROLE OF THE ENDOTHELIUM IN INFLAMMATION

The alteration in the surface expression of adhesion molecules and the functional changes in endothelial cells induced by cytokines are referred to as "endothelial activation."[54] While much of the evidence for the changes in the endothelium induced by cytokines has come from *in vitro* experiments using cultured endothelial cells, cytokine-induced endothelial activation occurs *in vivo* and may contribute to immune and vascular injury.

A. CYTOKINE ACTIVATION

Acute inflammation is associated with neutrophil accumulation at the site of antigen recognition. Neutrophil accumulation involves the delivery of additional neutrophils to the site of the antigen, adhesion of the delivery neutrophils to the endothelial cells of the local venules, and subsequent neutrophil action. IL-1 and TNF promote neutrophil attachment to endothelium by inducing the expression of ELAM-1. Cytokine-mediated induction of ELAM-1 is probably involved in the early stages of neutrophil adhesion.[55] Recall that peak ELAM-1 expression on cultured endothelial cells occurs at 4 to 6 h after exposure to cytokines.

Although IL-1 and TNF appear to be involved in the process of acute inflammation, IFN-γ appears to be uniquely involved in those aspects of endothelial activation related to immune inflammation. IFN-γ can act synergistically with TNF and LT to modulate endothelial cell function. The fact that this combination of cytokines is released concomitantly by the same population of T-cells suggests that they are likely to appear together *in vivo*. This has led to the hypothesis that IFN-γ is the signal that converts acute inflammation to immune inflammation,[56] which is initiated by T-cell recognition of foreign antigen. Recognition of antigen by T-cells results in the release of IFN-γ, which subsequently induces the activation of local venular endothelium.[56] The enhanced expression of Class I MHC and Class II MHC molecules on the surface of these endothelial cells allows them to participate in the presentation of foreign antigen to additional T-cells. This has two effects on the inflammatory process. First, the endothelial cells can use the antigen-MHC complex to selectively bind additional circulating T-cells specific for that antigen. Second, the response can be amplified by endothelial expression of IL-1. This phenomenon would serve to activate additional T-cells and enhance cytokine secretion. The additional level of cytokine would add to the inflammatory response. Increased ICAM-1 expression on the endothelial cells would promote adhesion of additional T-cells and monocytes. Thus, cytokine-activated T-cells may play a number of pivotal roles in the development and enhancement of cell-mediated immune inflammation.

B. DELAYED-TYPE HYPERSENSITIVITY

If endothelial activation is a necessary part of cell-mediated immunity, then it should be observable whenever cell-mediated immune reactions occur. Delayed-type hypersensitivity is a local inflammatory reaction mediated by antigen-stimulated helper T-cells.[57] The delayed-type hypersensitivity phenomenon is often used as a model in which to study the cell-mediated immune response. The T-cells that are responsible for the delayed-type hypersensitivity response are activated by the recognition of a specific antigen presented on the surface of accessory cells in association with Class II MHC molecules. The activated T-cells secrete Interleukin-2 (IL-2), TNF, LT, and IFN-γ. IL-2 feeds back on the T-cell of origin to amplify cytokine secretion.[58] IL-2 also induces proliferation and cytokine secretion from other T-cells that do not specifically recognize the particular antigen in question. These cytokines (TNF, LT, and IFN-γ) combine to mediate the local recruitment and activation of mononuclear phagocytes. Thus, the characteristic cellular infiltrate of delayed-type hypersensitivity reactions is a mixture of activated helper T-cells and mononuclear phagocytes. Peak cellular infiltration into the postcapillary perivenular tissue occurs 24 to 48 h after an antigenic challenge in a previously sensitized host, thus the term delayed-type hypersensitivity. The mononuclear cell infiltrate occurs at the time when there are plasma protein extravasation and structural changes in the endothelial cells themselves. The leakage of fibrinogen leads to fibrin deposition in the perivascular space, which accounts for the characteristic induration of the delayed-type hypersensitivity response.

The action of cytokines on endothelial cells may contribute to several aspects of the delayed-type hypersensitivity response. As mentioned above, the delayed-type hypersensitivity response is initiated by T-cell recognition of antigen. The T-cells that respond to a specific antigen may reside within a particular tissue or the antigen may be carried via the lymphatics to lymph nodes where the antigen sensitive T-cell may reside. Antigen may also be presented to circulating T-cells on the luminal surface of postcapillary venular endothelial cells at or near the site of actual antigenic challenge.[58] Endothelial cells induced to express Class II MHC molecules by the action of IFN-γ may act as antigen-presenting cells under these conditions.

In summary, cytokine-inducible endothelial cell changes play an important role in several aspects of the delayed-type hypersensitivity response. These include T-cell recognition of antigen, activation of antigen-specific T-cells, adhesion of circulating lymphocytes to the endothelium, diapedesis of the various leukocyte subpopulations, and the development of macromolecular leakiness leading to tissue edema.

IV. ROLE OF THE ENDOTHELIUM IN AUTOIMMUNITY AND VASCULAR INJURY

Immunologic self reactivity can lead to tissue damage. Frank autoreactive processes directed at the endothelium itself can lead to vasculitis and vascular injury. More subtle processes such as gradual vascular scarring and sclerosis may be initiated by immune-mediated focal endothelial necrosis with resulting thrombosis. The role of the endothelium itself as an initiator of these reactions is unclear. However, cytokine-induced alterations in endothelial cells may play an important role in this process. While cytokines have not been shown to be directly toxic to vascular endothelial cells, they may alter the potential of endothelial cells to initiate an anti-self immune response by increasing the expression of molecules, such as Class I and Class II MHC antigens, IL-1, and ICAM-1, that serve to activate and localize lymphocytes.[59] It is also possible that by modifying the surface of the endothelial cell, cytokines may alter the ability of the effector phase of the immune system to recognize the endothelium itself. This last phenomenon may be involved in two autoimmune vascular disorders, Kawasaki's disease and hemolytic uremic syndrome.

A. KAWASAKI'S DISEASE

Kawasaki's disease is a childhood disorder characterized by fever, mucocutaneous manifestations, and panvasculitis of unknown cause. A generalized immune activation involving increased T-cell and polyclonal B-cell activation is invariably seen. Skin biopsies of patients show evidence of cytokine-mediated activation as evidenced by the expression of ELAM-1 and Class II MHC molecules and enhanced expression of ICAM-1.[60] Patients with this disorder have serum complement-activating antibodies that lyse cultured endothelial cells after pretreatment with IL-1 or TNF for 4 h or IFN-γ for 72 h. Serum from patients in remission or from nonaffected individuals does not lyse endothelial cells.[61,62] These findings suggest that the autoantibodies are directed against an endothelial antigen induced by IL-1, TNF, or IFN-γ. The nature of this antigen is unknown. It is proposed that the enhanced T-cell activity in these patients results in the elevation of cytokines that activate the endothelium and induce new surface antigens, which in turn elicits an antibody response that results in endothelial cell lysis and eventual vascular injury.[11]

B. HEMOLYTIC UREMIC SYNDROME

Hemolytic uremic syndrome is a pediatric microangiopathic disorder that often arises after an episode of diarrhea caused by shiga or viro toxin-positive bacteria, which usually presents as renal injury secondary to occlusion of renal arterioles and glomerular capillaries. In contrast to Kawasaki's disease, patients with hemolytic uremic syndrome have circulating endothelial cell-specific autoantibodies directed against an antigen expressed on untreated but not IFN-γ-pretreated endothelial cells.[63] Thus, there are autoantibodies in both Kawasaki's disease and hemolytic uremic syndrome that recognize cytokine-modulated determinants.

To date there are no known examples of disorders in which cytokines induce endothelial cell antigens that are targets of cell-mediated immune reactions. (Both Kawasaki's disease and hemolytic uremic syndrome are examples of humorally mediated immune reactions.) However, it has been demonstrated *in vitro* that cytolytic T-lymphocytes specific for Class II MHC antigen lyse endothelium after exposure to IFN-γ.[48] It is likely that these events occur *in vivo* in certain types of vascular injury such as that which occurs during the rejection of foreign allografts.

V. SUMMARY

Vascular endothelial cells of the microcirculation play an important and critical role in inflammatory and immune reactions. Through the action of cytokines produced by a wide variety of circulating leukocytes, vascular endothelial cells can induce, promote, and augment the response to an antigen. While these actions are part of the normal response to a foreign antigen, they may also serve as the underlying mechanism responsible for autoreactive diseases. Presently these autoreactive processes are poorly understood. Further experimentation and conceptualization in the area of leukocyte-vascular endothelial cell interaction are necessary in order to clarify the mechanisms involved in these autoreactive phenomena and the role of the microcirculation in this process.

REFERENCES

1. **Cohen, S.,** Physiologic and pathologic manifestations of lymphokine action, *Hum. Pathol.,* 17, 122, 1986.
2. **Bevilacqua, M. P., Pober, J. S., Wheeler, M. E., Cotran, R. S., and Gimbrone, M. A., Jr.,** Interleukin 1 acts on cultured human vascular endothelium to increase the adhesion of polymorphonuclear leukocytes, monocytes and related leukocytic cell lines, *J. Clin. Invest.,* 76, 2003, 1985.
3. **Bevilacqua, M. P., Pober, J. S. Wheeler, M. E., Cotran, R. S., and Gimbrone, M. A., Jr.,** Interleukin 1 (IL-1) activation of vascular endothelium, effects on procoagulant activity and leukocyte adhesion, *Am. J. Pathol.,* 121, 393, 1985.
4. **Bochner, B. S., Peachell, P. T., Brown, K. E., and Schleimer, R. P.,** Adherence of human basophils to cultured umbilical vein endothelial cells, *J. Clin. Invest.,* 81, 1355, 1988.
5. **Dunn, C. J. and Fleming, W. F.,** The role of Interleukin-1 in the inflammatory response with particular reference to endothelial cell-leukocyte adhesion, in *The Physiological, Metabolic and Immunologic Actions of Interleukin-1,* Kluger, M. J., Oppenheim, J. J., and Powanda, M. C., Eds., Alan R. Liss, New York, 1985, 45.
6. **Lamas, A. M., Mulroney, C. M., and Schleimer, R. P.,** Studies on the adhesive interaction between purified human eosinophils and cultured vascular endothelial cells, *J. Immunol.,* 140, 1500, 1988.

7. **Pohlman, T. H., Stanness, K. A., Beatty, P. G., Ochs, H. D., and Harlan, J. M.,** An endothelial cell surface factor(s) induced in vitro by lipopolysaccharide, interleukin 1, and tumor necrosis factor α increases neutrophil adherence by a CDw18-dependent mechanism, *J. Immunol.,* 136, 4548, 1986.
8. **Schleimer, R. P. and Rutledge, B. K.,** Cultured human vascular endothelial cells acquire adhesiveness for neutrophils after stimulation with interleukin 1, endotoxin, and tumor-promoting phorbol diesters, *J. Immunol.,* 136, 649, 1986.
9. **Pober, J. S. and Cotran, R. S.,** Cytokines and endothelial cell biology, *Physiol. Rev.,* 70, 427, 1990.
10. **Pober, J. S., Bevilacqua, M. P., Mendrick, D. L., Lapierre, L. A., Fiers, W., and Gimbrone, M. A., Jr.,** Two distinct monokines, interleukin-1 and tumor necrosis factor, each independently induce biosynthesis and transient expression of the same antigen on the surface of cultured human vascular endothelial cells, *J. Immunol.,* 136, 1680, 1986.
11. **Cotran, R. S. and Pober, J. S.,** Effects of cytokines on vascular endothelium, their role in vascular and immune injury, *Kidney Int.,* 35, 969, 1989.
12. **Dustin, M. L. and Springer, T. A.,** Lymphocyte function-associated antigen-1 (LFA-1) interaction with intercellular adhesion molecule-1 (ICAM-1) is one of at least three mechanisms for lymphocyte adhesion to cultured endothelial cells, *J. Cell. Biol.,* 107, 321, 1988.
13. **Pober, J. S., Gimbrone, M. A., Jr., Lapierre, L. A., Mendrick, D. L., Fiers, W., Rothlein, R., and Springer, T. A.,** Overlapping patterns of activation of human endothelial cells by interleukin 1, tumor necrosis factor, and immune interferon, *J. Immunol.,* 137, 1893, 1986.
14. **Marlin, S. D. and Springer, T. A.,** Purified intercellular adhesion molecule-1 (ICAM-1) is a ligand for lymphocyte function-associated antigen 1 (LFA-1), *Cell,* 51, 813, 1987.
15. **Bussolino, F., Breviario, F., Telta, C., Aglietta, M., Mantovani, A., and Dejana, E.,** Interleukin 1 stimulates platelet-activating factor production in cultured human endothelial cells, *J. Clin. Invest.,* 77, 2027, 1986.
16. **Braquet, P., Hosford, D., Braquet, M., Bourgain, R., and Bussolino, F.,** Role of cytokines and platelet-activating factor in microvascular immune injury, *Int. Arch. Allergy Appl. Immunol.,* 88, 88, 1989.
17. **Kurt-Jones, E. A., Fiers, W., and Pober, J. S.,** Membrane interleukin 1 induction on human endothelial cells and dermal fibroblasts, *J. Immunol.,* 139, 2317, 1987.
18. **Warner, S. J. C., Auger, K. R., and Libby, P.,** Interleukin induces interleukin 1. II. Recombinant human interleukin 1 induces interleukin 1 production by adult human vascular endothelial cells, *J. Immunol.,* 139, 1911, 1987.
19. **Broudy, V. C., Kaushansky, K., Harlan, J. M., and Adamson, J. W.,** Interleukin 1 stimulates human endothelial cells to produce granulocyte-macrophage colony-stimulating factor and granulocyte colony-stimulating factor, *J. Immunol.,* 139, 464, 1988.
20. **Zsebo, K. M., Yuschenkoff, V. N., Schiffer, S., Chang, D., McCall, E., Dinarello, C. A., Brown, M. A., Altrock, B., and Bagby, G. C., Jr.,** Vascular endothelial cells and granulopoiesis, interleukin-1 stimulates release of G-CSF and GM-CSF, *Blood,* 71, 99, 1988.
21. **Varani, J., Bendelow, M. J., Sealey, D. E., Kunkel, S. L., Gannon, D. E., Ryan, U. S., and Ward, P. A.,** Tumor necrosis factor enhances susceptibility of vascular endothelial cells to neutrophil-mediated killing, *Lab. Invest.,* 59, 292, 1988.
22. **Carroll, M. C., Katzman, P., Alicott, E. M., Koller, B. H., Strominger, J. L., and Spies, T.,** Linkage map of the human major histocompatibility complex including the tumor necrosis factor genes, *Proc. Natl. Acad. Sci. U.S.A.,* 84, 8535, 1987.

23. **Granger, G. A. and Kolb, W. P.,** Lymphocyte in vitro cytotoxicity, mechanisms of immune and non-immune small lymphocyte mediated target L cell destruction, *J. Immunol.,* 101, 111, 1968.
24. **Ruddle, N. H. and Waksman, B. H.,** Cytotoxicity mediated by soluble antigen and lymphocytes in delayed hypersensitivity. III. Analysis of mechanism, *J. Exp. Med.,* 138, 1267, 1968.
25. **Matthews, N.,** Tumor-necrosis factor from the rabbit. II. Production by monocytes, *Br. J. Cancer,* 38, 310, 1978.
26. **Steffen, M., Oltman, O. G., and Moore, M. A. S.,** Simultaneous production of tumor necrosis factor α and lymphotoxin by normal T cells after induction with IL-1 and anti-T3, *J. Immunol.,* 140, 2621, 1988.
27. **Le, J. and Vilcek, J.,** Tumor necrosis factor and interleukin 1, cytokines with multiple overlapping biological activities, *Lab. Invest.,* 56, 234, 1988.
28. **Pober, J. S., Lapierre, L. A., Stolpen, A. H., Brock, T. A., Springer, T. A., Fiers, W., Bevilacqua, M. P., Mendrick, D. L., and Gimbrone, M. A., Jr.,** Activation of cultured human endothelial cells by recombinant lymphotoxin, comparisons with tumor necrosis factor and interleukin 1 species, *J. Immunol.,* 138, 3319, 1987.
29. **Cavender, D., Saegusa, Y., and Ziff, M.,** Stimulation of endothelial cell binding of lymphocytes by tumor necrosis factor, *J. Immunol.,* 139, 1855, 1987.
30. **Hughes, C. C. W., Male, D. K., and Lantos, P. L.,** Adhesion of lymphocytes to cerebral microvascular cells, effects of interferon γ, tumor necrosis factor and interleukin-1, *Immunology,* 64, 677, 1988.
31. **Libby, P., Ordovas, J. M., Auger, K. R., Robbins, A. H., Birinyi, L. K., and Dinarello, C. A.,** Endotoxin and tumor necrosis factor induce interleukin 1 gene expression in adult human vascular endothelial cells, *Am. J. Pathol.,* 124, 179, 1986.
32. **Locksley, R. M., Heinzel, F. P., Shepard, H. M., Agosti, J., Eessalu, T. E., Aggarwal, B. B., and Harlan, J. M.,** Tumor necrosis factor α and β differ in their capacities to generate interleukin 1 from human endothelial cells, *J. Immunol.,* 139, 1891, 1987.
33. **Nawroth, P. P., Bank, I., Handley, D., Cassimeris, J., Chees, I., and Stern, D.,** Tumor necrosis factor/cachectin interacts with endothelial cell receptors to induce release of interleukin 1, *J. Exp. Med.,* 163, 1363, 1986.
34. **Broudy, V. C., Kaushansky, K., Segal, G. M., Harlan, J. M., and Adamson, J. W.,** Tumor necrosis factor type α stimulates human endothelial cells to produce granulocyte/macrophage colony-stimulating factor, *Proc. Natl. Acad. Sci. U.S.A.,* 83, 7467, 1986.
35. **Munker, R. J., Gasson, J., Ogawa, M., and Koeffler, P.,** Recombinant human TNF induces production of granulocyte-monocyte colony-stimulating factor, *Nature (London),* 323, 79, 1986.
36. **Sieff, C. A., Niemeyer, C. M., and Faller, D. V.,** Interleukin 1, tumor necrosis factor and the production of colony-stimulating factors by cultured mesenchymal cells, *Blood,* 72, 1316, 1988.
37. **Bussolino, F., Camussi, J. G., and Baglioni, C.,** Synthesis and release of platelet-activating factor by human vascular endothelial cells treated with tumor necrosis factor or interleukin 1α, *J. Biol. Chem.,* 263, 11856, 1988.
38. **Messadi, D. V., Pober, J. S., Fiers, W., Gimbrone, M. A., Jr., and Murphy, G. F.,** Induction of an activation antigen on post-capillary venular endothelium in human skin organ culture, *J. Immunol.,* 139, 1557, 1987.
39. **Munro, J. M., Pober, J. S., and Cotran, R. S.,** Tumor necrosis factor and interferon-γ induce distinct patterns of endothelial activation and leukocyte accumulation in skin of *Papio anubus, Am. J. Pathol.,* 135, 121, 1989.

40. **Lapierre, L. A., Fiers, W., and Pober, J. S.,** Three distinct classes of regulatory cytokines control endothelial cell IMHC antigen expression, interactions with immune (γ) interferon differentiate the effects of tumor necrosis factor and lymphotoxin from those of leukocyte (α) and fibroblast (β) interferons, *J. Exp. Med.,* 167, 794, 1988.
41. **Gamble, J. R., Harlan, J. M., Klebanoff, S. J., and Vadas, M. A.,** Stimulation of the adherence of neutrophils to umbilical vein endothelium by human recombinant tumor necrosis factor, *Proc. Natl. Acad. Sci. U.S.A.,* 82, 8667, 1985.
42. **Demaeyer, E. and Demaeyer-Guignard, J.,** *Interferons and Other Regulatory Cytokines,* John Wiley & Sons, New York, 1988, 221.
43. **Brooimans, R. A., Hiemstra, P. S., Van Der Ark, A. A. J., Sim, R. B., Van Es, L. A., and Daha, M. R.,** Biosynthesis of complement factor H by human umbilical vein endothelial cells. Regulation by T cell growth factor and IFN-γ, *J. Immunol.,* 142, 2024, 1989.
44. **Luster, A. D., Unkeless, J. C., and Ravetch, J. V.,** γ-Interferon transcriptionally regulates an early-response gene containing homology to platelet proteins, *Nature (London),* 315, 672, 1985.
45. **Ripoche, J. J., Mitchell, A., Erdei, A., Madin, C., Moffatt, B., Mokoena, T., Gordon, S., and Sim, R. B.,** Interferon γ induces synthesis of complement alternative pathway proteins by human endothelial cells in culture, *J. Exp. Med.,* 168, 1917, 1988.
46. **Collins, T., Lapierre, L. A., Fiers, W., Strominger, J. L., and Pober, J. S.,** Recombinant human tumor necrosis factor increases mRNA levels and surface expression of HLA-A, B antigens in vascular endothelial cells and dermal fibroblasts in vitro, *Proc. Natl. Acad. Sci. U.S.A.,* 83, 446, 1986.
47. **Masuyama, J., Minato, N., and Kano, S.,** Mechanisms of lymphocyte adhesion to human vascular endothelial cells in culture. T lymphocyte adhesion to endothelial cells through endothelial HLA-DR antigens induced by γ interferon, *J. Clin. Invest.,* 77, 1596, 1986.
48. **Pober, J. S., Collins, T., Gimbrone, M. A., Jr., Cotran, R. S., Gitlin, J. D., Fiers, W., Clayberger, C., Krensky, A. M., Burakoff, S. J., and Reiss, C. S.,** Lymphocytes recognize human vascular endothelial and dermal fibroblast Ia antigens induced by recombinant immune interferon, *Nature (London),* 305, 726, 1983.
49. **Pober, J. S., Gimbrone, M. A., Jr., Cotran, R. S., Reiss, C. S., Burakoff, S. J., Fiers, W., and Ault, K. A.,** Ia expression by vascular endothelium is inducible by activated T cells and by human γ interferon, *J. Exp. Med.,* 157, 1339, 1983.
50. **Wagner, C. R., Vetto, R. M., and Burger, D. R.,** Expression of I-Region-Associated Antigen (Ia) and interleukin 1 by subcultured human endothelial cells, *Cell. Immunol.,* 93, 91, 1985.
51. **Yu, C.-L., Haskard, D. O., Johnson, A. R., and Ziff, M.,** Human γ interferon increases binding of T lymphocytes to endothelial cells, *Cell. Immunol.,* 62, 554, 1985.
52. **Thornhill, M. H., Williams, D. H., and Speight, P. M.,** Enhanced adhesion of autologous lymphocytes to γ-interferon-treated human endothelial cells in vitro, *Br. J. Exp. Pathol.,* 70, 59, 1989.
53. **Dewall, R. M. W., Bogman, M. J. J., Maass, C. I. N., Cornelissen, L. M. H., Tax, W. J. M., and Koene, R. A. P.,** Variable expression of Ia antigens on the vascular endothelium of mouse skin allografts, *Nature (London),* 303, 426, 1983.
54. **Cotran, R. S. and Pober, J. S.,** Endothelial activation, its role in inflammatory and immune reactions, in *Endothelial Cell Biology,* Simionescu, N. and Simionescu, M., Eds., Plenum Press, New York, 1988, 335.
55. **Bevilacqua, M. P., Pober, J. S., Mendrick, D. L., Cotran, R. S., and Gimbrone, M. A., Jr.,** Identification of an inducible endothelial-leukocyte adhesion molecule, *Proc. Natl. Acad. Sci. U.S.A.,* 84, 9238, 1987.

56. **Pober, J. S.,** Cytokine-mediated activation of vascular endothelium, physiology and pathology, *Am. J. Pathol.,* 133, 426, 1988.
57. **Greene, M. I., Schalten, S., and Bromberg, J. S.,** Delayed hypersensitivity, in *Fundamental Immunology*, Paul, W. E., Ed., Raven Press, New York, 1984, 685.
58. **Smith, K. A.,** Interleukin-2, inception, impact and implications, *Science,* 240, 1169, 1988.
59. **Pober, J. S., Collins, T., Gimbrone, M. A., Jr., Libby, P., and Reiss, C. S.,** Inducible expression of class II major histocompatibility complex antigens and the immunogenicity of vascular endothelium, *Transplantation,* 41, 141, 1986.
60. **Leung, D. Y. M., Cotran, R. S., Kurt-Jones, E. A., Burns, J. C., Newburger, J. W., and Pober, J. S.,** Endothelial activation and high interleukin-1 secretion in the pathogenesis of acute Kawasaki disease, *Lancet,* 2, 12982, 1989.
61. **Leung, D. Y. M., Collins, T., Lapierre, L. A., Geha, R. S., and Pober, J. S.,** IgM antibodies in the acute phase of Kawasaki syndrome lyse cultured vascular endothelial cells stimulated by γ interferon, *J. Clin. Invest.,* 77, 1428, 1986.
62. **Leung, D. Y. M., Geha, R. S., Newburger, J. W., Burns, J. C., Fiers, W, Lapierre, L. A., and Pober, J. S.,** Two monokines, interleukin 1 and tumor necrosis factor, render cultured vascular endothelial cells susceptible to lysis by antibodies circulating during Kawasaki Syndrome, *J. Exp. Med.,* 164, 1958, 1986.
63. **Leung, D. Y. M., Moake, J. L., Havens, P. L., Kim, J. M., and Pober, J. S.,** Lytic anti-endothelial cell antibodies are present in hemolytic uremic syndrome, *Lancet,* 1, 183, 1988.

Chapter 9

Thermal Injury

Daniel L. Traber, Christopher W. Lentz, Charles S. Cox, Jr., Lillian D. Traber, and David N. Herndon

CONTENTS

I. INTRODUCTION

Approximately 2 million people were injured in fire accidents in the U.S. from 1965 to 1986.[1] Over 130,000 of these individuals required hospitalization. Although statistics for thermal injury in the world are not available, the number of individuals who are burned annually is staggering. In addition to the debilitating aspects of thermal injury that result from fire accidents, a large number of individuals sustain first- and second-degree thermal injury as a result of ultraviolet radiation. If the number of victims who in addition to burn injury sustain an injury to their airway as a result of the inhalation of smoke are taken into consideration, then it becomes quite obvious that thermal injury is a very significant problem.

The immediate effect of the high temperatures that occur in fires is damage to the cutaneous areas. When the entire dermal thickness is destroyed it is difficult, if not impossible, for the skin to regenerate. This is a problem which has created a considerable interest at the time of this writing. Perhaps more important to the ultimate fate of the victim of fire accidents, thermal injury to the cutaneous areas produces a leakiness of the microcirculation so massive as to induce hypovolemic shock and probable death in the underresuscitated individual. In addition to the effects of hypovolemic shock and reperfusion, this thermally induced edema may likewise produce tissue damage and interfere with the healing processes.

0-8493-4547-2/94/$0.00+$.50

Victims of fire accidents, especially those who are injured in enclosed areas, sustain chemical injury to their respiratory tract as a result of breathing the toxic gases associated with the incomplete combustion of the burning materials, especially acrolein and formaldehyde.[2-4] A majority of the tissue injury and morbidity induced by inhalation injury is the result of microcirculatory changes in the systemic circulation to the airway as well as the pulmonary microvasculature. This chapter will describe the processes involved in inducing the microcirculatory pathophysiology associated with the edema formation which occurs with thermal damage and smoke inhalation.

II. EDEMA FORMATION IN THE BURN WOUND

Historically, one of the clinical hallmarks of thermal injury is the loss of body fluid. The primary appreciation of second-degree thermal injury is the appearance of a blister. The patient with large burns may manifest the fluid loss as hemoconcentration and subsequent hypotension. The treatment of this form of hypovolemia is the administration of intravenous fluids which has markedly improved survival of burn victims.[5-7] Fluid resuscitation is also associated with edema in both burned and unburned skin, internal tissues, and other organs.[8] These observations have led to investigations into the microvascular changes that induce the fluid shifts which occur with thermal injury.

A. STARLING-LANDIS FORCES

Edema in burned patients results from the loss of plasma fluid into the interstitium. The local and distant edema formation may result in (1) hypovolemia, (2) impairment of vital organ function, (3) conversion of viable second-degree burns to third-degree burns, and (4) impairment of local tissue perfusion. Edema is more pronounced in second-degree burns compared to full thickness burns which are completely devitalized. If burned areas exceed approximately 30% total body surface area (TBSA), then edema involving noninjured skin and internal tissues may occur.[9,10] To adequately review the microvascular changes that occur during and after burn injury, the Starling-Landis equation variables must be considered.[11,12]

$$J_v = K_f[(P_c - P_{if}) - \sigma(COP_p - COP_{if})]$$

This equation describes the physical forces and physiologic mechanisms which govern fluid transfer between vascular and extravascular compartments. The equation has been discussed in detail in earlier chapters in this book and it is presented here to focus on the possible mechanisms responsible for the transvascular fluid flux following thermal injury.

B. TRANSVASCULAR FLUID FLUX

Since the early experiments of Ernest Starling in 1896, investigators have used lymph flow as an index of transvascular fluid flux.[12] In an elegant series of experiments, Arturson and his group examined lymph flow from the scalded paws of anesthetized cats and dogs.[13-15] Cutaneous lymph flow changes have been evaluated in our laboratory following thermal injury.[16] We determined that there was a sevenfold increase in lymph flow from the cutaneous areas on the flank (prefemoral lymphatic) of sheep following a third-degree flame burn. This is illustrated in Figure 1. The change in lymph flow occurs almost immediately and is sustained for the 48-h period of observation. Similar changes in lymph flow were reported from the prefemoral lymphatic following a third-degree scald burn in sheep.[17] In the latter situations, the studies were accomplished in chronically prepared sheep and, although the injury was induced under anesthesia, the animals were fully awake within minutes of injury and during the period of study. This is possible since

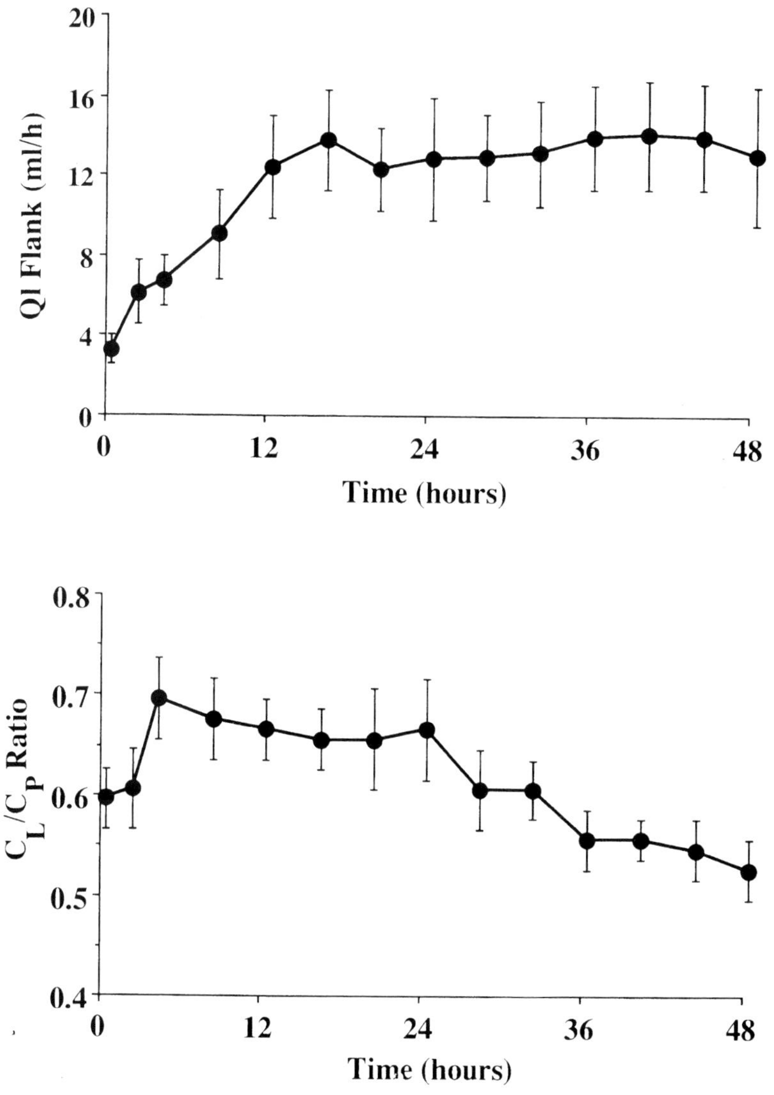

Figure 9-1 (Upper) After cutaneous thermal injury in sheep, the prefemoral lymph flow increases sevenfold, reaching a peak at 18 h post injury. (Lower) The lymph protein (C_L) to plasma protein (C_P) ratio quickly increased with concomitant increases in lymph flow indicative of an increase in microvascular permeability.

in both cases the injury was full thickness and thus the pain fibers were destroyed. These factors are emphasized to demonstrate the tremendous increase in transvascular fluid flux noted and the lack of probable experimental artifact. Similar changes in fluid flux have been demonstrated in thermally injured rats and guinea pigs using gravimetric and tracer techniques.[18,19]

Table 9-1 **Prefemoral lymphatic data 24 h after inhalation and thermal injury**

Group	Lymph Flow (ml/h)	C_L/C_P Ratio	Total Volume (ml)	Plasma (ml)	CI (L/min/m^2)
Sham	2.8 ± 0.6	0.33 ± 0.03	2480 ± 523	0	5.8 ± 0.5
Smoke (S)	8.0 ± 2.4*	0.25 ± 0.04	4386 ± 561*	140 ± 80	5.1 ± 0.4
Burn (B)	10.8 ± 2.3*	0.45 ± 0.05†	6122 ± 521*	1065 ± 223†	5.4 ± 0.8
S + B	19.8 ± 2.3*†‡	0.46 ± 0.03†	6277 ± 942*	805 ± 129†	6.0 ± 0.4

Note: Lymph protein to plasma protein ratio (C_L/C_P), total volume of resuscitation to maintain a urine output between 0.5 to 1.0 ml/kg/h (total volume), plasma infusion required to maintain plasma protein of 5.0 ± 0.05 g/dl (plasma), cardiac index (CI). Significant vs. sham group, † significant vs. smoke group, ‡ significant vs. burn group, $p < 0.05$ (ANOVA, Neuman-Keuls).

1. Reflection Coefficient

Historically, the edema formation seen in the burn wound has been attributed to a change in the microvascular permeability. This conclusion was reached as a result of the discovery that blister fluid contained high concentrations of proteins. The finding of protein in high concentrations in the lymph draining the burn wound has likewise been reported as proof that the changes in microvascular permeability was secondary to a change in the microvascular permeability to protein. The reflection coefficient (σ) is an index of the microvascular permeability to plasma proteins. A σ of 1.0 represents an impermeable membrane; a σ of 0 represents a completely permeable membrane. Montero and others noted an increase in prefemoral lymph flow with an increased lymph to plasma protein ratio in burned sheep.[16] The data of Montero are shown in Figure 1 and Table 1. The changes in lymph flow are immediate and occur with a relatively constant lymph to plasma protein concentration ratio. The lymph protein rises with time post burn, reaching a peak at about 4 h. These data support the concept that burn edema formation is due in part to an increased microvascular permeability.

Arturson and his group evaluated microvascular permeability in the thermally injured dog paw. They graded the depth of injury by controlling the temperature of the water which produced the injury.[15] Increased depth of burn was associated with a rise in lymph protein concentration. With second-degree burns, the lymph flow increased, however the protein level did not change. In other studies using the *canine* preparation they demonstrated that high molecular weight dextran would leak from the wound following injury. Using differing molecular weights of dextran, they showed that the capillaries were more permeable to smaller molecules in mild scald burns. Severe burn injury was associated with permeability of molecules up to 80,000 Da. The maximal protein flux across the microvasculature was determined to be at 2 to 3 h post burn. Techniques using radiolabeled albumin supported these findings, showing the maximal protein leakage post injury at 30 min and maximal tissue water content occurred at 3 h post burn.[18] As time post burn injury progressed in the dog and rat preparation, the permeability returned to the preburn level. This was not seen in sheep either in our studies or those of Demling et al.[20,21] In our studies we maintained plasma protein levels by the administration of fresh frozen plasma, a procedure not performed by Demling's group who resuscitated their animals with Ringer's solution. In the experiments performed in dogs and rats, the animals were not resuscitated to normal cardiac outputs and filling pressures. Perhaps the resuscitation process itself maintained the permeability phenomena.

Although the studies we have thus far discussed present data to support the increased permeability to protein, the actual reflection coefficient, σ, was not determined. Using an outflow occlusion technique, Pitt et al.[22] studied the lymph drainage from the dog paw and found σ to be 0.87 in control, nonburned animals, and this fell to 0.47 at 2 h after third-degree burn injury. They likewise determined the various protein fractions that were filtered and from these data calculated effective pore radii of the skin of the dog paw. Prior to thermal injury, there were two populations of pores, one at 50 Å and the other at 300 Å, with 13% of the pores being in the larger category. Two hours following thermal injury, the pore sizes changed to 70 and 400 Å and 49% of the pores were of the larger variety. These changes in large pore size accounted for the reduction in reflection coefficient. There was a 240% increase in filtration coefficient in these studies as well. These data were not determined at other times post injury since these were acute experiments. Additional evidence that the microvascular gaps are huge in the burned areas following third-degree burn can also be found in the works of Demling et al.[17,23] and Honeycutt et al.[24] These investigators resuscitated some of their sheep with high molecular weight starch compounds. In the case of Demling and his colleagues, this consisted of Dextran-70; Honeycutt et al. used pentafraction with an average molecular weight of 200,000. Neither of these compounds affected the lymph flow from the thermally injured soft tissue of the sheep. This more accurately quantified the permeability change in the microvasculature that contributed to the observed increase in lymph flow and protein flux in other experimental animal models.

The effect of changes in σ on transvascular fluid flux can be determined by examining the Starling-Landis equation. By decreasing σ, the colloid oncotic pressure (COP) gradient that promotes the resorption of fluid into the microvasculature markedly decreases. These decreases, however, can only increase net filtration pressure by approximately 10 mmHg, and this cannot explain the driving pressures of 250 mmHg calculated by Arturson that are required to produce the edema seen experimentally.[25] In the studies of Pitt et al., only 47% of the increased capillary filtration was attributable to permeability.[22] Permeability will not account for the changes in microvascular filtration seen with smaller burns. Therefore, other factors are at play in inducing edema formation.

2. Capillary Hydrostatic Pressure

Capillary pressures are influenced by the arterial and venous pressures and the capillary resistance. In the studies by Pitt et al., capillary pressures were estimated using the occlusion technique and found to be almost doubled following thermal injury — from 24 to 48 mmHg after thermal injury to the paw of the dog.[22] In these studies, the pre- and postmicrovascular resistances were calculated, and the changes in microvascular pressure were found to be attributable to a reduced precapillary resistance with the postcapillary resistance remaining virtually at the preburn level. In their calculations, they assumed that the interstitial hydrostatic pressure was negligible or zero. At 3 h after burn injury, the pressure gradient contribution to fluid filtration was considered to be 28%, with increased permeability accounting for 72%. Early after the burn injury the pressure contribution was higher, accounting for 69% of the fluid filtration.

It is most interesting to compare the findings of Pitt et al. with those of Arturson and Mellander.[25] In these latter studies, the Swedish group investigated the cat paw. At 1 h post thermal injury, they likewise found that a high pressure gradient was needed to produce the measured changes in net capillary filtration. Their data are virtually identical with those recorded by Pitt et al. at that time.[22] Although they did not measure the exact capillary pressures, as was the case with the Mobile investigators, the Swedes calculated the resistance changes in the paw and determined that such a large change in resistance would only be possible with a dilation of arterioles and venular constriction. Thus the increased microvascular pressure was attributable to reduced precapillary resistance by both groups of investigators using two different animal models, on two different continents, over 25 years apart.

Arturson and Mellander measured microvascular filtration within a minute of thermal insult. They estimated that the driving forces needed to produce the early changes in microvascular filtration had to be on the order of 250 to 300 mmHg.[25] This is much greater than can be accounted for by a change in microvascular pressure. Consequently, other forces must be involved.

3. Interstitial Fluid Hydrostatic Pressure

As mentioned above, permeability and microvascular hydrostatic pressure changes alone cannot explain the extravasation of fluid shifts which occur from the vasculature into the interstitial space following thermal injury. In the 1960s, Arturson and Mellander examined the acute changes in capillary filtration and edema formation in burned tissues.[25] From the increase in lymph flow, filtration coefficient should have increased by 1500% to account for the accumulation of edema fluid. However, they found that the filtration coefficient only increased by 100 to 300%; therefore, a transcapillary pressure gradient of approximately 200 to 300 mmHg must exist to account for the fluid shifts. Since this was impossible to develop on the vascular side, they suggested:

A transcapillary osmotic pressure gradient is immediately created by the thermic lesion. The mechanisms responsible for the increased extravascular osmolality are not clear. A plausible explanation is release of intracellular molecules into the interstitial fluid.[14]

More recently, Lund et al.[26] continuously measured interstitial pressure (P_{if}) with a micropipette in the burned dermis of rats. In an elegant group of experiments, they demonstrated an acute, early drop in P_{if} to –120 mmHg after a 40% TBSA burn injury, and –16 mmHg after a 10% TBSA burn injury. The extent of the drop in P_{if} correlated with the extent of burn injury, i.e., greater decreases in P_{if} were observed with larger TBSA burned. This discovery helps to account for the predictions of Arturson. The finding of a graded change in the interstitial pressure helps to explain the findings of Arturson and Soeda[15] that there was a graded increase in transvascular fluid flux without a significant change in filtration coefficient following small burns. The Norwegian investigators attribute the changes in pressure to a breakdown of collagen with an expansion of the interstitial matrix. The interstitial COP may rise due to formation of new macromolecules or collagen degradation products acting as newly generated colloids.[27] Using Arturson's estimates that a driving pressure of approximately 200 to 300 mmHg is required to quantitatively explain the edema formed after burn injury, Lund et al. state that the "imbibition pressure" would account for this difference. After this initial increase in the P_{if}, this pressure then returns to –8 to –10 mmHg after 2 h. These latter measurements are fairly consistent with assumptions that P_{if} is zero when calculating K_f and the relative contributions of pressure and permeability to increased microvascular fluid flux in the early period after burn injury.

In their studies, Lund et al.[27] found that the early rise in the interstitial oncotic pressure with thermal injury were proportional to the degree of injury. The larger the burn, the greater the reduction in interstitial pressure that was recorded. These data help to explain the phenomena, previously reported by Arturson and Soeda,[15] that with increasing size of burn there was an increase in lymph flow from the thermally injured dog paw. In addition, if one adds the findings of Lund and his group to the data from Arturson and Pitt and their colleagues, then all of the forces necessary to produce the changes in microcirculatory function needed to produce the transvascular fluid flux are seen in the first few hours following thermal injury.

4. Plasma Colloid Osmotic Pressure

In the above studies there were acute elevations in plasma osmotic pressure as the fluid rushed from the vascular to the interstitial space immediately after thermal injury.[13] Then, as the permeability to protein increased in the first hours after thermal injury, the colloid osmotic pressure falls as the protein flows into the interstitium. The degree of this fall is, of course, dependent on the total surface area which is burned. A reduction in plasma colloid osmotic pressures (COP_p) is a common finding in burned patients during their hospital course.[8] During the resuscitation phase, this is explained, from the standpoint of our early discussion, by the relative movement of the plasma protein into the interstitium. In addition, the fluid used for resuscitation is typically of a crystalloid nature, and thus will dilute plasma protein concentrations.[28-30]

In addition to these changes, there are also modifications in the synthesis of plasma proteins that affect their levels following thermal injury. With burns, the pain, fear, and regulatory events that surround the changes in plasma volume, cardiac output, and mean arterial pressure, induce a release of catecolamines into the circulation.[31,32] In addition to the cardiovascular changes that these neuronal mediators induce, they also have been shown to cause the release of interleukin-6.[33,34] This cytokine stimulates the synthesis of acute phase reactants and reduces the formation of albumin.[33,34] In addition, the thermally injured patients have a markedly elevated breakdown in body protein that can also contribute to a fall in plasma protein, especially albumin.[7,35]

5. Interstitial Colloid Osmotic Pressure

The contribution of the interstitial colloid oncotic pressure (COP_{if}) to edema formation has not been studied as extensively as vascular pressures and plasma COP due to the inherent difficulty in sampling interstitial fluid. Most investigators use subcutaneous wicks under burned tissue to measure COP in the interstitium.[27] As stated above, the observed reduction in the COP_p is thought to be accompanied by an increase in the COP_{if}. The Norwegian investigators demonstrated a reversal in the normal COP gradient with $COP_{if} > COP_p$ following thermal injury in rats[36] and humans.[37] Lund et al. likewise reported that the COP_{if} increased over time and with increasing duration of heat exposure.[27] They proposed that the increase in COP_{if} was due to the formation of split products of collagen acting as newly formed colloids together with extravasated plasma proteins. Heat exposure could also result in a change in the steric conformation of the collagen triple helix to provide a larger space for movement of water and small solutes into this space to increase COP_{if}. More recently, Onarheim and Reed[38] have reported that the plasma to interstitial oncotic pressure was reduced by thermal injury. This phenomenon was made worse by resuscitating the animals with Ringer's solution. The use of plasma for resuscitation restored the gradient once again.

To summarize, the edema formed in burned tissue is the result of an increased driving pressure that favors fluid entry into the interstitium. This pressure is primarily a "suction or imbibition pressure" immediately after burn. Increases in hydrostatic capillary pressures contribute about 20 to 30% of the driving pressure of fluid filtration. To a lesser extent, increased microvascular permeability contributes to the fluid filtration across the microvasculature after burn injury. The driving pressures that contribute to edema formation after thermal injury are summarized in Figure 2.

C. INFLAMMATORY MEDIATORS

There has been a great deal of research by the Ward and Till group at the University of Michigan at Ann Arbor on the mediation of the edema formation in the burn wound.[39] These investigators demonstrated a very strong link between changes in microvascular permeability, evaluated by flux of radioactively tagged albumin, and the release of oxygen free radicals.[40] The latter was determined by measuring lipid peroxidation products, and treatment with oxygen free radical scavengers from a number of sources and administration of iron chelating materials.[41] These latter have an effect since iron is a key catalyst in the formation of hydroxyl ion. These studies consequently demonstrated a strong correlation between the changes in microvascular permeability and oxygen free radical release.

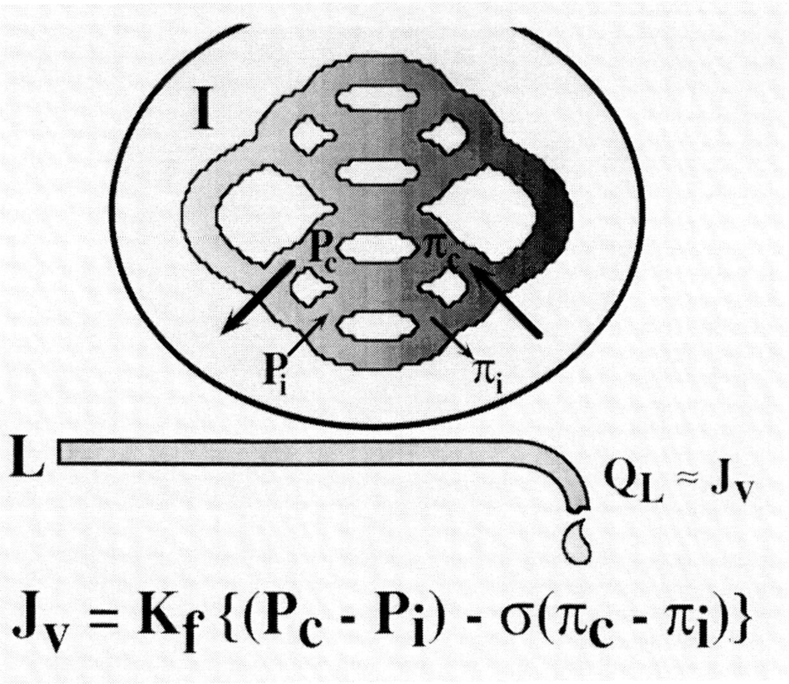

Figure 9-2 Diagram of the Starling-Landis forces after burn injury. The variables measured by different investigators account for the edema formation observed after thermal injury. Reflection coefficient (σ) decreases from 0.85 to 0.47 after thermal injuy. Interstitial pressure (P_i) decreases from 0 to –1 mmHg to –150 mmHg to create a negative pressure that pulls fluid into the interstitium. The capillary pressure (P_c) increases from 24 to 48 mmHg after thermal injury. Plasma colloid osmotic pressure (Π_p) decreases from approximately 25 to 10 mmHg after thermal injury. Interstitial fluid colloid osmotic pressure (Π_i) remains relatively constant, but can increase from 10 to 15 mmHg depending on the COP of the plasma. Capillary filtration coefficient (K_f) increases from 0.04 to approximately 0.1 ml (mmHg/min/100g tissue) Transvascular fluid flux (J_v) can be estimated by measuring lymph flow.

The most common phagocytic cell in the cutaneous area is the polymorphonuclear neutrophil. Yet when the Michigan group depleted their animals of these cells, it had no effect upon the formation of oxygen radicals.[41] They consequently evaluated other sources of oxygen free radical formation. In additional studies, they demonstrated that the inhibitor of xanthine oxidase, allopurinol, would block the formation of lipid peroxidation products and the changes in microvascular permeability seen with thermal injury.[41] This response was likewise affected by the administration of an antihistamine, in this case a H_2 receptor antagonist. The major source of histamine is the mast cell. The release of histamine and the edema formation was prevented by the use of the drug cromolyn, which stabilizes mast cells, and by depletion of complement.[42] They therefore proposed that histamine was released after thermal injury secondary to complement activation,[42] which this group also found to be elevated. Histamine caused the conversion of xanthine decarboxylase to xanthine oxidase.[43] The latter enzyme releases oxygen free radicals when it converts hypoxanthine to xanthine.[44,45] In the studies of the Michigan group, they demonstrated an elevation of plasma xanthine oxidase in parallel with a rise in histamine following thermal injury.[42]

These investigators also demonstrated that the oxygen free radicals formed at the site of thermal injury would also result in the further formation of hemolytic complement.[46] Hemolysis and complement release are common entities following thermal injury.[47,48] Histamine release from the burn wound was also reported by Arturson, who found an elevation in histamine in the lymph draining the burned paw of the dog following thermal injury.[49] In earlier work, Brimblecombe and Farrington[50] have also reported that they could antagonize burn edema in the rat with a histamine H_2 receptor blocker.

In support of the hypotheses that have been put forth by the Michigan group, Demling and LaLonde[51] have reported that there was an elevation of lipid peroxidation products in the lymph draining the burn wound of thermally injured sheep. The plasma levels of these materials were likewise elevated in these animals. They were able to prevent the rise in lipid peroxidation products and the elevation of lymph flowing from the burned skin by pretreating the animals with allopurinol, a drug that blocks xanthine oxidase.

There is ample evidence for a massive release of oxygen free radicals following thermal injury. In recent studies accomplished in human patients with severe thermal injury, we were able to demonstrate a massive release of oxygen free radicals, which was apparently related to polymorphonuclear (PMN) cell activation.[52] We measured elastase levels as a marker for PMN activation/degranulation. Nonsurviving patients had concomitant smoke inhalation injury and a more rapid consumption of circulating plasma antioxidants (vitamin E and total sulfhydryl groups). However, the nonsurvivors did not have higher circulating elastase levels compared to burned patients without smoke inhalation injury. Lipid peroxidation was recently reported in thermally injured patients by others.[53] Consequently, the concepts espoused by the Michigan group are of considerable interest. They have recently reported that they could reduce lipid peroxidation in thermally injured patients by treating them with superoxide dismutase, the enzyme which converts superoxide to hydrogen peroxide.[54]

In the above discussion concerning the changes in microvascular pressure which occur following thermal injury, we noted that there was a reduction in the precapillary microvascular resistance and that the postcapillary resistance remained unchanged. The mechanisms responsible for the precapillary vasodilatation noted with thermal injury are as yet uninvestigated. However, the concept of edema mediation by histamine release following thermal injury might also explain this phenomena. Since the time of Henry Dale, it has been known that histamine is an arteriolar dilator in dog and man.[55,56] Recently, it has been shown that the vasodilatation induced by the autocoid is mediated by the release of nitric oxide.[57] Thus, with thermal injury, activation of mast cells in the cutaneous areas, release of histamine, and subsequent release of nitric oxide by the endothelial cells results in vasodilation. This is an explanation for the precapillary dilation noted. The question to be answered is, why isn't there a vasodilatation of the postcapillary areas of the cutaneous microvasculature? This phenomenon may be related to the fact that histamine likewise induces the formation of oxygen free radicals. These have been demonstrated to inactivate nitric oxide by oxidation.[58] Thus, if one were to follow this line of reasoning, thermal injury histamine induces the release of nitric oxide in the precapillary areas, causing an arteriolar or precapillary dilation. Histamine also induces a release of nitric oxide in the postcapillary smooth muscle and or vascular endothelium, but this material is oxidized before it can induce a vasodilatation. Therefore, one can explain the phenomena observed following thermal injury, as summarized in Figure 3.

Eicosanoids, especially prostaglandins and thromboxanes, have likewise been implicated as probable mediators of burned wound edema since their presence in blister fluid was first reported by Arturson et al.[59] His group also reported the release of prostaglandin E_2 in the lymph draining the burn wound, and the administration of indomethacin, a cycloxoygenase inhibitor, would depress the elevation in burn lymph formation which

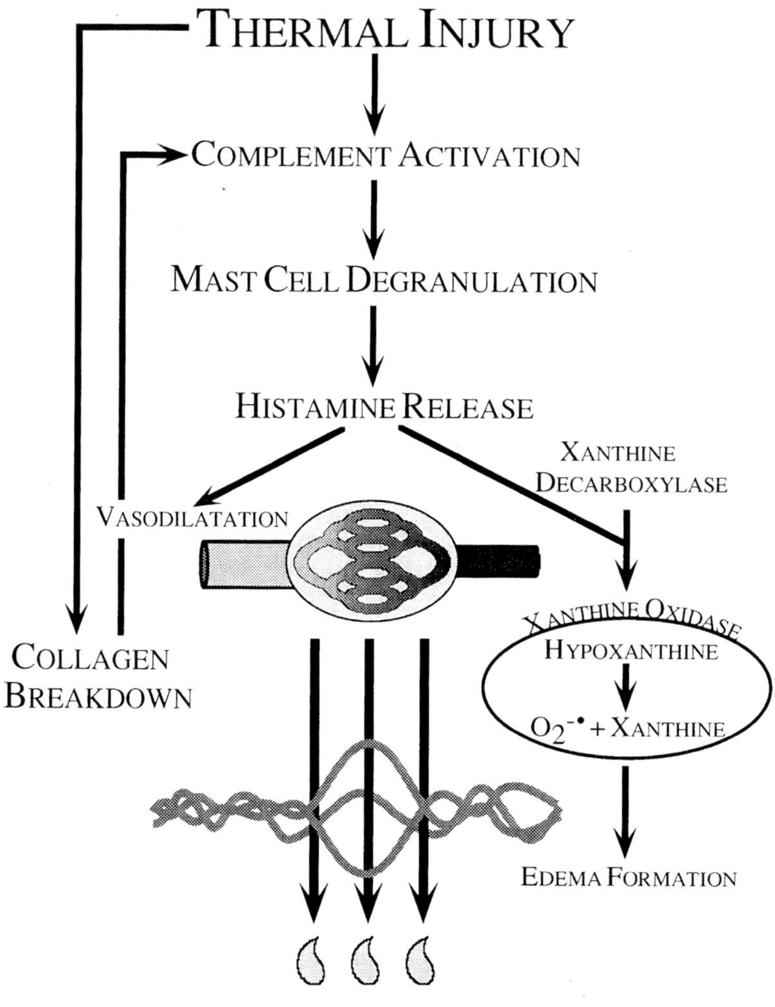

Figure 9-3 The mechanism of tissue edema following thermal injury. Thermal injury induces complement activation which results in histamine release through mast cell degranulation. Histamine produces arteriolar vasodilatation and is also responsible for the conversion of xanthine decarboxylase to xanthine oxidase. This ultimately results in formation of xanthine and oxygen free radicals which contribute to edema formation. Thermal injury directly injures tissue, denaturing collagen to produce the negative interstitial "imbibition" pressure described by Lund.[27] Exposed collagen fibers, in turn, perpetuate complement activation.

occurs following thermal injury without affecting the permeability of the tissue.[14] Hilton and Wells[60] also reported a reduction of burn edema in the dog with the administration of nicotinic acid, which they likewise attributed to the blockade of the synthesis of prostaglandins. Similarly, Demling and LaLonde[61] have reported that application of ibuprofen, a cyclooxygenase inhibitor, to the burn wound decreased early postburn edema and the lymph drainage from the burned wound without affecting the protein concentration, again suggesting an action of the eicosanoids on microvascular pressure. They demonstrated a moderate increase in thromboxane B_2, the stable metabolite of the potent vasoconstrictor thromboxane A_2, in the lymph drainage from the untreated burned wound. In a later study, this pair of investigators was unable to demonstrate an important effect of intravenously administered ibuprofen on the formation of protein-rich skin lymph, which is formed following burn injury in the sheep.[51] Herndon et al.[62] have reported elevated thromboxane B_2 levels in thermally injured patients. The exact role that it plays in the edema formation of the burn wound seems to be related to pressure mediation of edema formation. But apparently this is a minor effect.

In summary, the changes in microvascular permeability may be due to microvascular damage from oxygen free radicals produced by PMNs. The vasodilation phenomenon that contributes to the postburn microvascular pressure changes may also be explained by nitric oxide release in the burn wound.

III. EDEMA IN NONBURNED TISSUE

A. UNBURNED SKIN

Edema of the soft tissues of nonburned areas is a common finding in thermally injured patients. Edema in nonburned areas generally occurs after thermal injuries of greater than 25 to 30% TBSA. Carvajal et al.[9] studied the effects of edema in nonburned tissues of rats with burns ranging from 10 to 40% TBSA. Edema formation occurred in distant tissues only in burns of 30% TBSA or greater, and the edema disappeared 12 h after thermal injury. Demling's group examined edema formation in unburned tissue using the prefemoral lymph fistula model in sheep with 25% TBSA burns.[63] Their findings confirmed those of Carvajal, showing that there was a transient increase in lymph flow and increase in the lymph to plasma protein ratio lasting about 12 h. They also noted that the protein permeability was only to small (58 Å) molecules compared to the permeability in burned tissues (108 Å molecules). A criticism of the studies is that the sheep received a large volume of lactated Ringer's with 4 ml/kg/% body surface area burned plus an additional 1000 ml of fluid. Most clinicians do not fluid resuscitate burns of less than 30% TBSA. Although interesting, these data may not have clinical correlates.

The common practice of resuscitating thermally injured patients with exceptionally large volumes of a noncolloid-containing material may be a partial explanation for edema formation in unburned tissue, since this practice certainly reduces plasma protein concentrations and thus effective oncotic pressure. Studies by Arturson[14] and his group determined transvascular fluid flux using a cutaneous lymphatic. The vascular permeability was evaluated using dextran molecules of differing molecular weights. In these elaborate investigations, thermal injury was induced to the lower torso of the dog (approximately 50% TBSA) and cervical lymph was collected. They determined that the cutaneous lymph flow was elevated in both the burned and nonburned tissues. The lymph flow draining the burned areas likewise demonstrated an elevation in high molecular weight dextran materials. Lymph draining the nonburned areas, although demonstrating an elevation in permeability to dextran molecules, did not show an elevation in molecular weight species of the caliber of albumin. Thus, these studies demonstrate that edema in nonburned areas can likewise occur following thermal injury as a result of changes in the caliber of small pores. These investigations were accomplished in animals which were not fluid resuscitated, consequently they were not the result of the fall in oncotic pressure that would be associated with the dilution of plasma protein with fluid containing no protein. Although there are no reports of treatments on the effects of thermal injury on the nonburned skin, Kramer et al.[21] reported that the addition of colloid, in the form of dextran, to the resuscitation solution, reduced the amount of lymph flowing from the uninjured soft tissue following thermal injury.

B. THE LUNG

The changes to the microcirculation of the lung in thermally injured animals is somewhat controversial. For the most part, damage to the lung of burned patients without inhalation injury or some other form of pulmonary trauma is almost never observed.[64-66] In a similar fashion, Demling and his colleagues have reported a modest increase in protein-poor lung lymph following thermal injury. These changes are, as we have stated above, in animals heavily resuscitated with crystaloid solutions.[17,67,68] There is a suggestion that these changes may be the result of the large amount of fluid administered to their animals without colloid since the addition of colloid to the resuscitation mixture reduces the lung lymph flow.[17,23,68] On the other hand, these animals likewise showed an elevation in pulmonary microvascular pressure, and increased levels of thromboxane B_2. These changes can be reversed by the administration of ibuprofen, the cyclooxygenase inhibitor.[68]

Demling and his colleagues reported that, following cutaneous thermal injury, the lungs contained lipid peroxidation products and increased numbers of neutrophils but did not demonstrate tissue edema.[68,69] A controversy exists because Ward and Till and their colleagues have consistently reported increased pulmonary microvascular injury following thermal injury in rats.[70-72] They report that the injury is mediated by complement activation, the deposition of polymorphonuclear cells in the microvasculature, and the release of oxygen free radicals. As proof of their hypothesis, they were able to reverse these changes by depletion of complement, neutrophils, or the use of oxygen free radical scavengers.[70-74] Their findings are very similar to those which Granger[75] and his group have seen with reperfusion injury in the gut. One consequently wonders if these are the phenomena seen by Ward's group. The rat is extremely sensitive to volume loss and the rats were given little fluid resuscitation. Certainly they were not monitored in a way that would have ensured adequate fluid resuscitation. Lung damage, as a result of a reperfusion injury to the pulmonary circulation, has been reported in rabbits[76,77] and dogs.[78] In addition, peripheral ischemia can lead to lung damage and edema.[79,80] It is interesting to note that in these cases the lung damage appears to be resolved by agents which interfere with the action of thromboxane.[78,81]

IV. INHALATION INJURY

As was mentioned earlier, inhalation injury is a very serious problem in fire accident victims, and is responsible for significant morbidity and mortality.[82-84] This injury results in major pathologic changes in the microvasculature of the bronchial and pulmonary circulation.[65,85,86] In addition, various mediators released from the damaged tissue affect systemic capillary beds.[16,86] Host defenses, namely inflammatory cells, also contribute to the pathophysiology through the production of oxygen metabolites and the release of proteolytic enzymes.[87,88] The numerous effects on the microcirculation contribute to edema formation and tissue destruction.

The changes of the airway microcirculation are immediately apparent following smoke inhalation. The most widely accepted diagnosis of inhalation injury is bronchoscopic evidence of hyperemia and edema.[89,90] The responses of the pulmonary and bronchial circulation of the sheep and dog following inhalation injury have received considerable attention since these models mimic the response seen in man. The *ovine* model of inhalation injury is of particular interest because sheep have a single bronchial artery which supplies some 80% of the systemic circulation to the airway below the carina.[91-93] This facilitates evaluation of the systemic contribution to lung circulation. There is also a substantial pulmonary component to the circulation of the airway that apparently supplies the adventitial areas.[94] This latter has yet to be studied following inhalation injury. The sheep is also of great interest for studies of the microcirculation of the lung as a result of the development of pulmonary and systemic lymph fistula models. The study of lung and soft tissue lymph drainage enables the investigation of the microvasculature in chronically unanesthetized animals following inhalation injury.[95,96] A tracheal lymphatic has likewise been described in this animal that allows for the study of the proximal airway microcirculation.[97] Inhalation injury is induced in most of these studies by a technique originally developed by Walker et al.[98] and later refined in our laboratories.[99] The sheep are anesthetized and smoke from burning cotton toweling is insufflated into the lungs of the animals. The temperature of the smoke is monitored to ensure that the damage to the airway is the result of the smoke and not heat.

The study of these sophisticated animal models permits detailed evaluation of the microvascular pathophysiology following inhalation injury. The response to this insult is manifest in the airway and lung parenchyma as well as systemic vascular beds remote from the pulmonary system. Each response will be discussed in this section.

A. AIRWAY RESPONSE

Inhalation of caustic agents in smoke results in a rapid, immediate elevation of airway blood flow. This is such a common phenomenon that it is often used to diagnose the malady.[100,101] The majority of the blood flow increase is localized to the mucosal areas[102] and thus the engorgement of the vasculature can be visualized by broncoscopy. We have also been able to detect the increase in mucosal blood flow with a laser Doppler flow probe.[103] During the early part of the response to smoke insufflation, the hyperemia is restricted to the area of smoke exposure. Distal airway blood flow can also be measured continuously by placement of a transonic flow probe on the bronchial artery of sheep.[104,105] In these studies, the bronchial blood flow increased almost immediately by some 10- to 13-fold and remained elevated for at least 48 h. The degree of blood flow elevation in the bronchial artery appears to be proportional to the duration of smoke exposure (Figure 4).[104,106] We have likewise determined blood flow with the radioactive microsphere technique.[106-108] It appears that the majority of airway blood flow is distributed to the mucosa following inhalation injury.[107] The differences between the blood flow in the

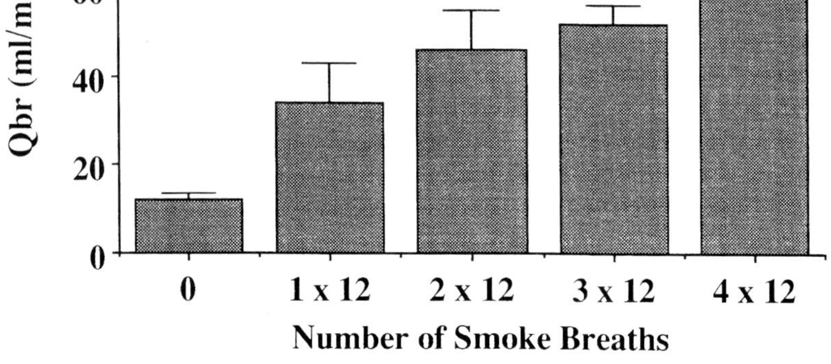

Figure 9-4 The dose response of bronchial artery blood flow (Qbr) to increasing smoke exposure in sheep after smoke inhalation injury. Increasing duration of smoke inhalation results in a progressive increase in bronchial artery blood flow. * Significant vs. baseline, $p < 0.05$.

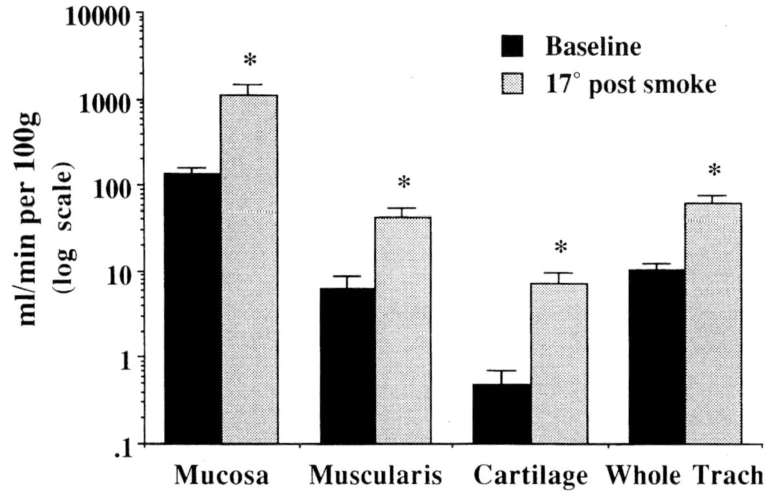

Figure 9-5 Blood flow distribution to the distal trachea in sheep after smoke inhalation injury as determined by radioactive microspheres. The blood flow to all portions of the trachea increased, however mucosal blood flow was exponentially higher after smoke inhalation. * Significant vs. baseline, $p < 0.05$.

mucosa, serosa, and cartilage are exponential (Figure 5). Since the blood flow to the cartilage is minimal, the flow in the larger cartilagenous airways is lower per unit weight than the smaller bronchi which have less cartilage.[107] Duration of smoke exposure does not affect the increase in blood flow except in the smallest airways.[106] Low dosages of smoke are not associated with an elevation in blood flow to 0.5- to 1.0-mm bronchi. But with increased duration of smoke exposure, the hyperemia becomes evident in these smaller airways (Figure 6). Thus, the increase in blood flow in the bronchial artery following inhalation injury, noted with the ultrasonic flow probe, results in the spread of the hyperemia down the airway.

Barrow et al., from our laboratories, have identified a lymphatic that drains the trachea.[97,109] In these studies, they used a modified endotracheal tube to induce a selective inhalation injury to the trachea by insufflating it with smoke from burning cotton toweling. They anesthetized these animals at various time intervals following injury and determined the flow of lymph from the tracheal lymphatic.[97] This was seen to increase approximately sixfold following inhalation injury.[97] The lymph from this vessel had a higher protein level following smoke insufflation suggesting that the increase in tracheal lymph flow was mediated by an increase in microvascular permeability.[97,109] We have also confirmed the elevation in transvascular fluid flux by determining the wet/dry ratio of the trachea following inhalation of cotton smoke and finding it was elevated compared to normal animals.[107] Hales and his group have studied inhalation injury in both dogs and sheep.[110-112] They have demonstrated that there is edema formation in the airway following inhalation of acrolein, one of the major compounds present in smoke.[111] They were likewise able to demonstrate that following the insufflation of the airway with acrolein it became permeable to monastral blue, a high molecular weight dye.[111] Histologically, they found edema and dye extravasation present in the airway from the trachea to bronchi as small as 1 mm in diameter.

Following the inhalation of smoke, there is light and electron microscopic evidence of upper airway denudation and formation of an exudative material in the tracheobronchial

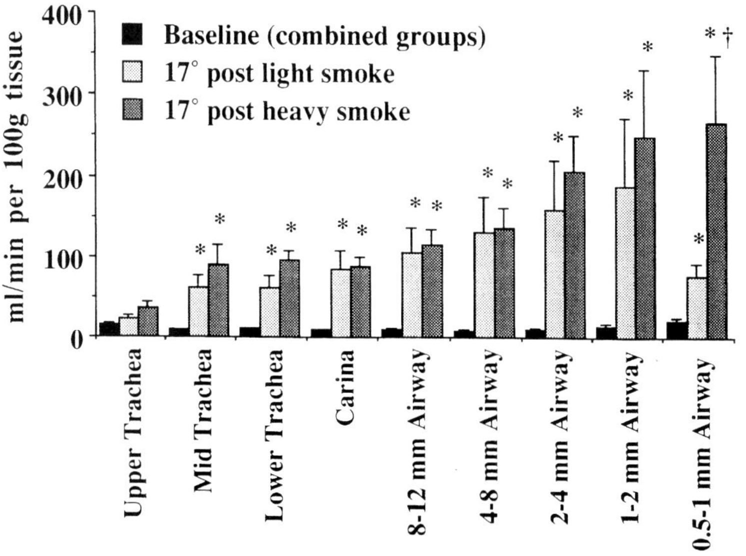

Figure 9-6 The blood flow to large and small airways after light and heavy smoke inhalation injury. A hyperemic airway response occurs after inhalation injury and increases in the more distal bronchi. This effect is seen to the same degree in the light and heavy smoke down to the 1- to 2-mm bronchi. The smaller bronchi (0.5 to 1.0 mm), however, developed increased hyperemia only after prolonged exposure to smoke. * Significant vs. sham, † significant vs. light smoke, $p < 0.05$.

areas.[113] This exudate is rich in protein, suggesting an increase in the permeability of the bronchial microvasculature. By comparing the protein composition of this exudative material with the plasma and lung lymph, we have found that the exudate is similar in composition to lymph fluid.[114] These data from the various studies give strong evidence of a microvascular permeability change having taken place in the airway following inhalation injury. The large increase in blood flow would likewise suggest an increased surface area perfusion in addition to a probable change in microvascular pressure. The latter has yet to be evaluated.

There have been numerous attempts to identify the mediators responsible for the increased bronchial artery blood flow which occurs with smoke inhalation. Since histamine is associated with vasodilatation and edema formation with burn injury, the effects of H_1 and H_2 histamine blockade in inhalation injury were investigated in sheep following inhalation injury. Neither the H_1 blocker diphenhydramine or the H_2 receptor antagonist ranitidine affected the increase in bronchial blood flow noted with smoke insufflation.[115]

In previous studies we had identified the fact that prostacyclin was increased in the blood and lymph following inhalation injury.[114] Since this material is a vasodilator, the effects of a cyclooxygenase inhibitor on the bronchial hyperemia was evaluated in our *ovine* model of inhalation injury. Despite pretreatment with the cyclooxygenase inhibitor ibuprofen, there was no noticeable effect on bronchial artery blood flow following smoke inhalation.[116] Therefore it appears that neither histamine nor prostanoids are putative mediators of bronchial hyperemia.

Since antihistamines and antiprostanoids failed to attenuate the increase in bronchial blood flow seen with the insufflation of smoke, our interest was directed to a neural source. The cervical vagosympathetic trunk is virtually the only source of innervation to the lung and airway vasculature. Thus, the first studies performed were to determine the effects of blocking this neural trunk with a local anesthetic. In acute preparations, a local anesthetic had markedly reduced the response in airway blood flow elevation following smoke inhalation.[117] The majority of motor fibers that vasodilate the bronchial microvasculature are parasympathetic in origin, with acetylcholine as the primary neurotransmitter. Consequently, we investigated the effect of atropine on the elevated bronchial blood flow seen with inhalation injury. The sheep that received the anticholinergic compound had an elevation in blood flow which was virtually identical with the untreated animals that were exposed to smoke.

The work of Martling et al.[118] has indicated that the majority of the bronchial circulatory vasodilation induced by vagal stimulation in the pig was mediated by sensory nerve afferents. The sensory C-fibers, which can be desensitized by the chronic administration of capsaicin, were present in abundance around the airway smooth muscle and microvasculature. These fibers contain the neuropeptides substance P and calcitonin gene-related peptide that produce changes similar to those seen in inhalation injury — namely vasodilitation, bronchoconstriction, and vasculature permeability.[119,120] Also, investigators have shown that the bronchial vasodilation induced by inhalation of cigarette smoke was prevented by the chronic administration of capsaicin.[118] Lundberg et al.[121] have also reported that cigarette smoke causes an increase in airway permeability, and that the permeability changes could be blocked by pretreatment with capsaicin. Therefore, sensory nerve afferents appear to be likely candidates as the mediators of bronchial hyperemia and microvascular permeability associated with inhalation injury. Preliminary data have been collected by our laboratory that demonstrate that the changes in airway blood flow noted with inhalation injury can be reduced by capsaicin desensitization.[122]

Some of the bronchial hyperemia noted with smoke inhalation may be mediated hemotogenously. We carried out experiments in which the trachea and right lung were injured with smoke, while the left lung was being ventilated with air. We demonstrated the usual hyperemia and edema in the smoke insufflated airway.[123] These changes occurred almost immediately as measured by both laser Doppler and radioactive microsphere techniques.[103,124] The air insufflated lung did not demonstrate a change in bronchial blood flow immediately, but by 24 h after the contralateral right lung and trachea had been injured, the small airways of the left lung began to show an increase in blood flow. Since, as we have seen above, the normal sequence of blood flow change in the smoke-injured lung is from trachea down, this hyperemic spread from the small airway up is evidence of a spread of injury from the pulmonary system.

B. PULMONARY MICROVASCULAR CHANGES

Following inhalation injury there is evidence of microvascular changes in the pulmonary microvasculature as well. There is a profound increase in lung lymph flow and extravascular lung water, measured by the thermal dilution technique, is elevated.[87,125,126] Also, postmortem histological and gravimetric analysis of the lung reveals an increased water content.[87,125] These increases in extravascular fluid formation are proportional to the duration of smoke exposure.[99] These changes are obviously related to alterations in the parameters of the Starling equation.

Pulmonary artery pressure and pulmonary vascular resistance increase between 4 and 12 h following inhalation injury.[104,127,128] Pulmonary capillary pressure, measured by the technique of Holloway et al.,[129] also rises by approximately 24 h after smoke inhalation.[128] The resistance changes noted appear to be secondary to a constriction of the venular side of the circulation. These changes in pulmonary microvascular pressures are obviously important in the formation of edema; however, changes in vascular permeability appear to be of much greater importance especially during the first 24 h after injury.[130]

As we have noted there is a change in lung lymph flow following inhalation injury. This phenomena differs somewhat from that seen in the tracheal areas, since it occurs with over a 4-h latency period after the airway exposure to smoke, suggesting that it is a mediated phenomena. These changes in lung lymph flow are associated with an elevation in lymph-to-plasma concentration ratio, and drop in the oncotic pressure gradient, supporting a change in microvascular permeability to protein.[104,126]

In an elegant study by Isago et al., both filtration and reflection coefficients were determined in an *ovine* model of smoke inhalation. Reflection coefficient in the pulmonary microvasculature was obtained by elevating capillary pressure using pneumatic occluders placed on the pulmonary veins.[131] Following inhalation injury, there was a marked reduction in the reflection coefficient and an elevation in the filtration coefficient (Figure 7).[130] Thus there was both an elevation in permeability to proteins as well as low molecular weight materials following smoke insufflation to these animals. The relative contributions of permeability and capillary pressure to transvascular fluid flux was calculated according to the method of Pitt et al.[22] They found that capillary permeability was responsible for the majority of the edema found during the first 24 h. During the next 24 h, the permeability and the lung lymph flow begin to return toward baseline values, and microvascular pressure appears to be responsible for the majority of the lymph flow changes noted at 48 h post smoke insufflation (Figure 8).[130]

These changes in microvascular fluid flux occur with the elevation of PMN cells in the lung, as evidenced by histology and bronchoalveolar lavage, and the release of materials associated with the PMN cells, such as proteases and oxygen free radicals.[87,99,114] With respect to the latter, Demling has reported that one of the lipid peroxidation products, conjugated dienes, were more abundant in the pulmonary arterial blood than the systemic arterial circulation suggesting a peripheral source for these materials.[132] On the other hand, we have seen high concentrations of conjugated dienes in the lung lymph and pulmonary tissues, suggesting the lung as a source of these materials.[133,134]

The role of the PMN cell as the vector of the cytotoxins responsible for pulmonary microvascular permeability changes has likewise been supported by a finding that the proteolytic enzymes, lipid peroxidation, and lung lymph flow changes are markedly reduced when the PMN cells are depleted using nitrogen mustard.[88] The changes in lung lymph flow seen with smoke inhalation may also be obtunded by administration of antiproteases[135] and oxygen free radical scavengers.[136,137] Both oxygen free radicals and proteases have been shown to be released by PMN cells.[138,139]

The delayed onset of the changes in transvascular fluid flux in the pulmonary bed suggests the release of mediators from other areas, perhaps the airway. It is difficult to conceive materials in the smoke traveling from the oral pharynx to the alveoli. Certainly, these materials come into contact with the airway circulation. The changes that occur in bronchial blood flow and the denudation of the tracheobronchial basement membrane are phenomena that occur almost instantaneously with smoke insufflation.[104,113] Consequently, this airway injury must in some way vector PMN cells to the parenchyma. The mechanisms by which cytokines might reach the pulmonary parenchyma from the airway may be related to the unique anatomy of the bronchial circulation. The systemic drainage from the intrapulmonary bronchi has been demonstrated to enter the pulmonary circulation at the precapillary level (Figure 9).[92,140] Consequently, chemotactic materials released in the airway could traverse this network and present themselves to the pulmonary microvasculature to attract PMN cells resulting in adherence to the microvasculature, transepithelial migration, and the release of their cytotoxins.

There have been several experiments that physiologically support a bronchopulmonary portal system. Using their dog model with acrolein inhalation, Hales et al. demonstrated an elevation in extravascular lung water using both the thermal dilution technique and gravimetric determinations.[110,111] In animals who had previously had their bronchial arteries ligated, the increase in edema was markedly reduced.[111] Similar experiments have been performed in chronically instrumented sheep. The sheep is unique from other animal

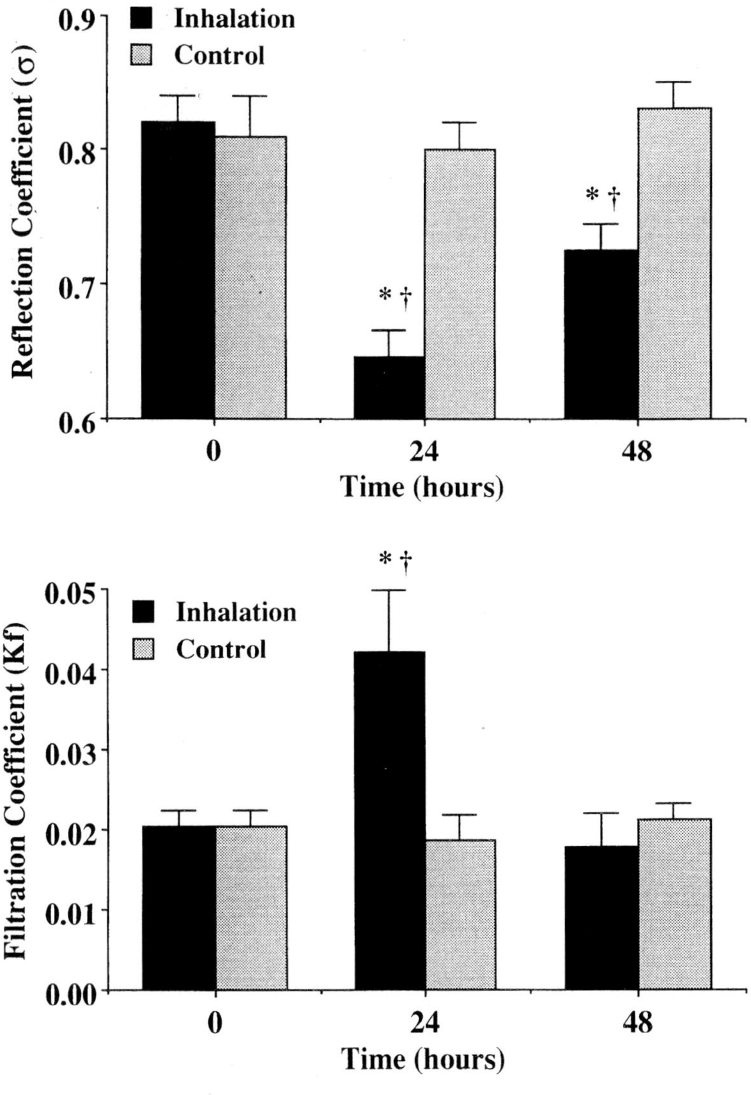

Figure 9-7 Reflection coefficient, σ, (upper) and filtration coefficient, K_f, (lower) after smoke inhalation injury in sheep. The reflection coefficient decreased from 0.81 to 0.64 and filtration coefficient increased from 0.021 to 0.042 ml/min/mmHg 24 h after smoke inhalation injury. K_f returned to baseline values by 48 h after insult. Although σ increased at 48 h, it was still lower than baseline values. * Significant vs. time 0, † significant vs. control, $p < 0.05$.

species, having only a single bronchial artery which supplies from 50 to 80% of the systemic circulation to the bronchial areas.[93] Occlusion of this vessel with a pneumatic device prior to inhalation injury resulted in a reduction in both lung lymph flow and extravascular lung water determined by the gravimetric technique (Figure 10).[105] Other experiments have been designed with confinement of smoke insufflation to a single lung. If the smoke injury was limited to the intrapulmonary airways the injury was localized

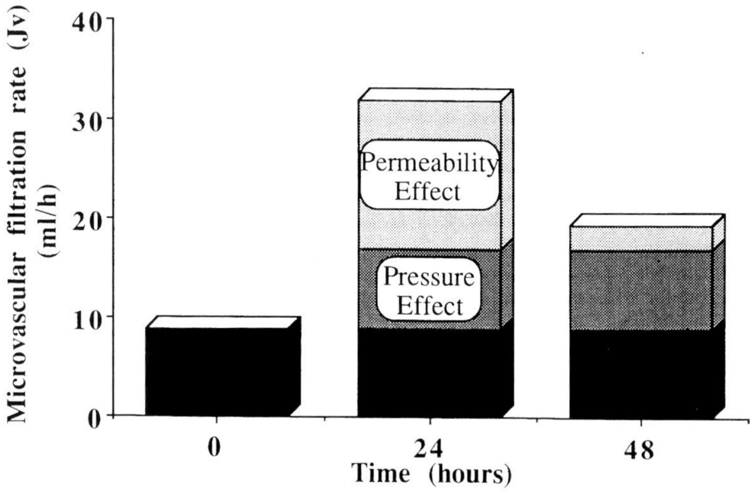

Figure 9-8 Relative contribution of increased capillary pressure and increased permeability to total capillary filtration 24 and 48 h after smoke inhalation as calculated using Pitt's method.

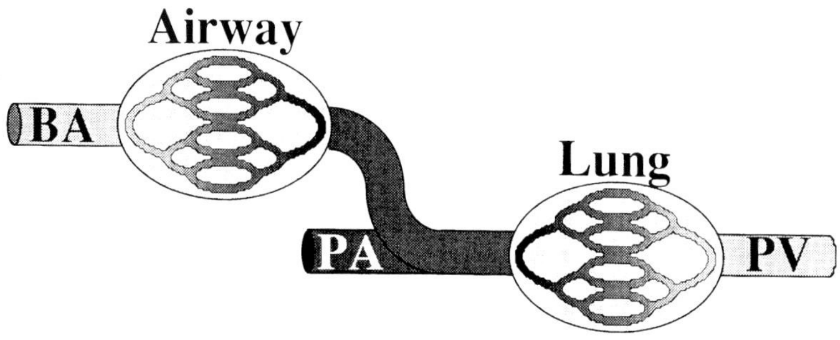

Figure 9-9 Diagram of the bronchopulmonary portal system. The systemic drainage of the intrapulmonary bronchi enters the pulmonary ciculation at the precapillary level. Bronchial artery (BA), pulmonary artery (PA), pulmonary vein (PV).

to the ipsilateral lung.[133,141] However, when the smoke damage included the trachea and bronchi (extrapulmonary airway), then the contralateral air-insufflated lung likewise demonstrated injury.[133] The changes in airway blood flow were also investigated using radioactive microspheres. With time, blood flow changes in the lung which was insufflated with smoke showed the greatest intensity in the upper airway with gradient down to the smaller airways.[106,107] These changes in blood flow occurred almost instantaneously. Interestingly, the blood flow changes to the air-insufflated lung occurred after a latency period and had a greater intensity in the smaller airways (unpublished data). This suggests a hematogenous origin for the vasodilating mediators. The venous drainage from the extra pulmonary airway enters into the azygos vein and thus the right atrium.[92] Therefore, mediators released from these airways outside the lung would enter into the heart and be distributed to both lungs. Bronchopulmonary pathophysiology is a fertile area for further investigation.

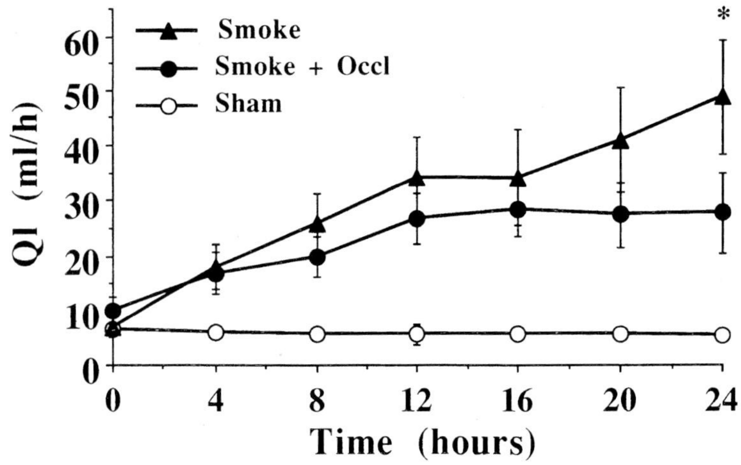

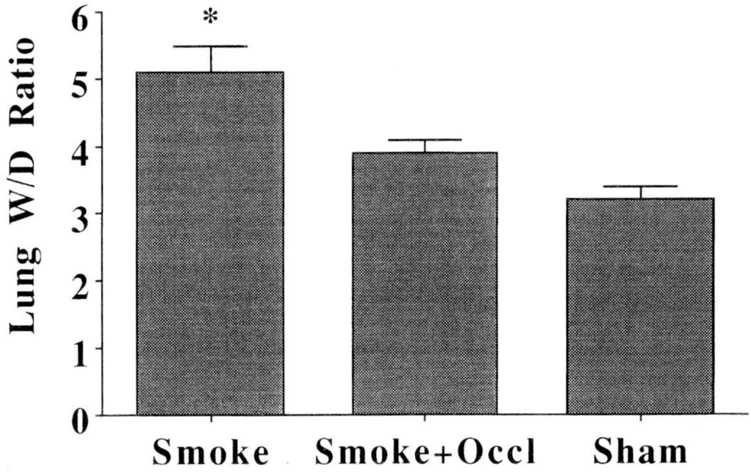

Figure 9-10 Lung lymph flow (upper) and lung wet-to-dry weight ratios (lower) after smoke inhalation injury, sham injury, or smoke inhalation with bronchial artery occlusion. Bronchial artery occlusion decreased the lung lymph flow and lung wet-to-dry weight ratios after smoke inhalation, emphasizing the importance of the systemic circulation in the pulmonary pathophysiology of smoke inhalation injury. * Significant vs. sham, $p < 0.05$.

C. SYSTEMIC CHANGES

With burn injury and other forms of trauma, mortality is usually the result of multiple organ system failure.[142,143] The contribution made by acute lung injury to this phenomena has, in the past, been considered the result of reduced oxygenation. Even with improved techniques of artificial restoration of arterial oxygenation saturation, it has now become obvious that other factors are involved since multiorgan system failure still occurs.

It has been recognized that individuals with the combination of thermal and smoke inhalation injury require greater fluid for resuscitation to nonpathogenic cardiovascular states than individuals with thermal injury alone.[144,145] This phenomena has been studied by cannulation of a lymphatic which drains the soft tissues of the skin on the lateral surface of sheep.[96] Inhalation injury induces a two-fold increase in the flow from this lymphatic vessel.[16,132] With thermal injury, this flow was much greater, reaching some 3- to 5-times the baseline levels.[16] When smoke inhalation was combined with the thermal injury, again the soft tissue lymphatic showed a several-fold increase in flow (Table 1).

These changes in peripheral microvascular fluid flux occur with a concomitant elevation in plasma lipid peroxidation products suggesting that they may be the result of the release of oxygen free radicals. The etiology of the formation of these cytotoxins is unknown.

We have reported that the lung releases peptidoleukotrienes following inhalation injury.[146] A similar finding has been made by the Hales and Quinn group.[112] They have likewise reported that there is a systemic vasoconstriction with inhalation injury and that this systemic vasoconstriction could be reversed by administration of a peptidoleukotriene antagonist. We have also reported an elevation in systemic vascular resistance with inhalation injury,[127] and likewise demonstrated a selective vasoconstriction in the distribution of the cephalic mesenteric artery of sheep following inhalation injury.[147] This vasoconstriction was on the order of 4 h in duration and was followed by reperfusion. Consequently, damage to the systemic circulation may be the result of an ischemia/reperfusion phenomenon. Further study is warranted in this area of investigation.

In summary, inhalation injury results in significant alterations in the microvasculature of various tissue beds. The airway changes occur immediately and are associated with edema and bronchial casts contributing to morbidity and mortality.[148] Secondly, latent changes in the lung parenchyma result in damage to the pulmonary microvasculature and tissue destruction from inflammatory mediators. Also, there is strong evidence to support the airway as a vector for the putative mediators causing the changes in the parenchymal microcirculation. Finally, vascular beds remote from the injury are similarly affected. It is obvious that inhalation injury is able to induce pathophysiology which results in acute respiratory distress syndrome and multiorgan system failure. Further investigation in the pathophysiology is essential to develop solutions to this challenging clinical entity.

REFERENCES

1. **Maley, M. P.,** Statistical data, in *Rekindle*, International Society of Fire Service Instructors, Ashland, MD, October 1985.
2. **Morikawa, T.,** Acrolein, formaldehyde, and volatile fatty acids from smoldering combustion, *J. Combust. Toxicol.,* 3, 135, 1976.
3. **Zikria, B. A., Ferrer, J. M., and Floch, H. F.,** The chemical factors contributing to pulmonary damage in "smoke poisoning", *Surgery,* 71, 704, 1972.
4. **Dost, F. N.,** Acute toxicology of components of vegetation smoke, *Rev. Environ. Contam. Toxicol.,* 119, 1, 1991.
5. **Townsley, M. I., Parker, J. C., Longenecker, G. L., Perry, M. L., Pitt, R. M., and Taylor, A. E.,** Pulmonary embolism: analysis of endothelial pore size in canine lung, *Am. J. Physiol.,* 255, H1075, 1988.
6. **Pruitt, B. A. and Goodwin, C. W.,** Current treatment of the extensively burned patient, *Surg. Annu.,* 15, 331, 1983.
7. **Wilmore, D. W.,** Pathophysiology of the hypermetabolic response to burn injury, *J. Trauma,* 30, S4, 1990.
8. **Zetterstrom, H. and Arturson, G.,** Plasma oncotic pressure and plasma protein concentration in patients following thermal injury, *Acta Anaesthesiol. Scand.,* 24, 288, 1980.
9. **Carvajal, H. F., Linares, H. A., and Brouhard, B. H.,** Relationship of burn size to vascular permeability changes in rats, *Surg. Gynecol. Obstet.,* 149, 193, 1979.

10. **Jelenko, C., III, Jennings, W. D., Jr., O'kelley, W. R., III, and Byrd, H. C.,** Threshold burning effects of distant microcirculation. II. The relationship of area burnt to microvascular size, *Arch. Surg.,* 106, 317, 1973.
11. **Landis, E. M. and Pappenheimer, J. R.,** Exchange of substances through the capillary walls, in *Handbook of Physiology,* Section 2, Vol. 2, Hamilton, W. F. and Dow, P., Eds., Williams & Wilkins, Baltimore, MD, 1963, 961.
12. **Starling, E. H.,** On the absorption of fluids from the connective tissue spaces, *J. Physiol. (London),* 19, 312, 1896.
13. **Arturson, G.,** The changes in capillary filtration, diffusion and permeability in experimental burns, *Bibl. Anat.,* 7, 453, 1965.
14. **Arturson, G.,** Microvascular permeability to macromolecules in thermal injury, *Acta Physiol. Scand. Suppl.,* 111, 1979.
15. **Arturson, G. and Soeda, S.,** Changes in transcapillary leakage during healing of experimental burns, *Acta Chir. Scand.,* 133, 609, 1967.
16. **Montero, K., Lübbesmeyer, H. J., Traber, D. L., Kimura, R., Traber, L. D., and Herndon, D. N.,** Inhalation injury increases systemic microvascular permeability, *Surg. Forum,* 38, 303, 1987.
17. **Demling, R. H., Kramer, G. C., Gunther, R., and Nerlich, M.,** Effect of nonprotein colloid on postburn edema formation in soft tissues and lung, *Surgery,* 95, 593, 1984.
18. **Brouhard, B. H., Carvajal, H. F., and Linares, H. A.,** Burn edema and protein leakage in the rat. I. Relationship to time of injury, *Microvasc. Res.,* 15, 221, 1978.
19. **Carvajal, H. F., Brouhard, B. H., and Linares, H. A.,** Effect of antihistamine-antiserotonin and ganglionic blocking agents upon increased capillary permeability following burn trauma, *J. Trauma,* 15, 969, 1975.
20. **Olson, N. C., Grizzle, M. K., and Anderson, D. L.,** Effect of polyethylene glycol-superoxide dismutase and catalase on endotoxemia in pigs, *J. Appl. Physiol.,* 63, 1526, 1987.
21. **Kramer, G. C., Gunther, R. A., Nerlich, M. L., Zweifach, S. S., and Demling, R. H.,** Effect of dextran-70 on increased microvascular fluid and protein flux after thermal injury, *Circ. Shock,* 9, 529, 1982.
22. **Pitt, R. M., Parker, J. C., Jurkovich, G. J., Taylor, A. E., and Curreri, P. W.,** Analysis of altered capillary pressure and permeability after thermal injury, *J. Surg. Res.,* 42, 693, 1987.
23. **Demling, R. H., Harms, B., Kramer, G., and Gunther, R.,** Acute versus sustained hypoproteinemia and posttraumatic pulmonary edema, *Surgery,* 92, 79, 1982.
24. **Honeycutt, D., Traber, L., Toole, D., Herndon, D., and Traber, D.,** Colloid resuscitation of *ovine* burn shock, *Circ. Shock,* 31, 72, 1991.
25. **Arturson, G. and Mellander, S.,** Acute changes in capillary filtration and diffusion in experimental burn injury, *Acta Physiol. Scand.,* 62, 457, 1964.
26. **Lund, T., Wiig, H., and Reed, R. K.,** Acute postburn edema: role of strongly negative interstitial fluid pressure, *Am. J. Physiol.,* 255, H1069, 1988.
27. **Lund, T., Onarheim, H., Wiig, H., and Reed, R. K.,** Mechanisms behind increased dermal imbibition pressure in acute burn edema, *Am. J. Physiol.,* 256, H940, 1989.
28. **Demling, R. H.,** Burns. Fluid and electrolyte management, *Crit. Care Clin.,* 1, 27, 1985.
29. **Herndon, D. N., Hilton, J. G., Traber, D. L., and Barrow, R. E.,** Burn shock and its resuscitation, *Prog. Clin. Biol. Res.,* 236, 539, 1987.
30. **Baxter, C.,** Fluid resuscitation, burn percentage, and physiologic age, *J. Trauma,* 19, 864, 1979.
31. **Herndon, D. N., Wilmore, D. W., Mason, A. D. J., and Pruitt, B. A. J.,** Humoral mediators of nontemperature-dependent hypermetabolism in 50% burned adult rats, *Surg. Forum,* 28, 37, 1977.

32. **Wolfe, R. R., Herndon, D. N., Peters, E. J., Jahoor, F., Desai, M. H., and Holland, O. B.,** Regulation of lipolysis in severely burned children, *Ann. Surg.,* 206, 214, 1987.
33. **van Gool, J., van Vugt, H., Helle, M., and Aarden, L. A.,** The relation among stress, adrenalin, interleukin 6 and acute phase proteins in the rat, *Clin. Immunol. Immunopathol.,* 57, 200, 1990.
34. **Nijsten, M. W., Hack, C. E., Helle, M., ten Duis, H. J., Klasen, H. J., and Aarden, L. A.,** Interleukin-6 and its relation to the humoral immune response and clinical parameters in burned patients, *Surgery,* 109, 761, 1991.
35. **Hartl, W., Jauch, K. W., Herndon, D. N., Cohnert, T. U., Wolfe, R. R., and Schildberg, F. W.,** Effect of low-dose bradykinin on glucose metabolism and nitrogen balance in surgical patients, *Lancet,* 335, 69, 1990.
36. **Lund, T. and Reed, R. K.,** Microvascular fluid exchange following thermal skin injury in the rat: changes in extravascular colloid osmotic pressure, albumin mass, and water content, *Circ. Shock,* 20, 91, 1986.
37. **Pitkanen, J., Lund, T., Aanderud, L., and Reed, R. K.,** Transcapillary colloid osmotic pressures in injured and non-injured skin of seriously burned patients, *Burns Incl. Therm. Inj.,* 13, 198, 1987.
38. **Onarheim, H. and Reed, R. K.,** Thermal skin injury: effect of fluid therapy on the transcapillary colloid osmotic gradient, *J. Surg. Res.,* 50, 272, 1991.
39. **Ward, P. A. and Till, G. O.,** Pathophysiologic events related to thermal injury of skin, *J. Trauma,* 30(12), S75, 1990.
40. **Hatherill, J. R., Till, G. O., Bruner, L. H., and Ward, P. A.,** Thermal injury, intravascular hemolysis, and toxic oxygen products, *J. Clin. Invest.,* 78, 629, 1986.
41. **Till, G. O., Guilds, L. S., Mahrougui, M., Friedl, H. P., Trentz, O., and Ward, P. A.,** Role of xanthine oxidase in thermal injury of skin, *Am. J. Pathol.,* 135, 195, 1989.
42. **Friedl, H. P., Till, G. O., Trentz, O., and Ward, P. A.,** Roles of histamine, complement and xanthine oxidase in thermal injury of skin, *Am. J. Pathol.,* 135, 203, 1989.
43. **Friedl, H. P., Till, G. O., Ryan, U. S., and Ward, P. A.,** Mediator-induced activation of xanthine oxidase in endothelial cells, *FASEB J.,* 3, 2512, 1989.
44. **Granger, D. N., McCord, J. M., Parks, D. A., and Hollwarth, M. E.,** Xanthine oxidase inhibitors attenuate ischemia-induced vascular permeability changes in the cat intestine, *Gastroenterology,* 90, 80, 1986.
45. **Granger, D., Rutili, G., and McCord, J.,** Superoxide radicals in feline intestinal ischemia, *Gastroenterology,* 81, 22, 1981.
46. **Oldham, K. T., Guice, K. S., Till, G. O., and Ward, P. A.,** Activation of complement by hydroxyl radical in thermal injury, *Surgery,* 104, 272, 1988.
47. **Judkins, K.,** Algorithm for managing injury from smoke inhalation, *Br. Med. J.,* 299, 1216, 1989.
48. **Ward, P. A., Till, G. O., Hatherill, J. R., Annesley, T. M., and Kunkel, R. G.,** Systemic complement activation, lung injury, and products of lipid peroxidation, *J. Clin. Invest.,* 76, 517, 1985.
49. **Arturson, G.,** The plasma kinins in thermal injury, *Scand. J. Clin. Lab. Invest.,* 24 (Suppl. 107), 1, 1969.
50. **Brimblecombe, R. W. and Farrington, H. W.,** Histamine H_2-receptor antagonists and thermal injury in rats, *Burns,* 3, 8, 1992.
51. **Demling, R. H. and LaLonde, C.,** Early postburn lipid peroxidation: effect of ibuprofen and allopurinol, *Surgery,* 107, 85, 1990.
52. **Gasser, H., Paul, E., Redl, H., Schlag, G., Traber, D., and Herndon, D.,** Loss of plasma antioxidants after burn injury, *Circ. Shock,* 34, 13, 1991.
53. **Bekyarova, G., Yankova, T., Yankov, D., and Kozarev, I.,** Erythrocyte rheology and lipid peroxidation in burns, *Biomed. Biochim. Acta,* 50, 71, 1991.

54. **Thomson, P. D., Till, G. O., Woolliscroft, J. O., Smith, D. J., and Prasad, J. K.,** Superoxide dismutase prevents lipid peroxidation in burned patients, *Burns,* 16, 406, 1990.
55. **Dale, H. H. and Laidlaw, P. P.,** The physiological action of β-imidazolylethylamine, *J. Physiol. (London),* 41, 318, 1991.
56. **Douglas, W. W.,** Histamine and 5-hydroxytryptamine (serotonin) and their antagonists, in *The Pharmacological Basis of Therapeutics,* Gilman, A. G., Goodman, L. S., Rall, T. W., and Murad, F., Eds., Macmillan, New York, 1985, 605.
57. **Leurs, R., Brozius, M. M., Jansen, W., Bast, A., and Timmerman, H.,** Histamine H1-receptor-mediated cyclic GMP production in guinea-pig lung tissue is an L-arginine-dependent process, *Biochem. Pharmacol.,* 42, 271, 1991.
58. **Furchgott, R. F. and Jothianandan, D.,** Endothelium-dependent and -independent vasodilation involving cyclic GMP, relaxation induced by nitric oxide, carbon monoxide and light, *Blood Vessels,* 28, 52, 1991.
59. **Arturson, G., Hamberg, M., and Jonsson, C. E.,** Prostaglandins in human burn blister fluid, *Acta Physiol. Scand.,* 87, 270, 1973.
60. **Hilton, J. G. and Wells, C. H.,** Nicotinic acid reduction of plasma volume loss after thermal trauma, *Science,* 191, 861, 1976.
61. **Demling, R. H. and LaLonde, C.,** Topical ibuprofen decreases early postburn edema, *Surgery,* 102, 857, 1987.
62. **Herndon, D. N., Abston, S., and Stein, M. D.,** Increased thromboxane B2 levels in the plasma of burned and septic burned patients, *Surg. Gynecol. Obstet.,* 159, 210, 1984.
63. **Harms, B. A., Bodai, B. I., Kramer, G. C., and Demling, R. H.,** Microvascular fluid and protein flux in pulmonary and systemic circulations after thermal injury, *Microvasc. Res.,* 23(1), 77, 1982.
64. **Taplin, G. V., Chopra, S., Yanda, R. L., and Elam, D.,** Radionuclidic lung-imaging procedures in the assessment of injury due to ammonia inhalation, *Chest,* 69, 582, 1976.
65. **Herndon, D. N., Langner, F., Thompson, P., Linares, H. A., Stein, M., and Traber, D. L.,** Pulmonary injury in burned patients, *Surg. Clin. North Am.,* 67, 31, 1987.
66. **Pruitt, B. A., Erickson, D. R., and Morris, A.,** Progressive pulmonary insufficiency and other pulmonary complications of thermal injury, *J. Trauma,* 15, 369, 1975.
67. **Demling, R. H., Niehaus, G., Perea, A., and Will, J. A.,** Effect of burn-induced hypoproteinemia on pulmonary transvascular fluid filtration rate, *Surgery,* 85, 339, 1979.
68. **Demling, R. H., Wong, C., Jin, L. J., Hechtman, H., LaLonde, C., and West, K.,** Early lung dysfunction after major burns: role of edema and vasoactive mediators, *J. Trauma,* 25, 959, 1985.
69. **Demling, R. H. and LaLonde, C.,** Systemic lipid peroxidation and inflammation induced by thermal injury persists into the post-resuscitation period, *J. Trauma,* 30, 69, 1990.
70. **Annesley, T. M., Till, G. O., and Ward, P. A.,** Cutaneous thermal burn and oxidant-mediated acute lung injury: appearance in serum of lung-related LDH isoenzyme, *J. Free Radic. Biol. Med.,* 1, 409, 1985.
71. **Till, G. O., Beauchamp, C., Menapace, D., et al.,** Oxygen radical dependent lung damage following thermal injury of rat skin, *J. Trauma,* 23, 269, 1983.
72. **Till, G. O., Friedl, H. P., and Ward, P. A.,** Antioxidant treatment in experimental thermal injury, *Adv. Exp. Med. Biol.,* 264, 543, 1990.
73. **Till, G. O., Hatherill, J. R., Tourtellotte, W. W., Lutz, M. J., and Ward, P. A.,** Lipid peroxidation and acute lung injury after thermal trauma to skin. Evidence of a role for hydroxyl radical, *Am. J. Pathol.,* 119, 376, 1985.

74. **Ward, P. A.,** How does the local inflammatory response affect the wound healing process?, *J. Trauma,* 24, S18, 1984.
75. **Granger, D. N.,** Role of xanthine oxidase and granulocytes in ischemia-reperfusion injury, *Am. J. Physiol.,* 255, H1269, 1988.
76. **Horgan, M. J., Lum, H., and Malik, A. B.,** Pulmonary edema after pulmonary artery occlusion and reperfusion, *Am. Rev. Respir. Dis.,* 140, 1421, 1989.
77. **Kowalski, T. F., Guidotti, S., Deffebach, M., Kubilis, P., and Bishop, M.,** Bronchial circulation in pulmonary artery occlusion and reperfusion, *J. Appl. Physiol.,* 68, 125, 1990.
78. **Haynes, J., Seibert, A., Bass, J. B., and Taylor, A. E.,** U74500A inhibition of oxidant-mediated lung injury, *Am. J. Physiol.,* 259, H144, 1990.
79. **Klausner, J. M., Paterson, I. S., Mannick, J. A., Valeri, R., Shepro, D., and Hechtman, H. B.,** Reperfusion pulmonary edema, *JAMA,* 261, 1030, 1989.
80. **Goldman, G., Welbourn, R., Klausner, J. M., et al.,** Ischemia activates neutrophils but inhibits their local and remote diapedesis, *Ann. Surg.,* 211, 196, 1990.
81. **Paterson, I. S., Klausner, J. M., Goldman, G., et al.,** Thromboxane mediates the ischemia-induced neutrophil oxidative burst, *Surgery,* 106, 224, 1989.
82. **Thompson, P. B., Herndon, D. N., Traber, D. L., and Abston, S.,** Effect on mortality of inhalation injury, *J. Trauma,* 26, 163, 1986.
83. **Herndon, D. N., Gore, D., Cole, M., et al.,** Determinants of mortality in pediatric patients with greater than 70% full-thickness total body surface area thermal injury treated by early total excision and grafting, *J. Trauma,* 27, 208, 1987.
84. **Shirani, K. Z., Pruitt, B. A. J. and Mason, A. D. J.,** The influence of inhalation injury and pneumonia on burn mortality, *Ann. Surg.,* 205, 82, 1987.
85. **Heimbach, D. M. and Waeckerle, J. F.,** Inhalation injuries, *Ann. Emerg. Med.,* 17, 1316, 1988.
86. **Traber, D. L. and Herndon, D. N.,** Pathophysiology of smoke inhalation, in *Respiratory Sequelae of Burns,* Haponik, E. F. and Munster, A. M., Eds., McGraw Hill, New York, 1990.
87. **Traber, D. L., Herndon, D. N., Stein, M. D., Traber, L. D., Flynn, J. T., and Niehaus, G. D.,** The pulmonary lesion of smoke inhalation in an ovine model, *Circ. Shock,* 18, 311, 1986.
88. **Basadre, J. O., Sugi, K., Traber, D. L., Traber, L. D., Niehaus, G. D., and Herndon, D. N.,** The effect of leukocyte depletion on smoke inhalation injury in sheep, *Surgery,* 104, 208, 1988.
89. **Robinson, L. and Miller, R. H.,** Smoke inhalation injuries, *Am. J. Otolaryngol.,* 7, 375, 1986.
90. **Herndon, D. N., Barrow, R. E., Linares, H. A., et al.,** Inhalation injury in burned patients: effects and treatment, *Burns Incl. Therm. Inj.,* 14, 349, 1988.
91. **Charan, N. B., Turk, G. M., and Ripley, R.,** Measurement of bronchial arterial blood flow and bronchovascular resistance in sheep, *J. Appl. Physiol.,* 59, 305, 1985.
92. **Charan, N. B., Turk, G. M., and Dhand, R.,** Gross and subgross anatomy of bronchial circulation in sheep, *J. Appl. Physiol.,* 57, 658, 1984.
93. **Magno, M. G. and Fishman, A. P.,** Origin, distribution, and blood flow of bronchial circulation in anesthetized sheep, *J. Appl. Physiol.,* 53, 272, 1982.
94. **Barman, S. A., Ardell, J. L., Parker, J. C., Perry, M. L., and Taylor, A. E.,** Pulmonary and systemic blood flow contributions to upper airways in canine lung, *Am. J. Physiol.,* 255, H1130, 1988.
95. **Staub, N. C., Bland, R. D., Brigham, K. L., Demling, R., Erdmann, A. J., and Woolverton, W. C.,** Preparation of chronic lung lymph fistulas in sheep, *J. Surg. Res.,* 19, 315, 1975.

96. **Demling, R. H., Smith, M., Gunther, R., Wandzilak, T., and Pederson, N. C.,** Use of a chronic prefemoral lymphatic fistula for monitoring systemic capillary integrity in unanesthetized sheep, *J. Surg. Res.,* 31, 136, 1981.
97. **Barrow, R. E., Morris, S. E., Linares, H. A., and Herndon, D. N.,** Tracheal venous blood and lymph collection: a model to study airway injury in sheep, *J. Appl. Physiol.,* 70, 1645, 1991.
98. **Walker, H. L., McLeod, C. G. J., and McManus, W. F.,** Experimental inhalation injury in the goat, *J. Trauma,* 21, 962, 1981.
99. **Kimura, R., Traber, L. D., Herndon, D. N., Linares, H. A., Lübbesmeyer, H. J., and Traber, D. L.,** Increasing duration of smoke exposure induces more severe lung injury in sheep, *J. Appl. Physiol.,* 64, 1107, 1988.
100. **Haponik, E. F., Crapo, R. O., Herndon, D. N., Traber, D. L., Hudson, L., and Moylan, J.,** Smoke inhalation, *Am. Rev. Respir. Dis.,* 138, 1060, 1988.
101. **Moylan, J. A. and Alexander, L. G. J.,** Diagnosis and treatment of inhalation injury, *World J. Surg.,* 2, 185, 1978.
102. **Stothert, J. C., Jr., Gbaanador, G. B., and Herndon, D. N.,** The role of autopsy in death resulting from trauma, *J. Trauma,* 30, 1021, 1990.
103. **Loick, H. M., Traber, L. D., Hurst, C., Herndon, D. N., and Traber, D. L.,** Endoscopic laser flowmeter — a valid method for detection and quantitative analysis of inhalation injury, *J. Burn Care Rehab.,* in press.
104. **Abdi, S., Herndon, D., Mcguire, J., Traber, L., and Traber, D. L.,** Time course of alterations in lung lymph and bronchial blood flows after inhalation injury, *J. Burn Care Rehab.,* 11, 510, 1990.
105. **Abdi, S., Herndon, D. N., Traber, L. D., et al.,** Lung edema formation following inhalation injury: role of the bronchial blood flow, *J. Appl. Physiol.,* 71, 727, 1991.
106. **Ashley, K. D., Stothert, J. C., Jr., Traber, D. L., Traber, L. D., Kramer, G., and Herndon, D.,** Airway blood flow following light and heavy smoke inhalation injury, *Surg. Forum,* 41, 293, 1990.
107. **Stothert, J. C., Jr., Ashley, K. D., Kramer, G. C., et al.,** Intrapulmonary distribution of bronchial blood flow after moderate smoke inhalation, *J. Appl. Physiol.,* 69, 1734, 1990.
108. **Kramer, G. C., Herndon, D. N., Linares, H. A., and Traber, D. L.,** Effects of inhalation injury on airway blood flow and edema formation, *J. Burn Care Rehab.,* 10, 45, 1989.
109. **Barrow, R. E., Morris, S. E., Basadre, J. O., and Herndon, D. N.,** Selective permeability changes in the lungs and airways of sheep after toxic smoke inhalation, *J. Appl. Physiol.,* 68, 2165, 1990.
110. **Hales, C. A., Barkin, P. W., Jung, W., et al.,** Synthetic smoke with acrolein but not HCl produces pulmonary edema, *J. Appl. Physiol.,* 64, 1121, 1988.
111. **Hales, C. A., Barkin, P., Jung, W., Quinn, D., Lamborghini, D., and Burke, J.,** Bronchial artery ligation modifies pulmonary edema after exposure to smoke with acrolein, *J. Appl. Physiol.,* 67, 1001, 1989.
112. **Quinn, D. A., Robinson, D., Jung, W., and Hales, C. A.,** Role of sulfidopeptide leukotrienes in synthetic smoke inhalation injury in sheep, *J. Appl. Physiol.,* 68, 1962, 1990.
113. **Abdi, S., Evans, M. J., Cox, R. A., Lubbesmeyer, H., Herndon, D. N., and Traber, D. L.,** Inhalation injury to tracheal epithelium in an ovine model of cotton smoke exposure. Early phase (30 minutes), *Am. Rev. Respir. Dis.,* 142, 1436, 1990.
114. **Herndon, D. N., Traber, L. D., Linares, H., et al.,** Etiology of the pulmonary pathophysiology associated with inhalation injury, *Resuscitation,* 14, 43, 1986.
115. **Traber, L. D., Herndon, D. N., Abdi, S., and Traber, D. L.,** Histamine does not mediate the increase in bronchial artery blood flow during inhalation injury, *FASEB J.,* 4 (Abstr.), A575, 1990.

116. **Abdi, S., Traber, L. D., Herndon, D. N., and Traber, D. L.,** Ibuprofen does not attenuate the increase in bronchial blood flow after inhalation injury, *Am. Rev. Respir. Dis.*, 143 (Abstr.), A785, 1991.
117. **Abdi, S, Maguire, J. P., Herndon, D. N., Traber, L. D., and Traber, D. L.,** Lidocaine attenuates bronchial artery response to inhalation trauma, *Crit. Care Med.*, 18 (Abstr.), S200, 1990.
118. **Martling, C. R., Matran, R., Alving, K., Lacroix, J. S., and Lundberg, J. M.,** Vagal vasodilatory mechanisms in the pig bronchial circulation preferentially involves sensory nerves, *Neurosci. Lett.*, 96, 306, 1989.
119. **Barnes, P. J.,** Neuropeptides in human airways: function and clinical implications, *Am. Rev. Respir. Dis.*, 136, S77, 1987.
120. **Barnes, P. J.,** Regulatory peptides in the respiratory system, *Experientia,* 43, 832, 1987.
121. **Lundberg, J. M., Martling, C. R., Saria, A., Folkers, K., and Rosell, S.,** Cigarette smoke-induced airway oedema due to activation of capsaicin-sensitive vagal afferents and substance P release, *Neuroscience,* 10, 1361, 1983.
122. **Traber, L. D., Herndon, D. N., Turner, J., Sant Ambrogio, G., and Traber, D. L.,** Peptide mediation of the bronchial blood flow elevation following inhalation injury, *Circ. Shock,* 31(Abstr.), 13, 1990.
123. **Prien, T., Traber, L. D., Herndon, D. N., Stothert, J. C., Jr., Lübbesmeyer, H. J., and Traber, D. L.,** Pulmonary edema with smoke inhalation, undetected by indicator-dilution technique, *J. Appl. Physiol.*, 63, 907, 1987.
124. **Loick, H. M., Traber, L. D., Theissen, J. L., Flynn, J., and Traber, D. L.,** Effect of thromboxane receptor blockade following inhalation injury in sheep, *Anesthesiology,* 75 (Abstr.), A224, 1991.
125. **Herndon, D. N., Traber, D. L., Niehaus, G. D., Linares, H. A., and Traber, L. D.,** The pathophysiology of smoke inhalation injury in a sheep model, *J. Trauma,* 24, 1044, 1984.
126. **Traber, D. L., Schlag, G., Redl, H., and Traber, L. D.,** Pulmonary edema and compliance changes following smoke inhalation, *J. Burn Care Rehabil.*, 6, 490, 1985.
127. **Sugi, K., Theissen, J. L., Traber, L. D., Herndon, D. N., and Traber, D. L.,** Impact of carbon monoxide on cardiopulmonary dysfunction after smoke inhalation injury, *Circ. Res.*, 66, 69, 1990.
128. **Isago, T., Fujioka, K., Traber, L. D., Herndon, D. N., and Traber, D. L.,** Derived pulmonary capillary pressure changes following smoke inhalation in sheep, *Crit. Care Med.*, 19, 1407, 1991.
129. **Holloway, H., Perry, M., Downey, J., Parker, J., and Taylor, A.,** Estimation of effective pulmonary capillary pressure in intact lungs, *J. Appl. Physiol.*, 54(3), 846, 1983.
130. **Isago, T., Noshima, S., Traber, L. D., Herndon, D. N., and Traber, D. L.,** Analysis of pulmonary microvascular permeability after smoke inhalation, *J. Appl. Physiol.*, 71(4), 1403, 1991.
131. **Isago, T., Traber, L. D., Herndon, D. N., Abdi, S., Fujioka, K., and Traber, D. L.,** Determination of pulmonary microvascular reflection coefficient in sheep by venous occlusion, *J. Appl. Physiol.*, 69, 2311, 1990.
132. **Demling, R. H. and LaLonde, C.,** Moderate smoke inhalation produces decreased oxygen delivery, increased oxygen demands, and systemic but not lung parenchymal lipid peroxidation, *Surgery,* 108, 544, 1990.
133. **Loick, H. M., Traber, L. D., Tokyay, R., Linares, H. A., Prien, T., and Traber, D. L.,** Mechanical alteration of blood flow in smoked and unsmoked lung areas after inhalation injury, *J. Appl. Physiol.*, 72, 1692, 1992.
134. **Isago, T., Traber, L. D., Herndon, D. N., and Traber, D. L.,** Pulmonary capillary pressure changes following smoke inhalation in sheep, *Anesthesiology,* 73, A1234, 1990.

135. **Niehaus, G. D., Kimura, R., Traber, L. D., Herndon, D. N., Flynn, J. T., and Traber, D. L.,** Administration of a synthetic antiprotease reduces smoke-induced lung injury, *J. Appl. Physiol.,* 69, 694, 1990.
136. **Brown, M., Desai, M., Traber, L. D., Herndon, D. N., and Traber, D. L.,** Dimethylsulfoxide with heparin in the treatment of smoke inhalation injury, *J. Burn Care Rehab.,* 9, 22, 1988.
137. **Kimura, R., Mlcak, R., Richardson, J., Desai, M., Herndon, D. N., Traber, L. D., and Traber D. L.,** Treatment of smoke-induced pulmonary injury with nebulized dimethylsulfoxide, *Circ. Shock,* 25, 333, 1988.
138. **Carlin, G. and Arfors, K. E.,** Peroxidation of liposomes promoted by human polymorphonuclear leucocytes, *J. Free Radic. Biol. Med.,* 1, 437, 1985.
139. **Guice, K. S., Oldham, K. T., Caty, M. G., Johnson, K. J., and Ward, P. A.,** Neutrophil-dependent, oxygen-radical mediated lung injury associated with acute pancreatitis, *Ann. Surg.,* 210, 740, 1989.
140. **Lakshminarayan, S., Kowalski, T. F., Kirk, W., Graham, M. M., and Butler, J.,** The drainage routes of the bronchial blood flow in anesthetized dogs, *Respir. Physiol.,* 82, 65, 1990.
141. **Prien, T., Linares, H. A., Traber, L. D., Herndon, D. N., and Traber, D. L.,** Lack of hematogenous mediated pulmonary injury with smoke inhalation, *J. Burn Care Rehab.,* 9, 462, 1988.
142. **Dinarello, C. A.,** The proinflammatory cytokines interleukin-1 and tumor necrosis factor and treatment of the septic shock syndrome, *J. Infect. Dis.,* 163, 1177, 1991.
143. **Cerra, F. B.,** The multiple organ failure syndrome, *Hosp. Pract. Off.,* 25, 169, 1990.
144. **Navar, P. D., Saffle, J. R., and Warden, G. D.,** Effect of inhalation injury on fluid resuscitation requirements after thermal injury, *Am. J. Surg.,* 150, 716, 1985.
145. **Herndon, D. N., Barrow, R. E., Traber, D. L., Rutan, T. C., Rutan, R. L., and Abston, S.,** Extravascular lung water changes following smoke inhalation and massive burn injury, *Surgery,* 102, 341, 1987.
146. **Traber, D. L., Sugi, K., Flynn, J. T., and Traber, L. D.,** Leukotrienes and lung response to inhalation injury, *FASEB J.,* 3, A695, 1989.
147. **Morris, S. E., Navaratnam, N., Townsend, C. M., Jr., and Herndon, D. N.,** Bacterial translocation and mesenteric blood flow in a large animal model after cutaneous thermal and smoke inhalation injury, *Surg. Forum,* 39, 189, 1988.
148. **Hubbard, G. B., Langlinais, P. C., Shimazu, T., Okerberg, C. V., Mason, A. D., and Pruitt, B. A.,** The morphology of smoke inhalation injury in sheep, *J. Trauma,* 31, 1477, 1992.

Chapter 10

Adjustments Associated with the Aging Process

Daniel R. Richardson

CONTENTS

I. GENERAL CONSIDERATIONS OF AGING

By the year 2000, the U.S. population age 65 years and over is predicted to grow from 4.1 to 11.9%.[1] Furthermore, by the year 2050, at least 5% of the U.S. population will be composed of persons over the age of 85.[2] These demographic statistics, coupled with the fact that many pathologic conditions that affect the microcirculation have a relatively high incidence among the aged population,[3] suggest that any text dealing with pathophysiology of the microcirculation should include a chapter on the "normal" adjustments of the microcirculation that attend the aging process. In this manner, changes in the microcirculation associated with pathological states, such as atherosclerosis, can be examined against a background of the microcirculation in a healthy elderly population.

0-8493-4547-2/94/$0.00+$.50

As many of the references cited in this chapter will bear out, there is little doubt that the structure and function of the microcirculation are modified with advancing age; however, it is not at all clear whether any particular modification is inherent to the aging process or an adaptive response of the microvessels to stress that occurs throughout an individual's lifetime. As Zweifach[4] has pointed out, the microcirculation has a phenomenal capacity to adapt to chronic stress situations and remodel itself so that homeostasis of blood-tissue exchange is maintained. In this regard, one of the challenges in aging research lies in separating changes that are inherent to the aging process from those that are adaptive in nature.

Another problem that affects aging studies of the microcirculation is that in humans the rate at which any given microcirculatory variable changes with age can be affected by a variety of lifestyle factors such as diet[5] and exercise.[6] The desirability of controlling such interactive variables is one reason animal models are used in aging research. Longitudinal studies over the life span of laboratory animals can also avoid many of the problems encountered in cross-sectional studies of specific age groups, such as differential survivorship.[7] However, Weindruch and Masoro[8] have cautioned that relying excessively on a particular animal model can lead to erroneous conclusions regarding the aging process. This note of caution suggests it would be best to use more than one species or strain of animal species to study a particular aging phenomenon.

With the above disclaimers in mind, this chapter will survey the structural and functional changes in the microcirculation that are associated with the aging process. The topic will begin with a description of some of the more salient age-related changes in the macro- and microcirculations. This description will be followed by a more detailed discussion of the microcirculations of those vascular beds which have been studied to the greatest extent with regard to age-related adjustments in humans. These are the cutaneous, skeletal muscle, myocardial, conjunctival, and cerebral circulations. To offer a comprehensive analysis, the review of these vascular beds will not be limited to human studies but will include animal model experiments as well.

II. DEFINITION OF AGE CATEGORIES

Since several microcirculatory studies have shown nonlinear changes in microvascular structure and/or function from young adulthood through old age,[9-12] any discussion of the aging process requires defining the age ranges involved. When human studies are discussed in this chapter, "young" will refer to ages 20 through 39 years. "Middle age" will refer to those 40 through 59, while "elderly", "old", and "older" will collectively refer to individuals above 60. These categories are reasonably consistent with those used in previous studies.[13,14] In describing animal model studies, the young and old categories will refer to a percentage of the life span of the organism equivalent to that of a human.

III. OVERVIEW OF THE CIRCULATORY CHANGES ASSOCIATED WITH AGING

A. THE MACROCIRCULATION

Several concise reviews of the changes that occur in macrovessels with advancing age have appeared over the past 30 years.[15-18] These reviews point out that age-related changes occur in virtually all segments of the arterial wall beginning with the intima where there is a generalized hypertrophy and shape irregularity of the endothelial cells. In addition, the connective tissue content of the intima increases and this is thought to be due to secretions from modified smooth muscle cells entering from the media. As aging progresses, the medial layer thickens, collagen deposits increase, and the outer surface of the muscle cells within the medium become irregular, thereby increasing the cell's surface area. However, Goldman[16] notes that after age 40, vascular smooth muscle cells tend to be replaced by connective tissue such that by the time old age is reached quite often only islands of muscle cells are discernible. Along these lines, Kojimahara et al.[19] have observed smooth muscle necrosis in cerebral arteries obtained from old rats, while Borchard et al.[20] have suggested that beyond middle age, vascular smooth muscle becomes less thick.

Throughout the vessel wall the percentage of collagen fibers increases, calcification progresses, and lipid deposits increase with advancing age. These effects are different from the classical plaques of atherosclerosis, which supports the notion that atherosclerosis is not an inherent aging process.[17]

The various effects of age on vessel cross-section collectively result in thicker, more rigid arteries which have a reduced luminal diameter and a modified endothelium. Yin[18] points out that similar changes occur in the pulmonary vessels, suggesting that age may affect veins and arteries similarly. However, as Kohn[17] has noted, the venous system has not received as much attention in aging studies as has the arterial tree.

In terms of vessel topography, the most characteristic age-related feature found at the macrocirculatory level is vessel tortuosity, a phenomenon which has been observed in both arteries[21-23] and veins.[17] Vascular coiling and spiraling, extreme forms of tortuosity, are observed primarily in the small arteries and arterioles of the senile brain,[24] but they have also been found in other tissues from older individuals including the myocardium[21] and bone.[22] Since vessel tortuosity is associated with several disease states,[25] it is unclear as to whether aging or some underlying disease process causes tortuous vessels to occur in older individuals. Nevertheless, vessel tortuosity is thought to be responsible for an altered distribution of tissue blood flow in the elderly and, in some cases, may be the cause of focal ischemia.[22] Arterial tortuosity may also be one of the factors responsible for the tendency for vascular resistance to increase in older individuals.[26,27]

B. THE MICROCIRCULATION

The salient qualitative changes in the macrocirculation associated with age, such as tortuosity,[21] extend into the microvessels.[24,28-32] However, the quantitative details and the mechanisms of age-related changes in the microvessels may be different from those seen at the macrovascular level. For example, in the cerebral circulation, the decrease in distensibility seen in the distributing arteries of older individuals[33] continues into the small arterioles.[34] However, in terms of mechanism, the increased rigidity of arteries seems to be due to an increase in collagen synthesis, whereas that of the corresponding arterioles may be due to an atrophy of distensible components.

Several studies have examined changes in the wall structure of microvessels as a function of age, but no consistent pattern can be gleaned from these various investigations. For example, some microvessels seem to become thinner with age[28,34-35] while others become thicker,[36-38] and some reports suggest that aging has no effect on the cross-sectional dimension of microvessels.[39] In a paper on the cutaneous circulation and aging, Braverman et al.[40] indicate that whether a microvessel in the skin becomes thicker or thinner with age depends upon the presence or absence of a perivascular fibroblast called a "veil" cell. Whether similar perivascular cells are responsible for maintaining microvessels in other tissues remains to be determined.

A distinct feature of the microcirculation is that it tends to atrophy with advancing age. This is evidenced by diffuse acellularity[41] and general loss of microvessels[23,29,42-44] including both blood capillaries[23,31,43,45-48] and lymph capillaries.[49] In this context, it is tempting to assume capillary rarefaction is inherent to the aging process, because it is found in a variety of tissues and animal species with advancing age. However, in some tissues, such as skeletal muscle, the reported effects of aging on capillary density are equivocal and appear to be associated more with age-related changes in tissue cell size and composition than to the effects of age on the circulation.[6,50,51] Furthermore, some capillary networks, such as the papillary capillaries of the skin, show age-related rarefaction in some regions of the body, such as the toes,[32] forearms,[52] and scalp,[53] but not in others, including the fingers.[32,54] Thus, capillary rarefaction in older individuals may be elicited by age-related changes in the parenchymal cell environment, not by aging of the blood vessels themselves. This notion is consistent with results from a variety of studies. For example, Braverman[36] has noted that the integrity of the superficial cutaneous microvessels depends upon the functional state of the veil cells. Mann et al.[55] suggested that the loss of cerebral capillaries with age is secondary to the loss of nerve cells. Finally, de Mignard and Bernick[56] demonstrated parallel vascular and osteocytic dysfunction with advancing age in bone tissue. They attributed the osteocytic abnormalities to an interruption in the vascular supply; however, the reverse scenario is just as likely.

Another characteristic of the aging microcirculation is the presence of dilated capillaries and/or venules,[28,52,54,57,58] which in certain instances take the form of microaneurysms.[41,59] Ryan's work[58] suggests that such phenomena may be elicited more by a breakdown of support tissue than by aging of the vessels. Thus, although it has been suggested that microcirculatory dysfunction plays an important role in the process of tissue aging,[23] the evidence discussed above indicates that the opposite may be the case. That is, age-related changes in tissue cells proper may elicit structural and functional changes in the attended microvessels.

C. BLOOD RHEOLOGY

Since aging is attended by an increase in plasma fibrinogen,[60] it is tenable that the tendency for peripheral resistance to be elevated with age[26,27] is at least in part mediated by an increase in blood viscosity. However, in a meticulous study of this question, *Lowe et al.*[61] *found only a 3% increase in blood viscosity over the age range of 20 to 80.* Giansanti et al.[62] found 68-year-old individuals to have about a 4% higher blood viscosity than 28-year-old subjects. These differences are well short of Amery et al.'s[26] estimate of a 56% increase in total peripheral resistance over the same age span. This suggests that viscosity would not significantly contribute to the age-related increase in peripheral resistance. However, both Lowe et al.[61] and Giansanti et al.[62] measured the viscosity of whole blood *in vitro*, a procedure which does not necessarily reflect conditions at the level of individual microvessels. In this regard, the reduced red cell deformability present in older individuals[63-66] could inhibit red cell aggregation, resulting in a lower viscosity (as measured by rotational viscometry) while simultaneously "plugging" capillaries in the circulatory system and effectively increasing blood flow resistance. Such plugging of capillaries may be in part responsible for the decrease in the density of patent capillaries observed in the skin of older men by *in vivo* microscopy.[32] Thus, while changes in the composition of rheological factors in the blood do occur with advancing age, it is uncertain what effect, if any, these changes may exert on peripheral resistance.

D. VASCULAR FUNCTION

Since peripheral vascular resistance increases and cardiac index slightly decreases in healthy older individuals,[27] it could be predicted that peripheral blood flow would be modified in the older individual. While this is generally held to be true in a qualitative sense, quantitative information from different reports on aging and tissue blood flow vary considerably. In one of the earliest studies of this subject, Bender[67] noted that, while splanchnic, renal, and cutaneous blood flow decreased markedly with age, flow through resting skeletal muscle showed virtually no aging effect. Some of these results are consistent with more recent findings while others are not. For example, Tsuchida[68] has confirmed that skin blood flow is decreased with age in several anatomical sites, while Richardson[13] reports that an age-related decrease in cutaneous blood flow occurs only under conditions of heat stress. Tuma et al.[69] found either no difference or a slight increase in skeletal muscle blood flow when they compared 24-month-old against 12-month-old rats. In contrast, Korkushko et al.[31] have shown a 25% decrease in resting muscle blood flow between 20- and 80-year-old humans and the difference between these two groups was even more pronounced during exercise.

It is not at all clear why different laboratories report different quantitative effects of aging on tissue blood flow. Nevertheless, the collective evidence suggests that aging results in a hypokinetic circulation (i.e., one in which blood flow is lower either at rest, during an increase in tissue function, or both).

In considering possible mechanisms for the effects of aging on peripheral blood flow, the discussion up to this point has considered only the structural determinants of flow. In this context, it is highly likely that some of the age-related changes in microvascular structure, such as tortuosity, contribute to an increase in "fixed" resistance to the flow of blood in the older organism. In addition, it is possible that an increase in vascular smooth muscle tone further contributes to a change in vascular resistance with age. This notion is consistent with the observation of an age-related increase in sympathetic tone.[70] However, an increase in sympathetic tone per se does not necessarily mean that constrictor tone of the innervated blood vessels is increased. In this regard, the direct application of alpha adrenergic agonists to blood vessels from different age groups of animals has shown either no age difference in the constrictor effect[71] or a blunted response in blood vessels from older animals.[71-73] Furthermore, postjunctional adrenergic responses are depressed in the hind limbs of old rats.[74] Collectively these results indicate that reduced peripheral blood flow in the aged is not likely to be mediated by an increase in the response to vasoconstrictor substances, such as catecholamines, even though sympathetic motor tone may be elevated.

Although aging may not attenuate the degree of vasoconstriction elicited by the administration of a constrictor substance, it is possible that a reduced response to dilatory agents could increase the effective degree of ongoing constrictor tone. This possibility is consistent with reports of reduced vascular effects of acetylcholine in older humans[75] and with the fact that blood vessels isolated from old rats show reduced relaxation in response to the application of dilator compounds.[76,77] Furthermore, the diminished dilatory responses of vessels from old animals has been shown to be dependent upon an intact vascular endothelium.[76,77] This observation suggests that altered endothelial cells may be responsible for reduced dilatory effects in old animals. This notion is consistent with a variety of studies which have shown age-related alterations in vascular endothelial cells.[36,37,77,78] In this regard, an altered vascular endothelium may be the mechanism which mediates the attenuated dilatory response observed in collateral vessels of older organisms,[79] since dilation of collateral vessels is thought to be endothelial cell dependent.[80]

Collectively, the results discussed in this section suggest that resting constrictor tone may be increased in blood vessels from older organisms and that the mechanism may be blunted dilatory effects due to altered endothelial cells. However, while it may be attractive to speculate that age-related changes in tissue blood flow are mediated by altered endothelial cells, it should be emphasized that the role of the endothelial cell in regulating vascular tone is an area of intense investigation in which physiologists are not at all clear as to the "normal" state of affairs let alone possible modifications due to conditions such as aging. These considerations emphasize the fact that the progress of aging research in the microcirculation is linked to our understanding of basic mechanisms of circulatory control.

E. BLOOD-TISSUE EXCHANGE

Ironically, the plethora of studies on age-related changes in the microcirculation contain very little information concerning its ultimate function — blood-tissue exchange. Undoubtedly, the surface area available for exchange must be depressed in those tissues which experience a decrease in capillary density with advancing age. However, if capillary rarefaction occurs in proportion to a loss of parenchymal cells, as some aging studies suggest,[55] then the ability of capillary networks to supply nutrients to the functional cells of a tissue would be modified only if the exchange characteristics of the remaining capillaries are affected by the aging process. On this point, what little evidence is available suggests that exchange is not impaired in the existing capillaries of an older person. For example, Van Best et al.[81] showed that vascular permeability was unaffected by age in the anterior chamber of the eye. Korkushko et al.[82] examined oxygen diffusion in the cutaneous circulation of elderly subjects and, although they did not have a young group for comparison, their data indicate that oxygen diffusion is not impaired with old age. Yamaguchi et al.[83] studied albumin permeability in cerebral capillaries of different aged subjects and found that, if anything, this variable is increased in elderly individuals. Prior to this work, Mooradian[84] had reviewed the subject of aging and the blood-brain barrier and noted that most studies up to that time had failed to show a significant age-related alteration in blood-brain barrier permeability to water soluble substances and high molecular weight solutes in healthy individuals.

In brief, there is no convincing evidence that aging has any detrimental effect on blood-tissue exchange at the level of single capillaries. It is possible that this lack of an aging effect is at least in part the result of compensatory adjustments that offset any age-related structural changes that could be detrimental to capillary exchange. In support of this notion, Stablein and Meyer[37] found that the age-related increase in the thickness of blood capillaries in the oral mucosa of rats is attended by an increase in the number of pinocytotic vesicles within the capillary endothelium. They suggested that this aging effect compensates for impaired exchange due to thickened capillary basement membranes in the older animals. It is unknown if similar changes in capillary structure occur elsewhere in the circulatory system of older organisms, but the study of Stablein and Meyer[37] points out the possibility of compensatory adjustment in capillary morphology geared toward maintaining normal blood-tissue exchange in the tissues of older individuals.

F. SUMMARY

In the macro- and microcirculations, advancing age is associated with peripheral arteries and veins that become narrower, more tortuous, and less compliant, and which take on a modified endothelium. In a qualitative sense the age-related changes observed in the arterial system continue through the arteriolar network and into the capillaries. There is a general rarefaction of capillaries, but the presence and extent of this phenomenon may be due more to the effects of aging on tissue function than to aging of the blood vessels. In terms of circulatory function, most vascular beds in older organisms seem to be hypokinetic with regard to resting blood flow and/or blood flow responses to physiological perturbations. However, at present there is little direct knowledge as to the exact mechanisms responsible for the age-related changes in circulatory function. Finally, the ultimate function of the microcirculation — blood-tissue exchange — has been studied very little with regard to age adjustments. However, what evidence is available suggests that any structural and/or functional changes which threaten to compromise exchange may be offset by compensatory adjustments in the remaining capillary vessels.

IV. AGE-RELATED CHANGES IN SPECIFIC VASCULAR BEDS

A. THE CUTANEOUS CIRCULATION

Since the cutaneous circulation participates in the regulation of blood pressure and body temperature,[85] investigation of the cutaneous microcirculation offers one approach to examining the modifications, if any, of these homeostatic systems with advancing age. Furthermore, a wide variety of pathologic disorders such as atherosclerosis, diabetes, and congestive heart failure are attended by structural changes in the cutaneous microcirculation.[28] In this context, the superficial microvessels of the skin offer a valuable diagnostic and prognostic tool in the detection and management of these and other pathological conditions.

1. Structural Considerations

The structure of the cutaneous circulation is relatively complex consisting of superficial and deep vascular plexes interconnected by ascending vessels.[85,86] Although age-related structural changes such as a decrease in vascular density have been reported to occur in the deep cutaneous vascular networks,[53] the most pronounced, and most widely studied, changes occur within the superficial vessels. Ryan and his colleagues[43,58,87] have extensively investigated the structure of these vessels in both development and aging. With regard to the former, they note that the redness of the newborn skin is due to a dense network of capillaries in the upper dermis which are covered by a relatively thin epidermal layer. This network is disorganized and contains relatively few looped capillaries. Over the first 4 months of life, it becomes more organized, the epidermis thickens, the dermis pushes up to form papilla, the looped papillary capillaries become distinct, and the low-resistance pathways (e.g., arteriovenous anastomoses — AVA) begin to form. However, the most complex shunt vessels, the highly innervated AV glomi, do not fully develop until about the age of four.[58]

According to Marinov and Tzvetkova,[88] between the ages of 3 and 20 the papillary capillaries take on "local peculiarities" such as lengthening and twisting of the vessels. These peculiarities become more numerous in the skin of the lower limbs, suggesting that environmental factors such as intravascular pressure may be responsible for local differences in cutaneous microvascular structure. This notion is consistent with the evidence of Perera et al.[87] to the effect that the development of the cutaneous microcirculation is governed by dynamic processes ranging from the formation of skin creases to the generation of blood pressure. In the same light, Syme and Riley[89] showed that the appearance of papillary capillaries in infants is determined more by body weight than by age. Thus, to a large degree the development of the superficial microvessels of the skin is determined by external factors some of which are peculiar to a particular region of skin. By the same token, the collective evidence to date suggests that the rate at which the cutaneous microcirculation changes with advancing age is to a large degree determined by factors other than aging per se.

One of the characteristic changes in the cutaneous circulation of the elderly is a reduction in the number of capillaries that supply the epidermal papillae.[29,32,52,53,58,90] The disappearance of these vessels and a concurrent thinning of the epidermis[91] results in an exposure of the subpapillary plexus — the vessels of which then tend to become dilated. This condition, termed Telangiectasis,[58] gives rise to the characteristic redness in certain skin areas of an older person. Figure 1 gives an example of these vascular changes as viewed in the forearm by videomicroscopy in a young and an old subject who had participated in one of our studies.[52] Note the generally wider horizontal plexus vessels and lack of looped capillary tips in the sample from the older subject. Also, as indicated, the older subjects tended to have more branching of the plexus vessels. This observation is in contrast to the results of Gilchrest et al.,[92] who reported a decrease in the number of venular crossings from vertical sections obtained from the buttock skin of elderly subjects. However, it not certain how much of the subpapillary plexus was represented in their biopsied sections. On the other hand, our results are consistent with those of Korkushko and Sarkisov,[90] which indicate that the diminution in the number of surface capillaries in the skin of older individuals is attended by development of the subpapillary vascular plexus. In this context, the "aging" effect on the cutaneous microcirculation may

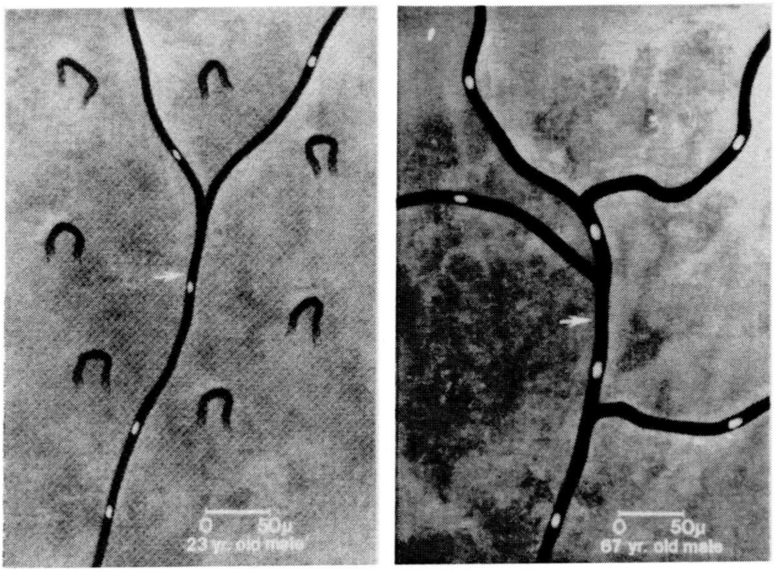

Figure 10-1 Sketch of the superficial vessels of the forearm as seen by videomicroscopy in a 23- (left) and a 67-year-old male (right). The horizontal vessels are those of the subpapillary plexus, whereas the ascending looped vessels are papillary capillaries. Note the lack of papillary capillaries in the older person.

be just the reverse of what happens in neonatal development, where the appearance of looped capillaries seems to be attended by a reduction in the number of plexus vessels.[58,87]

Although an age-related reduction in the number of papillary capillaries has been observed in a variety of skin sites by several independent investigators, it is not a ubiquitous finding. For example, de Nicola et al.[54] found the number of capillaries in the finger nailfold to be "within normal limits," and Richardson and Schwartz[32] found no significant difference in nailfold capillary density in the fingers of 27-year-old compared to 62-year-old men. However, the younger subjects in the Richardson and Schwartz study had a higher capillary density in their toe nailfolds relative to that of the older men and relative to the capillary density in their own fingers, whereas toe and finger capillary densities were the same in the elderly group.

A possible explanation for these findings is that cutaneous capillary rarefaction elicited by external factors, such as sun exposure (e.g., on the fingers), has a pronounced effect that occurs early in life. This notion is consistent with the observation that actinic damage exacerbates age-related changes in the cutaneous circulation.[29] However, since a variety of external factors affect the structure of the superficial cutaneous vessels,[88] other explanations are possible (e.g., a greater tendency towards mechanical trauma to the finger nailfolds). The point to be made here is that although there may be no clear aging effect within the circulation of a particular portion of skin (e.g., the finger nailfold), this does not necessarily mean that the associated vessels have remained unchanged throughout an individual's life.

Although a wide variety of factors may be responsible for the rarefaction of cutaneous capillaries with advancing age, they all may have a common denominator in altered veil cells. Braverman's laboratory[35,36,40] has shown that these fibroblast-like cells surround dermal blood vessels and secrete basement membrane-like substances that support the vessel wall. The thinning of the vessel walls and reduced papillary capillaries in older individuals are associated with a paucity of the veil cells. However, it is not known if these phenomena are in any way causally linked. Thus, although the evidence points away from aging per se as the cause of cutaneous capillary rarefaction in the elderly,[58,88] the exact mechanisms have yet to be clearly elucidated.

In addition to a reduction in the number of papillary capillaries in the elderly, those that remain have an increase in tortuosity.[29-32,54,93] In terms of causal factors, evidence suggests that external forces (e.g., gravity) play the major role in determining the degree of tortuosity seen in superficial microvessels.[32,88] That the inherent aging process itself probably has very little influence on vessel tortuosity is suggested by Ryan,[58] who stated that a given nailfold vasculature can be viewed periodically over many years with no apparent change in pattern or shape of the vessels.

In addition to the cutaneous capillaries tending to be tortuous in the elderly, several investigators have reported that the capillaries are longer and/or that the venous limb is dilated.[30,31,54,93] An increase in the length of cutaneous capillaries with age is consistent with what has been observed in the oral mucosa,[12] a tissue similar to skin.

A somewhat controversial finding in the cutaneous circulation of the older person relates to the low resistance AV pathways. An earlier report by Popoff[44] suggested that the number of AV glomi is decreased in the elderly, while a more recent study by Merlen[93] states that, owing to the atrophy of the dermis and hypodermis, the glomi seem to be more numerous in old age. In keeping with Merlen's findings, other reports suggest that flow through AV vessels is enhanced in the elderly. For example, Korkushko and Sarkisov[90] report the development of intercapillary anastomoses in the superficial vessels of older individuals, while Haimovici et al.[94] suggest that flow through preferential channels is increased in the aged skin. Thus, the weight of the evidence favors the notion that AV shunt flow is enhanced in the skin of the elderly person.

In terms of functional significance, investigations which address the role of arterio-venous anastomoses in vascular diseases[94,95] suggest that increased flow through shunt vessels may exacerbate problems of ischemia by reducing nutritional perfusion to tissue cells. In contrast, the development of AV anastomoses in the subepidermal plexus of healthy elderly could serve to compensate for the loss of papillary capillaries with regard to heat exchange, since cutaneous AVAs are thought to serve a thermoregulatory function.[96]

In contrast to the voluminous amount of information on the structure of the cutaneous microcirculation in aging humans, very little is known about this subject in animal models frequently used in aging research (e.g., the laboratory rat). Stablein and Meyer[12] made a very detailed study of the changes in capillaries within the oral mucosa of young, middle-aged, and old Sprague-Dawley rats. They noted a general increase in the length of the capillaries between young and old animals in a manner similar to what has been reported for capillaries of the human skin.[30,31,54,93] However, the age relationships were quite complex, with the middle-aged rats showing the greatest changes in some of the regions sampled. In rodent studies more directly related to the effects of aging on the cutaneous microcirculation, Holm-Pedersen et al.[97] and Yamaura and Matsuzawa[98] have studied the effects of aging on microvascularization of cutaneous lesions. The rate of vascular growth into the lesioned areas, and hence vascular density, was significantly reduced in old rats. In a similar manner, Kreisle et al.[99] have shown that the rate of capillary growth into melanomas and fibrosarcomas was reduced in old mice. These findings suggest that the rarefaction of cutaneous capillaries in the skin of older persons may be due more to reduced angiogenesis than to accelerated vessel absorption.

Our laboratory has studied the subepidermal vascular plexus in tails of young and old, Fischer-344[100] and Sprague-Dawley[101-102] rats by light microscopy. These animals do not have any looped capillaries in the skin,[103] and the subepidermal plexus can easily be viewed in all age groups. Although we have not made a detailed study of the vascular structure, there does not seem to be any overt structural modifications in vessels from the old rats, and vessel diameters are not significantly changed as a function of age.[100,102] Our major finding with regard to microcirculatory structure is in the density of plexus capillaries, and, in this context, there are differences between the Fischer-344 and Sprague-Dawley strains. In the Fischer-344 rats, there were no aging differences in capillary density at normothermic temperature, but the recruitment of capillaries during heat stress was modified.[100] By contrast, the Sprague-Dawley groups demonstrated a significant age-related decrease in capillary density but essentially no age differences in the ability to recruit vessels during heat stress.[102] These findings are discussed in more detail in the section dealing with the functional changes in the cutaneous circulation associated with aging.

2. Functional Considerations

a. *The Cutaneous Microcirculation and Skin Moisture Content in the Aged*

The structural alterations of the cutaneous microcirculation and rarefaction of superficial capillaries with old age give rise to the notion that such changes may be responsible for the altered appearance of the skin in elderly individuals. Along these lines, it would be reasonable to propose that an age-related decrease in capillary density would reduce interstitial volume, thus eliciting a dry and/or wrinkled appearance to skin.[104] However, it has been shown that water content of the skin increases rather than decreases with age.[105,106] In considering these findings, Kligman[105] suggests that it is the altered architecture of the tissue matrix, not the water content, that is responsible for the dry appearance of elderly skin. He further suggests that the increase in water content with age may be only relative owing to a decrease in structural constituents, such as collagen. On the other hand, if the subepidermal venous plexus tends to proliferate with age, as some studies indicate,[90] then the increase in dermal water content in the elderly could be absolute. This is particularly so considering that the filtration coefficient tends to increase towards the venous end of a capillary.[107]

Thus, in contrast to the perception that the aging skin may be "dry," the evidence indicates that the exact opposite is the case. However, it has yet to be determined what, if any, role the cutaneous microcirculation plays in the appearance of elderly skin.

b. *Percutaneous Absorption*

The classic procedure for quantifying percutaneous absorption in humans is the McClure-Aldrich test.[108] To administer this test, 0.2 ml of saline are injected intradermally on the volar side of the forearm, and the time required for the resultant wheel to dissipate is measured. Using this method, Aschner[109] and later Kligman[105] showed wheel disappearance time to be prolonged in the elderly. Sodium fluorescein[110] and radiolabeled sodium[111,112] studies have confirmed these findings by showing prolonged ion clearance times in older subjects.

In more recent studies, Roskos et al.[113] found that the reduced percutaneous absorption with aging occurs primarily with hydrophilic compounds, suggesting to these authors that this age-related defect is due to increased barrier function as opposed to reduced clearance by the circulation, a conclusion consistent with earlier observations.[111,112] To address the role of the cutaneous circulation in reduced percutaneous absorption in the elderly, the same group of investigators[114] later studied dynamic responses of blood flow to methyl nicotinate applied to the ventral forearm and found no significant age differences in the cutaneous circulatory response to this vasoactive compound. These results suggest that altered barrier function plays a more important role than any alterations in the microcirculation in determining the effects of aging on percutaneous absorption. Furthermore, the fact that the methyl nicotinate in Roskos et al.'s study[114] was topically applied suggests that the loss of superficial capillaries in the forearms of the elderly[52] is compensated for by adjustments elsewhere in the cutaneous circulation.

Thus, while percutaneous absorption may be reduced with advancing age, there is no evidence to suggest that this phenomenon is due to attenuated cutaneous microcirculatory function.

c. *Wound Healing*

The delay in wound healing in older individuals is a well-established phenomenon.[115] The observation that vascular proliferation is generally reduced in wounds from older organisms[97,116] gives rise to the notion that microcirculatory dysfunction in older individuals plays a significant role in the attenuation of the wound healing process. Evidence clearly favoring this notion has been provided by Holm-Pedersen et al.,[97] who noted that not only was the rate of vascular growth into wound areas reduced in old rats, but the vascular network in the wounds of the old animals was characteristically different from that of the young. For example, vascular permeability tended to increase during the first 3 or 4 days of the healing process in the young rats, whereas permeability of vessels from the old animals showed little if any change over the same time period. Collectively these findings suggested to the authors that the microvascular system in wounds from young animals was better suited for the promotion of wound healing compared to that of the older animals. Thus, differences in microvascular structure and/or function between young and old animals no doubt plays some role in the delayed wound healing of older individuals. However, it is probably not aging of the vessels per se that is responsible for this difference, but rather other age-related factors, such as a depressed immune system,[117] that result in a lack of support for new vessel growth. Along these lines, Ryan and Kurban[118] have shown that the growth of new vessels in traumatized skin is dependent upon the support of local factors. One such factor may be the reticulo-endothelial system, since it has been shown that this system becomes depressed with age.[43] Such depression may be responsible for the sluggish growth of vessels in wounds of elderly individuals. Alternatively, the tissue matrix from elderly individuals could be lacking in a number of angiogenic factors responsible for the development of new vessels.[119]

d. *Resting Vascular Dynamics*

Measurements of total blood flow in apical extremities (e.g., digits, hands, and feet) have shown that cutaneous blood flow in these regions is decreased in older persons.[68,120-124] In general, the same has been found for the superficial capillaries although reported aging effects are somewhat variable. For example, early data from Brown and Roth[30] show at least a 50% lower blood cell velocity (BCV) in finger nailfold capillaries from 70-year-old compared to 30-year-old subjects. In more recent studies, Ostergren and Fagrell[10] found only an 18% lower BCV in finger nailfold capillaries in old compared to young men, while Richardson and Schwartz[32] reported a 27% difference in BCV of finger nailfold vessels between these two groups with the elderly men having the lower value.

The reasons for the quantitative differences in the effects of aging on capillary flow velocity in same type of cutaneous blood vessels is not clear. Quite possibly differences in experimental conditions and/or methods can account for at least some of the variability. In this regard, the data from Ostergren and Fagrell[10] indicate that a lack of standardization in skin temperature could modify, or even mask, age differences in nailfold capillary BCV. Another experimental condition of importance in assessing the effects of age on flow dynamics in cutaneous microvessels is the position of the skin relative to heart level. In this context, Richardson and Schwartz[32] noted a 40% lower BCV in toe nailfold capillaries of elderly compared to young males when the subjects were in a seated posture. However, when the toes were placed at heart level in a subsequent study,[11] absolute flow values were higher in both groups, and there was only a modest, 10% difference between the old and young subjects. The mechanism of this apparent difference in orthostatic sensitivity of cutaneous capillary blood flow between young and old subjects has yet to be elucidated.

Thus, while in general old age in humans is attended by a decrease in blood flow through superficial capillaries of the skin, the magnitude of the aging effect depends on a variety of external factors (e.g., temperature and gravity loading). Nevertheless, even a slightly lower capillary blood flow, vis-a-vis a reduced capillary density in the elderly, could result in a marked reduction in total capillary flow in the region. For example, in one of our previous studies,[32] we multiplied the density of flowing capillaries by the measured blood flow per capillary to obtain an estimate of total capillary flow in the toenailfolds of young and old men. Respective values for these two groups averaged 27 and 10.5 cubic micra/sec/mm^2 × 10^4. In other words, the estimated capillary flow in the elderly was about 60% lower than that of the young when both capillary density and flow per capillary were taken into consideration.

Our laboratory has also found a similar aging effect on estimated capillary flow in the subepidermal vascular plexus of the rat tail. As mentioned previously, we have examined this vascular bed in young, middle aged, and old Sprague-Dawley rats.[102] At a thermoneutral skin temperature (25°C), capillary blood flow in single vessels was the same in all three groups, but there was an age-dependent decrease in capillary density. Multiplying the capillary density by capillary blood flow gave respective values of 8.9, 7.6, and 6.1 cubic micra/sec/mm^2 × 10^4 for the young, middle aged, and old groups. Thus, in the human nailfold and the subepidermal plexus of the rat tail, the decrease in density of cutaneous capillaries in older individuals does not seem to be compensated for by an increase in flow through remaining vessels at a thermoneutral skin temperature. As will be discussed subsequently, this is not the case with heat stress.

From the above discussion it can be concluded that, as a general trend, cutaneous blood flow in the extremities of humans is decreased with advancing age in regard to both total flow[68,120-124] and flow through the superficial capillaries.[10,30,32] This observation raises the question as to whether these two phenomena may be linked. That is, is the age-related reduction in capillary blood flow mechanistically connected to the decrease in total flow? On this point, recent studies in our laboratory[125] have shown a tighter coupling between laser Doppler measurements of total cutaneous blood flow and videomicroscopic measurements of nailfold capillary flow in the fingers of old compared to young men under thermoneutral conditions. This finding is consistent with the notion that age-related changes in total and capillary flow in the skin may be coupled. However, responses to physiological perturbations do not support this hypothesis. For example, the reduction in total digital flow elicited by isometric exercise in young men is attended by no change in nailfold capillary flow,[126] and, in both young as well as old men, orthostasis elicits opposite changes in total and capillary blood flow in the toe.[11] Furthermore, the nailfold vascular bed in atherosclerotic limbs is characterized by an increase in capillary blood flow and capillary density.[127] This suggests that, if anything, the microcirculation of the skin may compensate for abnormalities in arterial input. Thus, while both total and capillary flow in the cutaneous circulation of the extremities may decrease with age, the balance of present evidence suggests that the two are not connected.

In addition to the apical extremities, the cutaneous circulation of the human forearm has been relatively well studied with regard to aging effects. However, apical and forearm cutaneous circulations differ somewhat in both structure and function. Whereas the circulation in apical regions is rich in arteriovenous anastomoses and heat stress elicits vasodilation via sympathetic withdrawal, that of the forearm is relatively lacking in AVAs and heat elicited vasodilation occurs by way an active neurogenic mechanism.[85]

Early reports on age differences in forearm blood flow, as measured by venous occlusion plethysmography under thermoneutral conditions, indicate that in older men this variable is either higher than[128] or about equal to[129] that of younger subjects. However, collectively these studies had only two subjects over the age of 60, and the mean ages for the older groups were in the middle age range (40 to 60). In this regard, studies in apical areas of skin have indicated that circulatory results obtained with middle-aged subjects are not necessarily reflective of those obtained in the elderly.[10,11]

More recent reports, in which the older subjects were at least age 55, showed plethysmographic measurements of forearm blood flow to be slightly less in old compared to young subjects in thermoneutral conditions, but the elderly had a reduced dilatory response to heat stress such that the magnitude of the difference between young and old subjects became greater with increasing skin temperature.[130-132] Our laboratory has shown similar results using laser Doppler flowmetry (LDF) to measure cutaneous blood flow in the forearms of young and old subjects before and during direct heat applied to the arm.[13] Thus, the weight of the evidence suggests that cutaneous blood flow in the forearm is less in old compared to young individuals with the extent of the difference being dependent upon environmental temperature.

In terms of the microcirculation, our laboratory has investigated the subepidermal vascular plexus in the forearms of young and old subjects by videomicroscopy.[52] We could find no papillary capillaries in the forearms of the elderly, but their existing subpapillary plexus vessels were somewhat wider compared to the young (Figure 1). In terms of flow dynamics, the old subjects had a 23% lower blood cell velocity in single plexus vessels at a thermoneutral skin temperature, but this was more than offset by the wider diameter. The estimated volume flow through individual plexus vessels was respectively 7500 and 9400 cubic micra per second for the young and old subjects. These data, vis-a-vis the observation that there may have been a proliferation of plexus vessels in the forearms of the elderly (Figure 1), suggest that in the human forearm the subpapillary vascular plexus compensates for an age-related loss of papillary capillaries. The possible relevance of this to heat exchange will be considered subsequently.

e. Response to Heat Stress

A number of studies have shown a reduced cutaneous blood flow response to heat stress in elderly men,[13,130,131,133,134] and the effect seems to be related primarily to subject age and not to extrinsic factors such as health status[130] or exercise capacity.[133] Since an increase in cutaneous blood flow plays a major role in maintaining body temperature in the face of a heat load,[85,135] it would be reasonable to predict that thermoregulatory capacity is reduced in the elderly. However, in spite of a plethora of information on the relationship between aging and body temperature regulation, there is very little consensus as to what effects, if any, aging itself has on the ability of an organism to maintain body temperature. It is generally held that the thermoregulatory system is not qualitatively modified in the elderly, but there is a reduced ability to adjust to extremes of temperature.[136,137] Even so, evidence points toward associated factors, such as health status and fitness level, instead of aging in the ability of the older person to adjust to temperature stress. For example, in an earlier study, Drinkwater and Horvath[138] indicated that the sweat rate of females in response to a given heat load is diminished with age, whereas the same group showed, in a later investigation, that sweat rate among physically fit elderly women is not diminished relative to the young.[139] In a similar manner, Yousef's group showed that sweat rate among men has a much stronger relationship to fitness level than to age,[140] and that at similar fitness levels there is virtually no effect of age on thermoregulatory capacity of men in a desert environment.[141]

Thus, in spite of the fact that the cutaneous blood flow response to heat stress is reduced in elderly who are healthy and physically fit, such individuals seem to have no measurable loss in their ability to regulate body temperature in the face of a heat load. One possible explanation for this seeming paradox is that the distribution of cutaneous blood flow is modified in the elderly such that, while total blood flow to the skin may be reduced in these individuals, flow in the superficial microvessels where heat exchange occurs is not. This notion is consistent with data from our laboratory showing that, while the response of regional cutaneous blood flow in the forearm to heat stress is reduced in elderly men,[13] the response of individual vessels within the subepidermal plexus of the forearm is slightly higher than that of the young in terms of percent change.[52]

To further investigate the effects of aging on the response of superficial cutaneous microvessels to heat stress, our laboratory has recently turned to examining the subepidermal plexus within the rat tail as an experimental model. The rat's tail is a major thermoregulatory organ for this species,[142,143] and its cutaneous circulatory structure is similar to that of human apical skin in being rich in arteriovenous anastomoses.[144] Furthermore, the cutaneous dilatory response to heat stress is mediated by sympathetic withdrawal in both human digits[85] and the rat tail.[145]

Our first series of experiments investigated the response of total blood flow to the tail and blood flow in individual capillaries within the subepidermal plexus to body (indirect) heat stress in young (6 to 8 months) and old (22 to 24 months), unanesthetized Fischer-344 rats.[100] The only significant microcirculatory effect was that the degree of capillary recruitment during heat stress was less in the older animals. However, this was offset by a slightly greater response of total blood flow such that the ratio of the capillary perfusion index (flow per capillary × capillary density) to the total blood flow was reduced during heat stress in the old rats. This suggests that, in the Fischer-344 rat, macrocirculatory adjustments compensate for microcirculatory deficiencies with regard to the cutaneous circulatory response to heat stress (i.e., the opposite from what might be the case for the human circulation).[13,52] This observation, taken in conjunction with the fact that the Fischer-344 has a relatively low tolerance to heat stress compared to the Sprague-Dawley,[146] prompted a second aging study using the Sprague-Dawley strain.

The animals used in our second study[102] consisted of groups of young (4 months), middle-aged (16 months), and old (27 months) male rats. These ages represent approximately 13, 25, and 85% of the life span of a male Sprague-Dawley.[147] Experiments were performed on unanesthetized animals situated so that their bodies and tails could be housed in separate environmental chambers for respectively indirect and direct heat stress studies. In both cases, heat stress consisted of increasing environmental temperature in the body (indirect) or tail (direct) chambers from 25 to 35°C for a period of 40 min. Each animal underwent both direct and indirect heat stress trials each on a separate day. Microcirculatory variables which were measured included the density of flowing capillaries (DFC) within the subepidermal plexus, BCV of single capillaries within the subepidermal plexus, and the width of the capillary red cell column (WRC), an index of inside diameter. The BCV and WRC data were obtained by the same videomicroscopic system used in human studies.[52] Both parametric (1-way ANOVA) and nonparametric (U Test) statistics were used to analyze for significant age differences at a given environmental temperature.

We found that, during indirect heat stress, the rise in the colonic temperature of the old rats (+0.4°C) was less than that of the young (+1.0°C) or middle-aged (+1.0°C) animals. A reduced core temperature response to heat stress has also been found in other strains of old laboratory rats[100,148] and in elderly human subjects under certain experimental conditions.[141] It is not known why the core temperature response to heat stress seems to be reduced in older organisms, but Blake et al.[148] suggested that this phenomenon may be due to a more efficient heat dissipation system. Evidence in favor of this notion is presented in Figure 2, which gives the main findings of our study with the Sprague-Dawley rats. As indicated by WRC, there were no significant age differences in capillary diameter, meaning that the measurements of BCV (middle panel) are reflective of volume flow. Note that, at the thermoneutral temperature of 25°C, there were no significant age differences in BCV, but there was a definite age-related decrease in the DFC. During body heating there was an age-related increase in the response of BCV. This elevated response of individual subepidermal vessels to indirect heat stress no doubt compensated to a certain degree for the age-related decrease in the density of flowing vessels, although

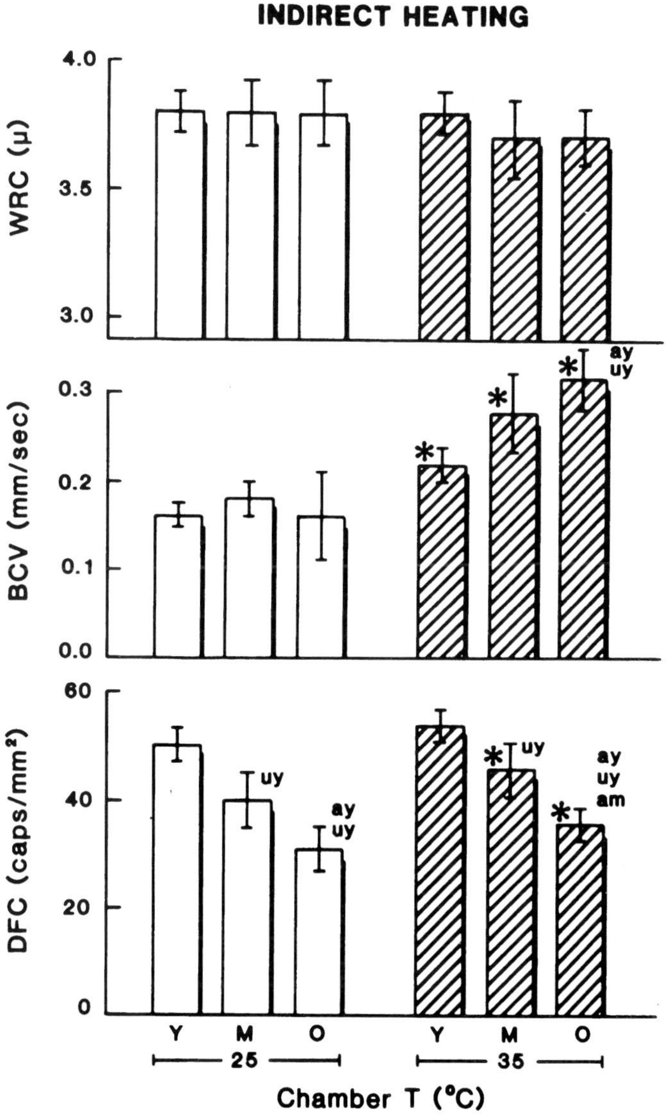

Figure 10-2 Group means ± SEM for width of the red cell column (WRC), blood cell velocity (BCV) of individual capillaries, and the density of flowing capillaries (DFC) before (25°C) and during (35°C) indirect heat stress. Tests for significance at $p < 0.05$. (*) Significant from pre-heat; (ay) significant from young group by ANOVA; (am) significant from middle age group by ANOVA; (uy) significant from young group by U-test; and (um) significant from middle age group by U-test. *(From Richardson, D., Shepherd, S., and Tyra, J., Endoth. Lymph., 7, 305, 1991. With permission.)*

a 2-way ANOVA indicated that DFC significantly increased during heat stress in these animals ($p < 0.006$).

For the old rats, the more pronounced rise in BCV during heat stress, vis-a-vis a lower increase in colonic temperature (Figure 2), clearly implies a more sensitive response of the cutaneous vessels to heat stress. In quantitative terms, the changes in BCV per degree

C change in colonic temperatures respectively 0.070, 0.091, and 0.385 mm/sec/°C for the young, middle-aged, and old rats. In other words, the old rats averaged over five times greater increases in BCV per °C than the young rats.

Figure 3 shows the effects of direct heating of the rat tail on BCV in subepidermal capillaries in the young, middle-aged, and old groups. For this procedure, colonic temperature did not significantly change in any of the groups, and the rise in skin temperature of the tail (Ts) was same in all animals — 10°C. Again note that there was an age-related increase in the response to heat stress. These results are consistent with what we have observed in the human forearm,[52] where the subpapillary plexus vessels in elderly subjects showed a greater response to direct heating in terms of a percent change in BCV.

The results with direct heating of the rat tail (Figure 3) indicate that the greater rise in BCV during indirect heating in the older animals (Figure 2) was in part due to an increase sensitivity of the blood vessels to local heat fluxes elicited by warming of the blood.

Collectively, our most recent rat[102] and human microcirculatory studies,[52] indicate that any effects of the aging process on the superficial microvessels (e.g., loss of papillary capillaries[52] or subepidermal vessels[102]) are compensated for by increased sensitivity of the remaining vessels to whatever mechanism(s) are responsible for the heat stress response. In this manner the heat exchange function of the skin may be well maintained with advancing age even though the response of total skin blood flow to heat stress is depressed in the older person.[13,130,131,133,134]

f. Reactive Hyperemia

Interestingly, the effects of age on the cutaneous circulatory response to heat stress are

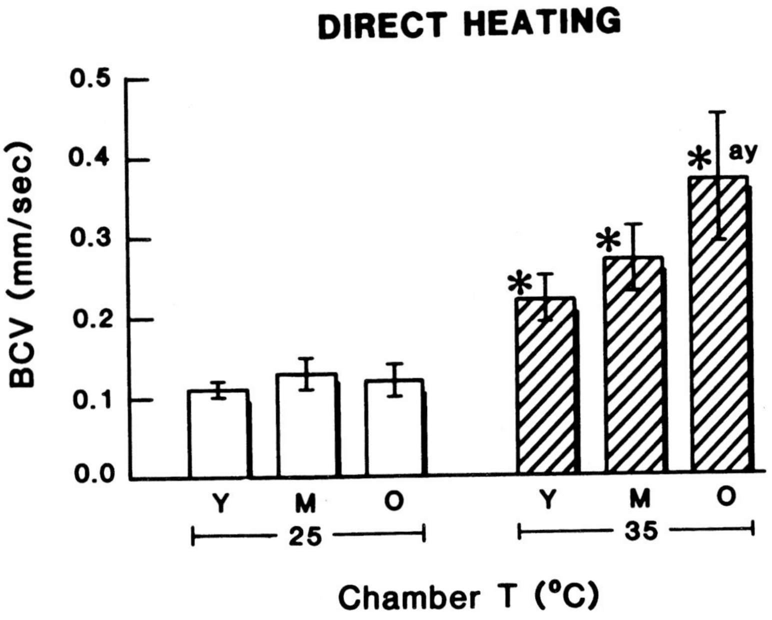

Figure 10-3 Group means ± SEM for blood cell velocity (BCV) of individual capillaries before (25°C) and during (35°C) direct heating of the tail. Symbols same as in Figure 2. *(From Richardson, D., Shepherd, S., and Tyra, J., Endoth. Lymph., 7, 305, 1991. With permission.)*

quite similar to the changes in the reactive hyperemic response noted in the older person. For example, as judged by LDF, postischemic hyperemia of total flow in a specific region of skin is depressed in elderly subjects,[149] whereas peak reactive hyperemia of cutaneous capillaries is elevated in older men.[10] An enhanced capillary blood flow response in the face of a depressed regional cutaneous circulatory response to two entirely different vasodilatory stimuli, heat and ischemia, suggests that microcirculatory compensation for reduced responses of the macrocirculation may be "built in" to the general schema of cutaneous circulatory control. In this regard, the appearance of such adjustments in the cutaneous circulation of the elderly may simply be manifestations of normal circulatory control and not a characteristic of aging per se.

g. Response to Cold Stress

It has been well demonstrated that the risk for developing hypothermia is increased among elderly populations.[150,151] The mechanisms which maintain body temperature in the cold consist of a combination of thermogenesis and heat conservation, and it is the latter in which the cutaneous circulation plays a role via sympathetic induced vasoconstriction and/or the direct constrictor effects of cold itself.[85] While there is ample evidence that cold-induced thermogenesis is reduced in older organisms,[152-155] the effect of age on heat conservation has received very little attention. Sowers and Mohanty[132] showed a reduced forearm vasoconstrictor response to a cold pressor test, suggesting a diminished reflex cutaneous vasoconstriction in response to a cold environment. Similar results have been provided by Collins et al.,[156] who showed that the elderly who are "at risk" for developing hypothermia fail to demonstrate cutaneous vasoconstriction when presented with a cold challenge. However, they presented their data in a semiquantitative manner as the percentage of subjects with which skin blood flow was reduced during cold exposure. Since at least two thirds of the elderly subjects in Collins et al.'s study fell into this category, it is unclear if, as a group, the elderly would be quantitatively different from the young in terms of the magnitude of the cutaneous blood flow response to cold. Furthermore, even if the elderly do have a diminished total cutaneous circulatory response to cold, this does not necessarily mean that flow in the superficial microvessels would also show a diminished response to cold. However, there have been no studies in which the response of cutaneous microvessels to cold stress have been examined in elderly subjects.

To address these issues, we recently measured total cutaneous blood flow in the tip of the finger, by LDF, and BCV in the nailfold capillaries of the same finger, by videomicroscopy, in ten young (mean age 25) and ten old (mean age 71) consenting male subjects before and during submersion of the contralateral hand and arm in a 15°C water bath for a period of 5 min. In a study by Fagrell et al.,[157] this procedure elicited a significant decrease in nailfold capillary BCV in a group of young male and female subjects.

The results of our study are presented in Figure 4. The young group showed an initial decrease in both LDF and BCV, and, although there was some rebound over the last 4 min of cooling, the values during cold stress remained significantly lower than control (by repeated measures ANOVA). By contrast, the elderly showed an initial decrease in LDF, but as the cold stress progressed, this variable showed almost complete recovery. Furthermore, BCV did not significantly change at all in the elderly, although there was a tendency in this direction over the first minute of cooling. To determine if the modest changes in cutaneous blood flow during cold stress in the elderly could have been the result of an elevated arterial blood pressure, seven young and seven old subjects had systemic blood pressure measured before and during the cold exposure. Mean arterial blood pressure increased during the cold test by an average of only 3.9 mmHg in the young subjects and 2.7 mmHg in the old group. The difference was not significant (*p*

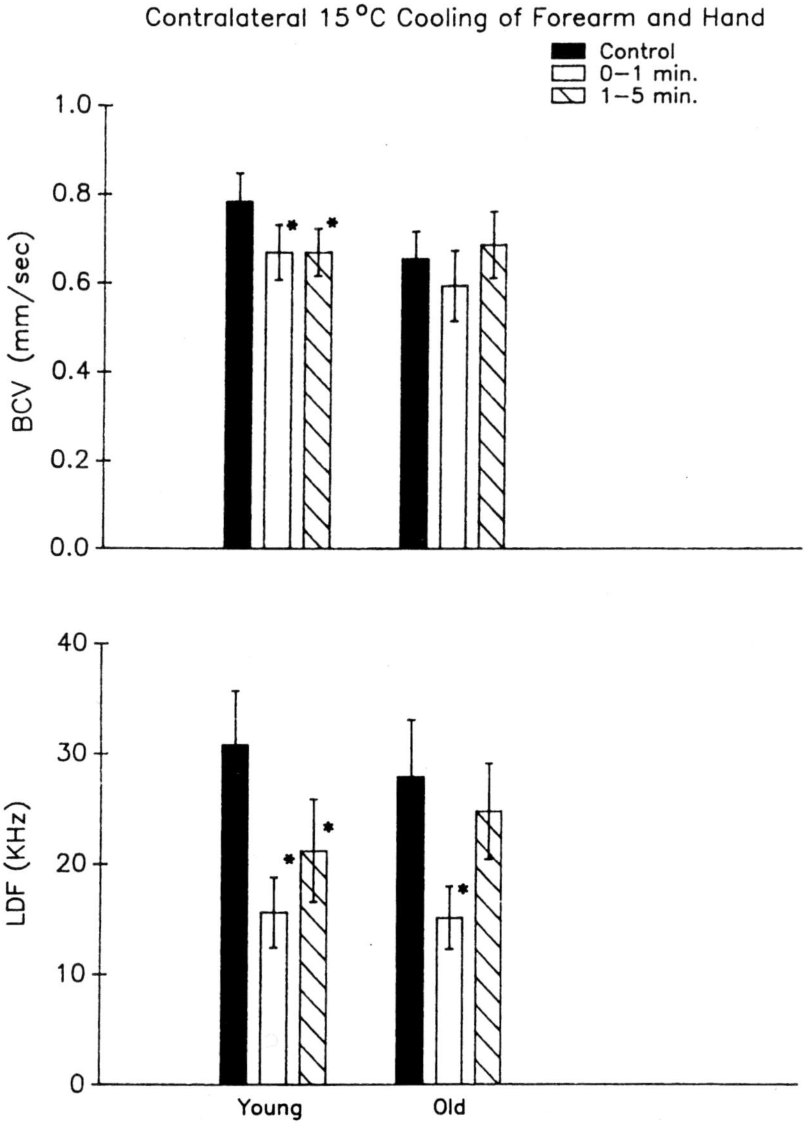

Figure 10-4 Effects of contralateral cooling of the forearm on blood cell velocity (BCV) in nailfold capillaries and laser Doppler flow of the fingertip in young and old male subjects. (*) Significant from pre-cooling control ($p<0.05$). *(From Richardson, D., Tyra, J., and McCray, A.,* J. Gerontol., *47 (6), M211, 1992, © 1992 Gerontological Society of America, with permission.)*

>0.41). These results indicate that the reduced cutaneous blood flow response to cold stress in the elderly was not due to a more pronounced pressor effect in this group.

Thus, our findings support those of Collins et al.[156] and indicate that heat conservation, as reflected by a decrease in total cutaneous blood flow in the finger tip during contralateral arm cooling, is compromised in the elderly. Furthermore, unlike what seems to be the case for the cutaneous circulatory response to heat stress in the elderly, the diminished macrocirculatory response to cold is not compensated for by adjustments in the superficial microvessels. Thus, the tendency toward hypothermia in the elderly[150,151] may in part be due to a diminished cutaneous vasoconstrictor response to cold.

h. Postural Stress

It is well known that the cardiovascular responses to orthostasis are blunted in older individuals[14,131,158-160] and that this defect is probably responsible for the increased incidence of orthostatic hypotension among the elderly.[161,162] There is evidence that at least a part of the orthostatic intolerance of the older person is due to diminished peripheral vasoconstriction in the upright posture. For example, several groups of investigators have demonstrated a diminished forearm vasoconstrictor response to orthostasis in older individuals.[131,132,163] Of these studies, those by Lipsitz et al.[163] showed that the lack of a vasoconstrictor response was similar in healthy and impaired old individuals, suggesting that the defect is related to aging and not health status.

Based on the results of lower body negative pressure, the cutaneous circulation plays the dominate role in the vasoconstrictor response of the human forearm to baroreceptor unloading.[164] Since this is the case, most of an older person's reduced forearm vasoconstrictor response to orthostasis is probably due to diminished reflex cutaneous vasoconstriction.

Although there is considerable controversy as to where the defect(s) responsible for the reduced baroreflex response in the elderly may be located, the collective evidence with regard to peripheral vasoconstriction suggests that reduced responsiveness occurs "...some place between (plasma membrane) receptor activation and the end organ (vascular smooth muscle) response."[160] This notion is consistent with the results of Hruza and Zweifach,[72] which show diminished constrictor responses of microvessels to topical application of catecholamines in mesenteric preparations from old rats, and recent studies by Minaker et al.,[165] which indicate that the effect of hypotension on sympathetic activity is not diminished in the elderly. Both of these very different lines of inquiry point towards a defective end organ response in the attenuated vasoconstrictor response to orthostasis in the elderly. However, as evidenced by the effect of orthostasis on capillary blood flow in the toes of young and old men,[11] the myogenic sensitivity of cutaneous precapillary arterioles is well maintained in older individuals. This observation, vis-a-vis the evidence discussed above, suggests that any age-related decrease in the cutaneous circulatory response to orthostasis would be due to a defect in signal transduction at the cellular level as opposed to a reduced vasoconstrictor capability of the vascular smooth muscle cells.

i. Exercise Response

No single area of aging research has captured more attention than has the relationship between aging and physical activity. The health benefits of regular exercise for the elderly have been well documented,[17,166-169] and it has become clear that the decrease in physical capacity that is associated with aging[170] is elicited by reduced levels of activity, not chronological aging.[171-172] In this regard, recent studies[173] suggest that physical performance assessments are much better indicators of functional age than is the number of candles on a person's birthday cake.

The cutaneous circulatory response to exercise is quite complex, consisting of an initial vasoconstriction, presumably due to exercise induced sympathetic drive, followed by vasodilation as thermoregulatory demands come to the fore.[174-177] Recent studies indicate that the dilatory phase of this response is decreased in healthy elderly subjects.[178] In this regard, it would be interesting to learn if this diminished total flow response is in any way compensated for by increased flow in the superficial cutaneous microvessels as seems to be the case for the cutaneous microvascular response to heat stress in older organisms (Figure 2). However, such studies have yet to be conducted. This void in our understanding of the effects of age on the cutaneous circulation begs to be filled, particularly in light of the marked influence of exercise on the aging process.

B. THE SKELETAL MUSCLE CIRCULATION

As a review of age-related changes in skeletal muscle points out, there is a wealth of information indicating that muscle performance declines with age.[179] However, once again it is not at all clear how much, if any, of this decremental process is due to aging itself as opposed to other factors such as reduced physical activity. This consideration, vis-a-vis the aforementioned benefits of physical exercise to the older person, makes studies of the skeletal muscle circulation an important topic to review within the context of age-related changes in the microcirculation.

1. Structural Considerations

General: Wiedeman[180] has provided concise descriptions of the circulatory architecture found in several skeletal muscle preparations commonly used in biomedical research, and although there are variations from one preparation to the next, there does seem to be a common structural framework. The distributing arteries and their attending veins run parallel to the muscle fibers from where the arteries give off transverse arterioles, which extend obliquely or at right angles to the axis of the muscle fibers. These arterioles subdivide into the terminal arterioles, which give rise to the capillaries. The precapillary sphincter is not a distinct anatomical entity but rather is simply the smallest division of the arterioles prior to the capillaries. In this regard, some investigators have defined the precapillary sphincter within the skeletal muscle circulation as the "last smooth muscle cell on a terminal arteriole".[181,182]

Capillary Supply: Like the supply arteries, the capillaries also run longitudinal to the muscle fibers; however, frequent anastomotic branchings transverse across the fibers, giving a "ladder-like" appearance to the capillary networks.[180] In this regard, Brotzu et al.[183] have presented evidence suggesting that the relative distribution of longitudinal and transverse capillaries is age dependent, albeit they examined only young and mature rats, not old animals. Nevertheless, since only longitudinal capillaries are generally observed in histological cross-sections, the study by Brotzu and his group casts a note of caution in interpreting capillary density data in different age groups of subjects.

Although on the average one longitudinal capillary attends each muscle fiber,[85] the exact number varies in different types of fibers in accordance to oxidative capacity. The slow oxidative (SO) and fast oxidative glycolytic (FOG) fibers have the most capillaries per cell and the fast glycolytic (FG) fibers the fewest.[184,185] However, the range of capillaries per fiber is relatively narrow,[185] and muscle fiber diameter is what seems to account for the variability in capillary density (capillaries per unit area of tissue). Oxidative fibers have smaller diameters compared to the glycolytic type,[185] and, therefore, a higher capillary density exists in muscles made up primarily of SO and/or FOG fibers. To paraphrase Plyley and Groom,[186] nature seems to prefer to increase oxygen supply by decreasing the diameter of a muscle fiber rather than by increasing the number of capillaries around the perimeter of the fiber. These considerations are of concern in assessing the effects of aging on the capillary supply in skeletal muscle since aging, exercise conditioning, and aging-exercise interactions affect muscle fiber size.[187]

To examine the role of muscle capillarization in the age-related decrease in maximal oxygen consumption, Parizkova et al.[51] measured overall capillary density (CD) and the number of capillaries per fiber (CF) in the lateral quadriceps muscles (vastus lateralis) of young and old healthy men. This muscle is a mixed type with predominately oxidative fibers.[188] Parizkova and his group found no age differences in CD, but the older men had a higher number of muscle fibers per square millimeter of tissue and therefore a lower CF. The latter finding supported their notion that the reduced aerobic capacity of the older person is, in part, due to a reduced muscle capillary supply. These results are somewhat different from those of Grimby et al.,[189] who reported that both CD and CF of the vastus lateralis and biceps brachii of 78- to 81-year-old subjects were within the range of values found in young subjects. However, their values for young individuals came from reports of previous studies in the literature, whereas Parizkova's group directly compared young and old subjects in the same study.

To determine if the lower CF in their older subjects could be related to physical inactivity, Parizkova et al.[51] subdivided the old subjects into groups that were physically active and inactive. The inactive group had smaller CD and CF values than the active older men, indicating that sedentary existence is in part responsible for the loss of muscle capillarization with age.

Expanding on Parizkova's study, Denis et al.[6] examined the effects of endurance training on the capillary supply of oxidative fibers (SO and FOG) within the vastus lateralis of young and old men. The results were quite complex. They found that no difference existed between the groups in CD either before or after training and that training improved CD in each group. Therefore, age did not attenuate the angiogenic response to aerobic conditioning as some animal studies have suggested.[50] Before training, the number of capillaries in contact with a muscle fiber (CC) was higher in Denis et al.'s older subjects, and training had no effect on CC in this group, whereas CC did increase with training in the young men. However, since training elicited a *decrease* in muscle fiber area in the elderly and a slight *increase* in this variable in the young, the relative CC (CC per fiber area) improved with training in the old subjects but not in the young.

From the above it can be surmised that in humans the effect of aging on skeletal muscle capillarization is a complex interaction of several factors including angiogenic control of overall capillary density, the effects of age on muscle fiber type and size, and the "training" effects of physical activity on both angiogenesis and muscle fiber size. Animal models have been used in attempts to sort out the relative importance of the various factors that seem to determine muscle capillary supply. Ripoll et al.[190] used Sprague-Dawley rats over a wide range of ages to examine relationships between body weight, fiber cross-sectional area, and capillary density in gastrocnemius and soleus muscles. Their results indicate that CD bears a tight inverse relationship to fiber cross-sectional area irrespective of animal age. These findings are consistent with the results of Brown,[191] who showed that the capillary per fiber ratio in the soleus and extensor digitorum longus muscles of rats remains remarkably constant with advancing age in spite of an age-related atrophy of the muscle fibers (i.e., an increase in CD with decreasing fiber diameter). In a study not directly related to aging, Myrhage[185] measured capillary to fiber ratios in a variety of muscles obtained from cats and found that this variable correlated quite well with oxidative capacity. This comparison of results suggests that the effects of age on CD, if any, are dependent upon changes in fiber size, whereas changes in the capillary to fiber ratio in the older person, if any, are governed by muscle oxidative capacity. In this regard, it is interesting to note that Young et al.[192] could find no effects of age on the capacity of muscle tissue for oxidative metabolism or the response of muscle mitochondrial enzymes to exercise conditioning in Long-Evans rats. These results favor the notion that aging by itself does not affect the capillary to fiber ratio in skeletal muscle.

To summarize this section, if that is possible, the structural aspect of muscle circulation that has captured the most investigative attention in aging research is the degree of capillarization; however, results are most equivocal. Some studies show only subtle differences between young and old subjects.[6] Others indicate no change in CD but a decrease in CF in the elderly,[51] while the results from yet other studies suggest that CD increases but CF remains constant.[191] In contrast, some studies point to lower CD and a higher CF with aging.[50] There are also some investigators who hold that aging has no effect at all on muscle capillarization.[189] Finally, any differences in muscle capillarization between the young and old may be dependent upon the level of physical activity of the subjects tested.[6,50,51]

2. Capillary Dynamics in Living Muscle Preparations

One of the difficulties with the muscle capillarization studies cited above is that for the most part histological procedures were used in which capillaries were identified on the basis of staining techniques. While appropriate for determining the total number of capillaries in a vascular bed, fixed tissue staining gives little indication as to how many of these vessels may have had active flow in the *in vivo* state. This problem is of particular concern in attempts to examine capillary recruitment as a mechanism in the skeletal muscle circulatory response to exercise. Using an *in vivo* microscopic approach, Gorczynski et al.[193] and Hudlicka et al.[194] examined living muscle preparations in attempts to address the problem; however, these two groups could not agree on the issue of capillary recruitment. One of the difficulties seems to have been in whether a nonflowing capillary is to be defined in absolute or relative terms (i.e., no flow or extremely low flow).

Using the zero flow definition for a nonflowing vessel, Tyml[195] determined the density of flowing and nonflowing capillaries on the surface of the sartorius muscle in anesthetized frogs. In addition, BCV was measured in flowing capillaries by a "flying spot" method. Measurements were made at rest and during an active hyperemic response to direct muscle stimulation. Although the emphasis of this study was not on aging, Tyml did examine two age groups of animals, mature (3-month captivity) and old (18-month captivity) frogs, and analyzing the data presented for these two groups did reveal some differences. At rest, both the 3- and 18-month animals had about the same total capillary density as identified by the presence of red cells. However, whereas less than 2% of the capillaries in the 3-month group had stationary red blood cell counts (i.e., zero flow) about 30% of the vessels in the 18-month group were nonflowing. Muscle stimulation (i.e., active hyperemia) had little effect on the number of capillaries with and without flowing red cells in the 3-month group; however, in the 18-month animals the total number of capillaries increased and the fraction of vessels with zero flow decreased to only 9% during stimulation. Also at rest, BCV values in Tyml's study respectively averaged 0.19 and 0.05 mm/sec for the 3- and 18-month frogs. Corresponding values during active hyperemia were 0.50 and 0.43 mm/sec. In other words, the older animals had an improved capillary flow response to muscle contraction in terms of both capillary recruitment and the degree of flow increase per vessel. These phenomena would probably have gone unnoticed in fixed tissue preparations.

The obvious criticism of this study is that it is difficult to determine if the differences between the two groups represent aging or physical inactivity due to a longer period of captivity for the older frogs. However, based on what is known about the effects of long-term muscle activity (i.e., training),[196] it is highly unlikely that long-term inactivity would have improved the active hyperemic response of muscle capillaries.

Recently Tyml's laboratory has turned to skeletal muscle preparations in middle-aged (12-month) and old (28-month) Fischer-344 rats.[197,198] At rest, the extensor digitorum longus muscle had about the same capillary density in both groups (30.2 caps/mm^2 in the middle aged and 33.1 caps/mm^2 in the old rats). In the middle-aged rats, 89% of the capillaries were flowing, while the corresponding figure for the old animals was 85%. Thus, in this particular muscle preparation, there appears to be no significant effect of age on the capillary supply in terms of either overall vessel density or the number capillaries with active flow.

The capillary BCV at rest in Tyml's study[198] was about three times higher in the old (0.32 mm/sec) compared to the middle-aged (0.11 mm/sec) animals. However, the higher capillary flow in the old rats appears to have been due to a "clustering" of groups of fast-flowing vessels around an arteriole. Exclusion of these clustered capillary groups resulted in a resting BCV of only 0.19 mm/sec for the old animals, a value much closer to that seen in the younger rats. Why such clustering of capillaries, around what appears to be dilated arterioles, is more prominent in old than in middle-aged animals is uncertain.

As a functional perturbation, Tyml's group[198] performed a 30-min occlusion of the arterial supply to the muscle preparations. Upon release of occlusion, individual capillaries in the older rats had a tendency towards a delayed onset of reactive hyperemia, and, as a group, these vessels had a significantly slower return of flow to baseline levels in the postocclusion period. This suggests either an enhanced dilatory response of the arterioles from the old rats in terms of duration of the dilatory effect or ischemic damage of the blood vessels in the old animals, such that they could not recover vascular tone. Histological examination of the capillary endothelial cells upon termination of an experiment provided information related to the latter possibility. Only one capillary among 86 sampled in the middle age group and two of 91 vessels among the old rats showed evidence of ischemic damage to the endothelium. These findings suggest that 30 min of ischemia did not damage the blood vessels in Tyml et al.'s study and, therefore, that the prolonged postischemic dilatory effect observed in the old rats was reflective of an enhanced dilatory response of the microvessels in this group.

3. Possible Capillary Flow/Total Flow Interactions in Muscle Circulation of the Young and Old

Collectively, Tyml's studies indicate that, while the effects of age on capillary blood flow in resting muscle may be different in different species and/or muscle groups, the response of this variable to a vasodilatory drive seems to be slightly enhanced by the aging process.[195,197,198] This is quite different from what is observed at the level of total muscle blood flow, where several investigators using a variety of techniques have shown an age-related decrease in resting muscle flow, decreased flow responses to a vasodilatory drive, or both.[31,120,199-201] The age-related decrease in total muscle blood flow is probably due to interactive factors such as physical conditioning and muscle strength, not aging per se. This is evidenced by the fact that exercise conditioning can markedly improve vasodilatory capacity in the older person[202] and normalizing muscle contractions as a percentage of a subject's maximal contractile force gives similar active hyperemic responses in young and old men.[203] Nevertheless, the tendency towards enhancement of the skeletal muscle capillary flow response to a vasodilatory drive,[195,197] vis-a-vis a reduced total flow response in older organisms,[31,120,199-201] indicates that in the older individual the microcirculatory control of capillary blood flow may adjust to compensate for a deficient total flow input. This hypothesis is consistent with Wahren et al.'s studies,[201] which show that a larger arterial-venous oxygen difference compensates for the reduced muscle blood flow response to bicycle exercise in middle-aged men. Since aging seems to have no effect on muscle mitochondrial enzymes,[192] the greater oxygen extraction noted by Wahren's group was probably due to an improved capillary recruitment.

In summary, a substantial amount of evidence, cited above, indicates that total blood flow to a given skeletal muscle group in elderly subjects is reduced at rest and during active hyperemia. However, emerging *in vivo* microcirculatory data suggest that improved capillary recruitment and/or flow per vessel compensates for the deficient total flow response of muscle circulation in an older person. This age-related microcirculatory compensation for a macrocirculatory deficiency is similar to what is observed in the cutaneous circulatory response to heat stress in the older subject (Figure 2).

4. Cardiac Muscle

At the microcirculatory level, the vascular architecture of cardiac muscle is quite similar to that of skeletal muscle,[180] and the two tissues have about the same average number of capillaries per fiber.[196] However, since the myocardium is made up almost exclusively of oxidative fibers, there are more muscle fibers per unit area in cardiac muscle and, hence, a higher CD.[196]

Several investigators have shown that decreases in both myocardial CD[45,48,204,205] and the capillary to fiber ratio[48,205,206] attend aging. However, in a recent study, Tomanek et al. pointed out that, although CD is reduced in the myocardium of older dogs, capillary volume is maintained by an age-related increase in capillary diameter.[206]

With regard to possible mechanisms, Tomanek's studies contend that the age-related decrease in myocardial CD is due to a combination of capillary rarefaction and an increase in muscle fiber size.[48,205] An additional factor that might be responsible for a reduction in myocardial CD with age is a simple decrease in the percentage of lean mass. This possibility is consistent with data from Burch and Giles,[207] which show an age-related increase in neutral fat in cardiac muscle, and information from Anversa et al.,[208] which indicate that the heart loses myocytes with advancing age.

Regardless of whether the decrease in myocardial capillarization with age is absolute or relative, the older organism is capable of increasing CD in the heart through exercise conditioning;[48,204] and, electron micrographic studies indicate that this is a true angiogenic response[209] as opposed to an adjustment in muscle fiber size or density. Thus, skeletal and cardiac muscle are similar in that both exhibit an angiogenic response to exercise training, and this response is maintained with advancing age.

Notwithstanding the ability of an older organism to increase myocardial CD through exercise training, the CD of the older heart is still less than that of hearts obtained from young, training-matched animals, such as the guinea pig[204] and the rat.[48] This raises the issue about what are the possible effects of a reduced CD on coronary perfusion, myocardial function, or both. The most direct approach to this question would be to measure blood flow in individual myocardial capillaries of young and old subjects. Although microscopic techniques that enable these measurements are available,[210] there do not seem to be any examples in the literature in which they have been used to study capillary blood flow in older hearts. However, Rakusan and Korecky[211] have used *in vivo* microscopy to examine the effects of age on functional capillary density in the myocardium. They noted a slightly smaller intercapillary distance in 4-month-old compared to 24-month-old rats, suggesting a higher CD for the younger animals.

In contrast to the virtual lack of *in vivo* microcirculatory measurements in the aged myocardium, several investigators have measured total coronary blood flow in young and old animals. In the resting unstressed heart, coronary blood flow per gram of tissue declines with age at peak systole[212] but shows little or no age difference when averaged over several cardiac cycles.[213-217] However, when isolated hearts are presented a vasodilatory challenge such as hypoxia,[217] ischemia,[214] the administration of vasodilator agents,[213,215] or an increase in myocardial metabolism,[216] the flow increase is consistently lower in the older animals. A comparison of the coronary blood flow response to dipyridamole in middle-aged and old men[218] suggests that the coronary circulation of older humans has a similar vasodilatory deficiency.

If, as some of the above investigators contend,[213,217] the peak hyperemic responses of coronary blood flow represent maximal vasodilation, then the lower values observed in the older hearts should reflect structural differences between the coronary circulations of young and old animals. However, at the level of the small coronary arteries and large arterioles, it is unclear whether structural changes with age would be sufficient to cause a reduction in maximal blood flow. For example, although tortuosity has been noted in the coronary arteries of older hearts,[21] a meticulous investigation by Weisfeldt et al.[217] did not reveal any pronounced structural differences between precapillary vessels from the hearts of young and old rats. Furthermore, Tomanek et al.[206] found no reduction in the lumen diameters of coronary arteries from senescent dogs.

Alternatively, Lakatta[219] has pointed out that a decrease in oxygen consumption attends the age-related decrease in maximal coronary blood flow. He suggested that the two phenomena might be coupled through a reduced mitochondrial oxygen utilization since, unlike skeletal muscle, mitochondrial oxygen uptake in the heart does seem to be age dependent.[220] In this regard, it is possible that a decrease in the number of functional capillaries (those with flow) is attended by reduced respiratory activity in the myocardium of old organisms and that a reduction in capillary flow is in turn responsible for the decrease in maximal coronary blood flow.

If the number of functional capillaries is reduced in older hearts, then this condition should be reflected in functional parameters such as oxygen extraction. Information on this point has been provided by Toma et al.,[216] who increased myocardial oxygen consumption by catecholamine infusion into Langendorff perfused hearts from immature (1-month) and adult (18-month) guinea pigs. Maximal oxygen consumption and coronary blood flow were both lower in the older animals, but there were no age differences in calculated oxygen extraction at rest or during the metabolic challenge. These results are similar to those of Weisfeldt et al.,[217] who used an entirely different approach. They measured coronary blood flow and oxygen consumption over a wide range of arterial pO_2 values in Langendorff perfused hearts from middle-aged (12-month) and old (27-month) male Wistar rats. As pO_2 was lowered, blood flow increased in both groups, but the increment was much less in the old animals. However, over the entire range tested there were no age differences in the percentage of the arterial oxygen extracted from the blood. The results of these two studies suggest the following: (1) that the diminished hyperemic response of the coronary circulation in older organisms is not reflected at the capillary level, and (2) that, in spite of a lower total number of capillaries, the aging myocardium is able to maintain a sufficient supply of functional capillaries to meet metabolic demands. Thus, the lower "maximal" blood flow in the hearts of older animals is unlikely to be due to a reduced number of functional capillaries. In the absence of any clear evidence for age-related structural changes elsewhere in the coronary circulation,[217] the question of what mediates reduced maximal coronary blood flow in older animals remains unanswered.

In summary, the results of this section indicate that although overall CD in myocardial tissue is decreased in older animals, this condition probably does not contribute to age-related differences in physiological responses of coronary blood flow and does not seem to affect nutrient exchange. However, to put these notions on more solid ground will require additional studies like those of Rakusan and Korecky,[211] in which the coronary microcirculation is directly examined in functioning hearts of young and old animals.

C. THE BULBAR CONJUNCTIVA

Like the superficial microvessels in the skin, the circulation in the conjunctiva of the eye has been extensively investigated in human subjects largely because it can be viewed with relative ease by noninvasive means. Conjunctival examinations in the elderly have been most frequently used to investigate how diseases prevalent in old age (e.g., atherosclerosis, hypertension, diabetes mellitus, heart disease, and liver disease) modify a microcirculatory network.[25,221] Such studies have been quite valuable in establishing microcirculatory examinations as a prognostic and diagnostic tool for detecting and/or managing disease states. However, in reviewing the conjunctival circulation literature, it is often difficult to distinguish the effects of aging-disease interactions from those of aging alone. For example, Davis and Landau[222] examined the conjunctival circulation in atherosclerotic patients from age 45 to 89 and found certain vascular signs of atherosclerosis to be more prevalent in the older subjects. How much this finding represents a progression of the disease as opposed to a simple aging effect is uncertain.

Nevertheless, certain characteristic changes have been observed in the conjunctival microcirculation of healthy elderly individuals, suggesting that these changes are part of the aging process which occurs independently from any disease states. Such changes include an increase in the diameter of venous vessels relative to arterioles.[9] However, such dimensional changes are not uniform as diameter irregularities are common in all conjunctival microvessels.[28] This is particularly true on the venous side, where focal dilations can appear as sacculations and microaneurysms.[28,59,73,223,224] On the arterial side, Tassi et al.[28] mention the appearance of thin, thread-like arterioles, but it is unclear whether these are due to "normal" aging or blood vessel disease. Several teams of investigators have shown that conjunctival microvessels increase in tortuosity with advancing age and that this can be extreme with some vessels becoming quite serpentine in shape.[25,28,73,221,225]

Collectively, the structural changes that occur in the conjunctival microcirculation with age suggest that the capillary network should be poorly perfused. While this seems to be the case for elderly patients with various disease conditions,[28] it is not certain whether the conjunctival capillary network is underperfused in healthy individuals of old age. To the contrary, de Nicola et al.[54] noted several cases in their elderly subjects where the conjunctival capillary network seemed to be "particularly rich." However, capillary proliferation in other microcirculatory beds, such as that of the skin, have been shown to occur distal to atherosclerotic lesions.[127] Thus, the "rich" conjunctival capillary networks noted by de Nicola's group in their older subjects may be a compensatory response to an elevated vascular resistance in the tortuous arteries and arterioles (i.e., a microcirculatory adjustment to a macrocirculatory disturbance).

Clarifying how age-related structural changes in the conjunctival microcirculation affect blood flow will require dynamic measurements of flow through single microvessels in this vascular bed. While measurements such as flow velocity have been made in conjunctival vessels of healthy adults,[226,227] there has not been a comprehensive, quantitative aging study of hemodynamics in the conjunctiva. Considering the speed with which the technology of quantitative microscopy is advancing, this deficiency will certainly be corrected in the near future. Given the time lag between the first draft of a manuscript and final publication, it may already have.

There have been a few attempts to examine the effects of topically applied vasoactive agents on the diameters of conjunctival vessels in young and old subjects. So far, it has been shown that constrictor responses to topical neosynephrine are diminished in the structurally abnormal conjunctival vessels characteristic of the aged.[73] This finding is consistent with results from Hruza and Zweifach,[72] which show diminished constrictor responses of rat mesenteric microvessels to topical application of catecholamines in preparations derived from old animals. These data comparisons indicate that a diminished constrictor response to vasoactive agents may be a general property of vascular smooth muscle in older organisms. As discussed in the section on the cutaneous circulation, the defect may be at the level of signal transduction as opposed to the contractile machinery of the smooth muscle itself.

Summary: Examination of the conjunctival microcirculation in humans has proven to be a simple but very effective means of noninvasively assessing the effects of aging, diseases prevalent in the aged, and interactions between age and disease on the peripheral circulation. Aging itself seems to elicit certain characteristic structural changes, such as diameter irregularities and vessel tortuosity, and several pathological conditions seem to exacerbate these changes.[9,25,28,221,222] However, most of the studies to date have been based on subjective observations, and there have been few, if any, quantitative comparisons of hemodynamics in the conjunctival microvessels of young and old subjects.

D. THE CEREBRAL CIRCULATION

The high incidence of cerebrovascular disease among the elderly,[228] coupled with a desire to elucidate the mechanisms of senile dementia, has resulted in numerous investigations into the possible role of cerebral circulatory dysfunction in dementia. However, to stay within the framework of this chapter, we will review only those studies which address the effects of aging itself on the cerebral microcirculation. To those authors whose work has been omitted or overlooked, I can only offer my apologies and assurance that this is not a reflection on the quality or importance of their contributions.

1. Anatomy of the Cerebral Circulation

The adult brain has a high oxidative capacity in which about 150 g of glucose and 72 l of oxygen are consumed each day.[229] Yet brain tissue has virtually no substrate storage capacity, making it totally reliant on the circulatory system to meet its metabolic needs. Therefore, so as to assure adequate perfusion of any given region of the brain, the cerebrum has an intricate circulatory system with multiple arterial inputs and numerous arterial-to-arterial anastomotic connections.

Tool[229] and Heistad and Kontos[230] have provided concise accounts of the anatomy of the cerebral circulation, and the following is a summary of these descriptions, supplemented with additional information from *Gray's Anatomy*.[231] As these sources point out, the brain is supplied by four major arteries — two carotids and two vertebrals. The relative importance of each of these vessels (i.e., the amount of blood carried) varies considerably among mammalian species. In primates the carotid and vertebral arteries are relatively balanced, whereas in rats the vertebral vessels carry the greater burden of cerebral perfusion. Each carotid artery gives off an internal and external branch and, in humans, the internal branches are the main source of cerebral blood flow, while the external vessels supply the face and scalp.

At the pontomedullary junction, the vertebral arteries join to form the basilar artery, which gives off branches that supply the cerebellum, pons, and the inner ear. The basilar artery ends at the midbrain, dividing into the left and right posterior cerebral arteries. At this point, the posterior cerebral arteries link up, via the posterior communicating arteries, with the internal carotids to form the circle of Willis, one of the most elaborate anastomotic complexes in the circulatory system. In addition to the posterior vessels, two other pairs of cerebral arteries, the anterior and the middle, also connect with or arise from the circle of Willis. These arteries collectively supply the bulk of the cerebral tissues.

In addition to the circle of Willis, there are major anastomotic connections between the internal and external carotid arteries and between the external carotids and vertebrals. The pial arterial system on the surface of the brain is also a complex network with numerous anastomotic connections.

The small artery and arteriolar branches of the cerebral arteries that enter the brain parenchyma are enveloped by a perivascular space of cerebrospinal fluid, which eventually thins out near the terminal arterioles where vascular and parenchymal basal laminae coalesce.[230] The capillaries arise at this level and course near the cell bodies of neurons, where they are joined to the nerve cells by protoplasmic astrocytes — structures which are thought to regulate blood-tissue exchange.[229] Finally, venous drainage of the cerebrum occurs through the superficial venous sinuses for the more peripheral areas of the brain and through the internal cerebral veins for the internal structures. Both routes eventually empty into the internal jugular veins.

2. Structural Changes with Age

At the macrovascular level, one of the most ubiquitous changes in the structure of the cerebral arteries to occur with age is thickening of the intima; however, this phenomenon is not restricted to old age since it occurs gradually throughout an individual's lifetime. Klassen et al.[232] examined autopsied brains from individuals over a wide range of ages and noted that at age 5 about 15% of the cerebral arteries had thickened intima. They went on to show that the thickening increased linearly to over 80% by age 80. This phenomenon appeared more pronounced at arterial branch points than along the axis of a vessel, and in the older age groups (60–80 years), the intimal thickening became degenerative and indistinguishable from atherosclerosis. Klassen's group[232] noted other age-related changes in cerebral arteries, including splitting of the internal elastic membrane, fewer smooth muscle cells in the media, and more collagen in the medial layer.

Baker[233] has provided more complete descriptions of the effects of aging on the internal elastic membrane and the medial layer of cerebral arteries. He noted that as early as the third decade the internal membrane begins to show areas of "reduplication" (i.e., splitting). This process continues until by the sixth decade the membrane becomes fragmented and probably projects into the lumen. With progressing age, the vascular medium shows markedly fewer muscular elements and an increased fibrosis, such that the medial layer eventually becomes indistinguishable from the adventitia, and in some cases, the medial-adventitial region becomes calcified.

Sorbara's laboratory[234,235] has shown that these age-related changes usually occur in all arteries associated with the circle of Willis. However, according to their studies, the degree of degeneration varies considerably among the different cerebral vessels; the middle cerebral arteries showed the most age-related change and the posterior communicating artery the least. Furthermore, Sorbara's group found that age-related changes in the middle cerebral artery were less pronounced in comparison to other peripheral vessels (e.g., radial and coronary arteries).[235]

Collectively, these various studies indicate that with advancing age the cerebral arteries become narrower, more rigid, and less able to adjust diameter. These changes do not appear to be characteristically different from those occurring elsewhere in the peripheral circulation of older persons[18] and may even be less severe than those appearing in other peripheral arteries.[235]

In contrast, structural changes in the small artery/arteriolar branchings of the distributing arteries seem much more extreme compared to those found elsewhere in the aged circulation. This is particularly true with regard to vessel topography. For example, Akima et al.[236] examined what appeared to be first- or second-order arteriolar branchings from distributing arteries in the cerebrum and cerebellum. They found that after age 40 tortuous deformities, specifically intertwining, began to show up in cerebral vessels, whereas intertwining arteries and arterioles occurred much less in the cerebellum and did not appear until after age 70. Hassler[24] made a detailed angiographic study in the cerebrum and found three fundamental types of changes to occur with advancing age: glomerular loops, in which a microvessel would form at least one whole loop on itself; vascular bundles, in which four or more vessels would run parallel to each other in close proximity; and vascular wickerworks, in which at least two vessels became intertwined. He found that all three types of deformities were more common in specimens from old individuals than young and that the frequency of occurrence increased most markedly between ages 60 and 74. Hassler's study[24] indicated, but did not positively state, that these age-related deformities were confined to the arterial side and involved vessels distal to the distributing arteries. A later study by Ravens,[237] which supported this conclusion, noted that tortuosities of small arteries and arterioles were common in cerebral tissue samples obtained from individuals over age 70.

Besides cerebral arterioles tending to be tortuous with advancing age, other studies have indicated that their cross-sectional wall structure, although containing all elements of normal arterioles,[238] is modified in older individuals. The age-related structural changes include a reduction in the cross-sectional area of the vessel wall;[34] a tendency toward a reduced diameter at a given intravascular pressure;[34] lipid droplets in the endothelium, smooth muscle, and adventitia;[238] proliferation of the adventitia;[237] thickening of the basal lamina;[38,239-241] and a decrease in the fraction of smooth muscle and elastin[34] coupled with a tendency toward fragmentation of the remaining muscle cells.[241]

In addition to examining the effects of age on the shape and morphology of cerebral microvessels, other investigations have been directed towards examining the density of cerebral microvessels as a function of age. Bell and Ball found that capillary density decreased in sections from the hippocampus[242] and visual cortex[243] of elderly humans, but arteriolar density was either unaffected or increased in the older subjects. Mann et al.[55] noted a trend toward decreasing capillary density with age in the frontal and temporal cortexes of human brains. A decrease in capillary density with age has also been shown in the hippocampus[46] and sympathetic ganglia[239] of rats and around the human optic nerve.[47] Thus, even though the exact amount of change varies from region to region, a decrease in capillary density with age seems to be ubiquitous throughout the central and, perhaps, the peripheral nervous systems.

Since cerebral capillaries seem to be structurally connected to nerve cells,[229] age-related capillary rarefaction may be coupled to the loss of neurons that occurs with old age.[244] Mann and his group[55] have provided data which support this hypothesis. They measured the densities of capillaries and pyramidal nerve cells within the cerebrum from subjects of various ages and noted that the capillary surface area per unit volume of tissue correlated much better with the number of nerve cells than with subject age. This observation is consistent with the finding of Topple et al.,[38] who noted that the number of neurovascular "appositions" in the hippocampus of rats is independent of subject age. Thus, with advancing age the capillary/neuron ratio seems to remain relatively constant, and, therefore, the age-related decrease in cerebral capillary density appears to occur in tandem with a loss of nerve cells.

A very important question regarding the close temporal demise of both neurons and capillaries is whether there is a common mechanism in the degeneration of these structures. Hypoxia secondary to arteriolar tortuosity is of course a possibility. However, this is unlikely since, as Banchero[245] has cited, long-term hypoxia has been shown to elicit an increase in capillary density within the cerebral cortex. Tayarani et al.[246] considered the possibility that capillary rarefaction in the central nervous system (CNS) is due to elevated free radicals, but they failed to find an age-related decrease in antioxidant enzymes within cerebral capillaries. This finding argues against the notion that free radicals may be elevated in the CNS of elderly individuals.

A more likely common mechanism for both capillary and neuronal rarefaction is the formation of "senile plaques." These are neural lesions frequently consisting of amyloid deposits. Bell and Ball[243] have shown that senile plaques occur most readily in cerebral regions rich in capillaries, suggesting that their formation requires a blood-borne agent. However, once a plaque lesion is formed, the damaged neuron may then elicit destruction of nearby capillaries (e.g., by reducing release of angiogenic agents), amyloid deposits may occur in the vessels, or both. Miyakawa et al.[247] found capillaries adjacent to amyloid-bearing cerebral plaques to be degenerated to the point of being invisible to light microscopy.

In summary, a decrease in capillary density with age is a common finding within the CNS, and the phenomenon seems to be coupled to the loss of neurons. A common mechanism such as amyloid plaques may be involved; however, this notion cannot be accepted with certainty, because investigations into possible mechanisms for the loss of nerve cells and associated capillaries with age are just beginning.

3. Structural/Functional Considerations of the Aging Cerebral Circulation

It has been noted that with advancing age vascular resistance increases in regions of the brain supplied by the middle cerebral artery.[248] Since the middle cerebral artery becomes structurally modified with age,[235] it is tenable that lesions of distributing arteries are responsible for the decrement in gray matter blood flow that occurs in certain regions of the senile brain.[249-251] However, since age-related changes in cerebral arteries are relatively mild in comparison to other peripheral vessels,[235] it is questionable as to what, if any, role the distributing arteries play in the effects of age on the cerebral circulation. More than likely, any changes in cerebral blood flow that occur with advancing age are probably due to structural and/or functional changes in the cerebral arterioles.

Collectively, the topographical and cross-sectional changes that tend to occur in cerebral arterioles with advancing age suggest that resistance to blood flow should be increased and that these vessels should have reduced ability to adjust diameter in response to dilator or constrictor substances. To investigate the possible functional significance of vessel tortuosities on blood flow, Hassler[24] constructed hydraulic models by twisting tubing into the various shapes of the abnormal microvessels he observed in elderly individuals. His models suggested that looping in the arterioles could reduce blood flow by almost 40%. A paper by Cervos-Navarro et al.[238] cites evidence that looping of cerebral arterioles is due to an increase in vessel length mediated by recurrent hypoxic or ischemic conditions. This suggests a positive feedback cycle of reduced cerebral blood flow, vascular tortuosity, and further reduced blood flow.

Given the above considerations, it is quite tempting to hypothesize that cerebral vascular tortuosity is what elicits the reduction in cerebral blood flow observed in the aged brain.[252] However, arguments against this notion can be made. For example, whereas arteriolar deformities can be found throughout both gray and white matter in the cerebrum of elderly individuals,[237] positron emission tomography measurements showed that reductions of normalized blood flow (i.e., flow values expressed per gram or per unit volume of tissue) in the senile brain seem to be limited to specific regions of cerebral gray matter.[249-251] As a specific example, Hassler[24] found vascular tortuosities in the occipital poles of the aged brain, whereas data from Pantano et al.[250] indicate that there is no significant effect of age on blood flow in the occipital region. Thus, the simultaneous occurrence of vascular tortuosity and reduced blood flow in the senile brain may be coincidental rather than signifying a causal relationship. If this is the case, then the lower blood flow observed in the brain of older individuals may be due to a structurally reduced vascular lumen, an increase in constrictor tone, or both.

Given that a loss of smooth muscle in the cerebral circulation attends aging,[34,241] the idea that constrictor tone is increased in cerebral vessels of the elderly seems questionable. Hajdu et al.[34] have recently addressed whether or not age-related loss of arteriolar smooth muscle affects vessel tone in the CNS. They measured pressure in first-order pial arterioles in anesthetized young and old Fischer-344 rats by a servo-null micropipette system before and after maximal dilation with ethylenediaminetetraacetic acid (EDTA). At rest, there was no significant difference in the diameter of arterioles between the young (39 micra) and old (38 micra) rats; pial arteriolar pressure was 62% of systemic arterial pressure in both groups of animals. After dilation with EDTA, arteriolar diameter — at a pressure of 70 mmHg — was significantly greater in the young (81 micra) than the old (67 micra) animals. Finally, the diameter change for a 60-mmHg increment in arteriolar pressure was greater in the young than in the old groups (26 vs. 18 micra). These results collectively indicate the following: (1) at rest there is sufficient tone in the vascular smooth muscle of old rats to maintain a normal caliber in the pial arterioles; (2) only about $^1/_3$ of the resistance to cerebral blood flow is encountered proximal to the first-order arterioles in both young and old animals and, therefore, any age-related increase in resistance must occur distal to these vessels; (3) cerebral arterioles from old animals have reduced dilatory reserve; and (4) these arterioles have a reduced compliance.

Besides having limited maximal dilatory capacity, cerebral arterioles in older individuals also seem to have reduced responses to submaximal dilatory stimuli. Yamamoto et al.[253] found the cerebral vasodilator response to carbon dioxide to be "mildly impaired" in normal aging of humans. Studies from Tanahashi et al.[254] indicate that the cerebral circulation of old cats has a reduced "low perfusion" hyperemia and a reduced reactive hyperemia following occlusion of the middle cerebral artery.

Recent *in vivo* microcirculatory studies from Mayhan et al.[255] have shown that pial arterioles in aged rats have reduced dilatory responses to acetylcholine, bradykinin, and adenosine diphosphate (ADP). However, the dilatory response to nitroglycerine in the Mayhan study was not significantly different between young and old rats, and there was no between-group difference in the constrictor response to the thromboxane analogue U46619. Since, as Mayhan et al.[255] pointed out, acetylcholine, bradykinin, and ADP are thought to exert their dilatory effects by releasing endothelial cell relaxing factor (EDRF) from the endothelium, whereas nitroglycerine acts directly on the smooth muscle, these results suggested to this group that impaired vasodilation in the cerebral circulation of aged rats is related to an alteration in endothelial cell function, not a dysfunction of the smooth muscle itself. This hypothesis is consistent with the diminished endothelial-dependent vascular relaxation observed in carotid arteries from old rats,[256] basilar arteries from elderly humans,[257] and with a reduced degree of arteriolar dilation to adenosine, a substance thought to be in part mediated by EDRF,[258] applied to the pial circulation of old rats.[259]

Although histological studies show that reduced levels of vascular smooth muscle in cerebral arterioles attends aging,[34,241] direct *in vivo* microcirculatory studies suggest that these vessels can maintain both resting tone in the older organism[34] and normal responses to dilator and constrictor substances that act directly on smooth muscle (e.g., nitroglycerine and thromboxane).[255] However, responses to dilatory agents that act through endothelial cell factors (e.g., acetylcholine) are reduced in the older cerebral vessels.[255] It is not yet known whether a damaged endothelium is responsible for the reduced cerebral circulatory responses to ischemia[254] and carbon dioxide[253] in the older individual, although this is a tenable hypothesis. In this context, the increased "expression" of vasodilator neuropeptides in the aged brain[260] may be a compensatory response to a reduced vasodilatory capability in cerebral vessels of older organisms. Collectively, the studies discussed above suggest that the dilator/constrictor balance which influences vascular tone may be shifted towards constriction in the cerebral circulation of the older person. This supports the notion that an elevated constrictor tone may mediate the lower cerebral blood flow in certain regions of the senile brain.

One area of structural-functional relationships in the cerebral circulation, and their modifications with age, that has received considerable investigative attention is the relationship between angiogenesis, blood flow, and cerebral oxygen consumption. Cerebral blood flow (CBF) is linked to the metabolic demands of the brain[261] as evidenced from the fact that in young individuals CBF per gram of tissue is about twice as high in gray matter than in white and from the observation that regions of the brain showing high blood flow also show high oxygen consumption.[250] With regard to aging, Tuma et al.[69] found no difference in cerebral blood flow between young and old unanesthetized rats. In human studies, Yamaguchi et al.[251] showed that, in a healthy (i.e., nonhospitalized) population, cerebral gray matter consumption of oxygen as a whole has a significant inverse relationship to subject age. However, they found no significant relationship between age and total gray matter blood flow although CBF in certain specific gray matter regions did show a significant reduction with advancing age. Martin et al.[249] confirmed Yamaguchi et al.'s[251] results and also found regionally specific reductions of blood flow in healthy, nonhospitalized elderly subjects. However, they found no relationship between total gray matter blood flow and subject age. The results from these two groups are inconsistent with those from Pantano et al.,[250] who studied hospitalized patients — albeit ones free of brain disease and vascular risk factors — and found a significant inverse relationship between global gray matter blood flow and patient age. Since the Yamaguchi, Martin, and Pantano groups all used positron emission tomographical methods to measure

CBF, comparing these results suggests that CBF may be more susceptible to an age-related deterioration in patients than in healthy individuals, regardless of the particular illness involved in the former. This notion is consistent with the results of Rogers et al.,[262] which indicate that physical inactivity, a health risk factor,[166,168] can precipitate a reduction in cerebral blood flow in the elderly. Thus, the conservative conclusion from these various studies is that while a decrease in CBF in certain regions of the brain may attend aging, the gray matter blood flow as a whole does not decrease with age in healthy, active individuals.

The observation that a decrease in cerebral blood flow[251] does not attend the age-related decrease in cerebral oxygen consumption suggests that a defective cerebral circulation does not elicit the neural degeneration of aging. This notion is supported by the fact that cerebral oxygen extraction is maintained with advancing age.[250,251,263] These results collectively indicate that, although both neural and capillary rarefaction occur in the cerebrum of the elderly, the relationship between these two phenomena is such that blood-tissue exchange is able to keep pace with the brain's ongoing metabolic needs. Hunziker et al.[264] came to a similar conclusion when they compared cerebral capillary geometry between brain tissues from young and old persons.

In summary, a loss of neurons within the central nervous system and corresponding changes in cerebral circulatory structure and function attend the aging process. The age-related structural changes consist of atherosclerotic-like lesions in the distributing arteries, tortuosities of arterioles, loss of vascular smooth muscle, and rarefaction of capillaries. The salient functional changes include reduced blood flow in certain regions of the brain, a compromised ability to respond to endothelial dependent vasodilator stimuli, and reduced vasodilatory reserve. Interestingly, there is no evidence that the structural and functional changes in the cerebral circulation of the older person are in any way mechanistically linked, nor is there any solid evidence that the circulatory changes in the senile brain have any direct role in the age-related loss of neurons.

ACKNOWLEDGMENTS

The author gratefully acknowledges the editorial assistance of Andrew McCray in the processing of this chapter. Portions of the author's studies were supported by grants from the Kentucky Heart Association and the National Institutes of Health (AG-05802 & HL-36552).

REFERENCES

1. **Brody, J. A. and Brock, D. B.,** Epidemiologic and statistical characteristics of the United States elderly population, in *Handbook of the Biology of Aging*, Finch, C. E. and Schneider, E. L., Eds., Van Nostrand Reinhold, New York, 1985, 3.
2. **Geokas, M. C., Lakatta, E. G., Makinodan, T., and Timiras, P. S.,** The aging process, *Ann. Int. Med.,* 113, 455, 1990.
3. **Widmer, L. K., Greensher, A., and Kannel, W. B.,** Occlusion of peripheral arteries: a study of 6,400 working subjects, *Circulation*, 30, 836, 1964.
4. **Zweifach, B. W.,** Microvascular basis of disease, *Rec. Adv. Cardiovas. Dis.,* 8 (Suppl.), L-1, 1987.
5. **Bruckner, G., Webb, P., Greenwell, L., Chow, C., and Richardson, D.,** Fish oil increases peripheral capillary blood cell velocity in humans, *Atherosclerosis*, 66, 237, 1987.
6. **Denis, C., Chatare, J. C., Dormois, D., Linossier, M. T., Geyssant, A., and Lacour, J. R.,** Effects of endurance training on capillary supply of human skeletal muscle on two age groups (20 and 60 years), *J. Physiol. Paris*, 81, 379, 1986.

7. **Kenney, R. A.,** *Physiology of Aging: A Synopsis*, Year Book, Chicago, 1982, 3.
8. **Weindruch, R. and Masoro, E. J.,** Concerns about rodent models for aging research, *J. Gerontol.*, 46, B87, 1991.
9. **Chen, P. C. Y. and Zweifach, B. W.,** Network reorganization — human bulbar conjunctiva in aging and disease, in *Proc. 4th World Cong. Microcirc.* Vol. 2, Tsuchiya, M., Asano, M., Mishima, Y., and Oda, M., Eds., Elsevier, Amsterdam, 1987, 569.
10. **Ostergren, J. and Fagrell, B.,** Skin capillary blood cell velocity in man. Characteristics and reproducibility of the reactive hyperemia response, *Int. J. Microcirc. Clin. Exp.*, 5, 37, 1986.
11. **Richardson, D.,** Orthostatic responses of regional and capillary blood flows in the toe circulation of different age groups of men, *AGE*, 11, 142, 1988.
12. **Stablein, M. and Meyer, J.,** Age-related changes in the epithelial dimensions and capillaries of the oral mucosa of the rat, *Arch. Oral Biol.*, 31, 609, 1986.
13. **Richardson, D.,** Effects of age on cutaneous circulatory response to direct heat on the forearm, *J. Gerontol.*, 44, M189, 1989.
14. **Smith, J. J., Hughes, C. V., Ptacin, M. J., Barney, J. A., Tristani, F. E., and Ebert, T. J.,** The effect of age on hemodynamic response to graded postural stress in normal men, *J. Gerontol.*, 42, 406, 1987.
15. **Abramson, D. I. and Turman, G. A.,** Aging changes in blood vessels, in *Structural Aspects of Aging*, Bourne, G. H., Ed., Hafner, New York, 1960, 49.
16. **Goldman, R.,** Speculations on vascular changes with age, *J. Am. Geriatr. Soc.*, 18, 765, 1970.
17. **Kohn, R. R.,** Heart and cardiovascular system, in *The Biology of Aging*, Finch, C. E. and Hayflick, L., Eds., 1977, 281.
18. **Yin, F. C. P.,** The aging vasculature and its effects on the heart, in *The Aging Heart*, Weisfeldt, M. L., Ed., Raven Press, New York, 1980, 137.
19. **Kojimahara, M., Sekiya, K., and Ooneda, G.,** Age-induced changes of cerebral arteries in rats, *Virchows Arch. Abt. A. Pathol. Anat.*, 361, 11, 1973.
20. **Borchard, F., Borchard, H., and Huth, F.,** Beitrag zur lymphvasculaeren sklerose des ductus thoracicus: Morphometrische Untersuchungen von 88 Faellen, *Beitr. Pathol.*, 146, 145, 1972.
21. **Hassler, O.,** A senile vascular change resulting from excessive spiraling of arteries, *J. Gerontol.*, 24, 37, 1969.
22. **Ratcliffe, J. F.,** Arterial changes in the human vertebral body associated with aging: the ratios of peripheral to central arteries and arterial coiling, *Spine*, 11, 235, 1986.
23. **Johnsson, L. G. and Hawkins, J. E.,** Vascular changes in the human inner ear associated with aging, *Ann. Otol. Rhinol. Laryngol.*, 81, 364, 1972.
24. **Hassler, O.,** Arterial deformities in senile brains, *Acta Neuropathol.*, 8, 219, 1967.
25. **de Nicola, P., Maggi, G., and Tassi, G.,** *Microcirculation: An Atlas*, F. K. Schattauer Verlag, Stuttgart, 1983, 21.
26. **Amery, A., Wasir, H., Bulpitt, C., Conway, J., Fagard, R., Lijnen, P., and Reybrouck, T.,** Aging and the cardiovascular system, *Acta Cardiol.*, 33, 443, 1978.
27. **Lund-Johansen, P.,** The hemodynamics of the aging cardiovascular system, *J. Cardiovas. Pharmacol.*, 12 (Suppl. 8), S20, 1988.
28. **Tassi, G., Maggi, G., and de Nicola, P.,** Microcirculation in the elderly, *Int. Angio.*, 4, 275, 1985.
29. **Montagna, W. and Carlisle, K.,** Structural changes in aging human skin, *J. Invest. Dermatol.*, 73, 47, 1979.
30. **Brown, G. E. and Roth, G. M.,** Biomicroscopy of the surface capillaries in normal and pathologic subjects, *Med. J. Australia*, 1, 499, 1927.
31. **Korkushko, O. V., Sarkisov, K. G., and Frayfeld, V. E.,** Blood circulation in the lower extremities in people of various ages, *Romanian J. Gerontol. Geriatr.*, 5, 103, 1984.

32. **Richardson, D. and Schwartz, R.,** Comparison of capillary blood flow in the nailfold circulations of young and elderly men, *AGE*, 8, 70, 1985.
33. **Nagasawa, S., Handa, H., Okumura, A., Naruo, Y., Moritake, K., and Hayashi, K.,** Mechanical properties of human cerebral arteries. I. Effects of age and vascular smooth muscle activation, *Surg. Neurol.*, 12, 297, 1979.
34. **Hajdu, M. A., Heistad, D. D., Siems, J. E., and Baumbach, G. L.,** Effects of aging on mechanics and composition of cerebral arterioles in rats, *Circ. Res.*, 66, 1747, 1990.
35. **Braverman, I. M. and Fonferko, E.,** Studies in cutaneous aging. II. The microvasculature, *J. Invest. Dermatol.*, 78, 444, 1982.
36. **Braverman, I. M.,** Elastic fiber and microvascular abnormalities in aging skin, *Clin. Geriat. Med.*, 5, 69, 1989.
37. **Stablein, M. and Meyer, J.,** Age-related changes in capillaries of rat oral mucosa. A quantitative electron microscopic study, *Mech. Age. Dev.*, 45, 23, 1988.
38. **Topple, A., Fifkova, E., and Cullen-Dockstader, K.,** Effect of age on blood vessels and neurovascular appositions in the rat dentate fascia, *Neurobiol. Aging*, 11, 371, 1990.
39. **Morlock, C. G.,** Arterioles of the pancreas, liver, gastrointestinal tract and spleen in hypertension, *Arch. Int. Med.*, 63, 100, 1939.
40. **Braverman, I. M., Sibley, J., and Keh-Yen, A.,** A study of the veil cells around normal, diabetic and aged cutaneous microvessels, *J. Invest. Dermatol.*, 86, 57, 1986.
41. **Kuwabara, T., Carroll, J. M., and Cogan, D. G.,** Retinal vascular patterns, *Arch. Ophthalmol.*, 65, 124, 1961.
42. **Gilchrest, B. A., Murphy, G. F., and Soter, N. A.,** Effect of chronologic aging and ultraviolet irradiation on Langerhans cells in human epidermis, *J. Invest. Dermatol.*, 79, 85, 1982.
43. **Ryan, T. J.,** The microcirculation of the skin in old age, *Gerontol. Clin.*, 8, 327, 1966.
44. **Popoff, N. W.,** The digital vascular system, *Arch. Pathol.*, 18, 295, 1934.
45. **Rakusan, K. and Poupa, O.,** Capillaries and muscle fibers in the heart of old rats, *Gerontologia*, 9, 107, 1964.
46. **Jucker, M., Battig, K., and Meier-Ruge, W.,** Effects of aging and vincamine derivatives on pericapillary microenvironment: stereological characterization of the cerebral capillary network, *Neurobiol. Aging*, 2, 39, 1990.
47. **Stringa, M.,** Optic nerve microangioarchitecture in the aging eye, *Metabol. Pediat. Syst. Opthalmol.*, 12, 83, 1989.
48. **Tomanek, R. J.,** Effects of age and exercise on the extent of the myocardial capillary bed, *Anat. Rec.*, 167, 55, 1970.
49. **Jdanov, D. A.,** On senile changes in lymphatic capillaries and vessels, *Ann. Anat. Pathol.*, 7, 108, 1966.
50. **Adolfsson, J., Ljungqvist, A., Tornling, G., and Unge, G.,** Capillary increase in the skeletal muscle of trained young and adult rats, *J. Physiol.*, 310, 529, 1981.
51. **Parizkova, J., Eiselt, E., Sprynarova, S., and Wachtlova, M.,** Body composition, aerobic capacity, and density of muscle capillaries in young and old men, *J. Appl. Physiol.*, 31, 323, 1971.
52. **Richardson, D. and Shepherd, S.,** The cutaneous microcirculation of the forearm in young and old subjects, *Microvas. Res.*, 41, 84, 1991.
53. **Ellis, R. A.,** Ageing of the human male scalp, in *The Biology of Hair Growth*, Montagna, W. and Ellis, R. A., Eds., Academic Press, New York, 1958, 469.
54. **de Nicola, P., Maggi, G., and Tammaro, A. E.,** The small vessels of the skin and mucous membranes in presenile and senile age, *Bibl. Anat.*, 7, 498, 1965.
55. **Mann, D. M. A., Eaves, N. R., Marcyniuk, B., and Yates, P. O.,** Quantitative changes in cerebral cortical microvasculature in ageing and dementia, *Neurobiol. Aging*, 7, 321, 1986.

56. **de Mignard, V. A. and Bernick, S.,** Microvascular changes in aging human osseous tissue, *Microvas. Res.,* 17, S11, 1979.
57. **Keohane, S. G., Adams, C. W. M., and Poston, R. N.,** Coronary arterial dimensions and cell populations in ageing man, *Atherosclerosis,* 69, 103, 1988.
58. **Ryan, T. J.,** Structure, pattern and shape of the blood vessels of the skin, in *The Physiology and Pathology of the Skin,* Jarret, A., Ed., Academic Press, London, 1973, 577.
59. **Labram, C.,** Les micro-anevrismes du champ vasculaire de la conjonctive bulbaire en pathologie interne. Etude biomicroscopique, *Ann. D'Oculistique,* 197, 150, 1964.
60. **Hume, R.,** The relationship to age and cerebral vascular accidents on fibrin and fibrinolytic activity, *J. Clin. Pathol.,* 4, 167, 1961.
61. **Lowe, G. D. O., Drummond, M. M., Forbes, C. D., and Barbenel, J. C.,** The effects of age and cigarette-smoking on blood and plasma viscosity in men, *Scot. Med. J.,* 25, 13, 1980.
62. **Giansanti, R., Boemi, M., DeTommaso, G., Rosati, S., Pennesi, F., and Fumelli, P.,** Changes in hemorheological parameters during normal aging, *Arch. Gerontol. Geriatr.,* 2 (Suppl.), 397, 1991.
63. **Abe, H., Orita, M., and Arichi, S.,** Erythrocyte deformability in aging, *Mech. Aging Dev.,* 27, 383, 1984.
64. **Ciuffetti, G., Mercuri, M., Rizzo, M. T., Lennie, S. E., and Lowe, G. D. O.,** Age and blood cell rheology, *Gerontology,* 35, 31, 1984.
65. **Reid, H. L., Barnes, A. J., Lock, P. J., Dormandy, J. A., and Dormandy, T. L.,** A simple method for measuring erythrocyte deformability, *J. Clin. Pathol.,* 29, 855, 1976.
66. **Ward, K. A., Baker, C., Roebuck, L., Wickline, K., and Schwartz, R. W.,** Red blood cell deformability: effect of age and smoking, *AGE,* 14, 73, 1991.
67. **Bender, A. D.,** The effect of increasing age on the distribution of peripheral blood flow in man, *J. Am. Geriatr. Soc.,* 13, 192, 1965.
68. **Tsuchida, Y.,** Age-related changes in skin blood flow at four anatomic sites of the body in males studied by Xenon-133, *Plastic Reconst. Surg.,* 85, 556, 1990.
69. **Tuma, R. F., Irion, G. L., Vasthare, U. S., and Heinel, L. A.,** Age-related changes in regional blood flow in the rat, *Am. J. Physiol.,* 249, H485, 1985.
70. **Iwase, S., Mano, T., Watanabe, T., Saito, M., and Kobayashi, F.,** Age-related changes of sympathetic outflow to muscles in humans, *J. Gerontol.,* 46, M1, 1991.
71. **Docherty, J. R.,** Aging and the cardiovascular system, *J. Auton. Pharmacol.,* 6, 77, 1986.
72. **Hruza, Z. and Zweifach, B. W.,** Effect of age on vascular reactivity to catecholamines in rats, *J. Gerontol.,* 22, 469, 1967.
73. **Knisely, W. H., Barnes, R. H., and Satterwhite, W. M.,** In vivo observations on the bulbar conjunctival blood vessels and blood of functioning people 60 years of age and over, *J. Gerontol.,* 12, 429, 1957.
74. **Handa, R. K. and Duckles, S. P.,** Age-related changes in adrenergic vasoconstrictor responses of the rat hindlimb, *Am. J. Physiol.,* 253, H1566, 1987.
75. **Hollenberg, N. K., Adams, D. F., Solomon, H. S., Rashid, A., Abrams, H. L., and Merrill, J. P.,** Senescence and the renal vasculature in normal man, *Circ. Res.,* 34, 309, 1974.
76. **Lee, T. J. F., Shirasaki, Y., and Nickols, G. A.,** Altered endothelial modulation of vascular tone in aging and hypertension, *Blood Vessels,* 24, 132, 1987.
77. **Moritoki, H., Hosoki, E., and Ishida, Y.,** Age-related decrease in endothelium-dependent dilator response to histamine in rat mesenteric artery, *Eur. J. Pharmacol.,* 126, 61, 1986.
78. **Darmady, E. M., Offer, J., and Woodhouse, M. A.,** The parameters of the ageing kidney, *J. Pathol.,* 109, 195, 1973.

79. **Yamaguchi, S., Kobayashi, S., Murata, A., Yamashita, K., and Tsunematsu, T.,** Effect of aging on collateral circulation via pial anastomoses in cats, *Gerontology*, 34, 157, 1988.
80. **Smiesko, V., Lang, D. J., and Johnson, P. C.,** Dilator response of rat mesenteric arcading arterioles to increased blood flow velocity, *Am. J. Physiol.,* 257, H1958, 1989.
81. **van Best, J. A., Kappelhof, J. P., Laterveer, L., and Oosterhuis, J. A.,** Blood aqueous barrier permeability versus age by fluorophotometry, *Current Eye Res.,* 6, 855, 1987.
82. **Korkushko, O. V., Ivanov, L. A., and Sarkisov, E. G.,** Mechanism of the effect of various doses of lidase on capillary-tissue oxygen diffusion in old age, *Fiziologiya Cheloveka*, 11, 474, 1985.
83. **Yamaguchi, K., Tanaka, Y., Kubo, H., Takagi, Y., Tachikawa, S., and Katsunuma, H.,** Comparison between PVHIS on the MRI and the permeability of brain blood vessels in elderly patients, *Nippon Ronen Igakkai Zasshi*, 26, 624, 1989.
84. **Mooradian, A. D.,** Effect of aging on the blood-brain barrier, *Neurobiol. Aging*, 9, 31, 1988.
85. **Sparks, H.,** Skin and muscle, in *Peripheral Circulation*, Johnson, P. C., Ed., John Wiley & Sons, New York, 1978, 193.
86. **Tan, O. T. and Stafford, T. J.,** Cutaneous circulation, in *Dermatology in General Medicine*, Fitzpatrick, T. B., Eisen, A. Z., Wolff, K., Freedberg, I. M., and Austen, K. F., Eds., 3rd ed., McGraw-Hill, New York, 1987, 357.
87. **Perera, P., Kurban, A. K., and Ryan, T. J.,** The development of the cutaneous microvascular system in the newborn, *Br. J. Dermatol.,* 82 (Suppl. 5), 86, 1970.
88. **Marinov, G. and Tzvetkova, T.,** Age related differentiation in the local peculiarities of the terminal vascular bed of the lower limb skin, *Verh. Anat. Ges.,* 71, S689, 1977.
89. **Syme, J. and Riley, I. D.,** Nail-fold capillary loop development in the infant of low birth weight, *Br. J. Dermatol.,* 83, 591, 1970.
90. **Korkushko, O. V. and Sarkisov, K. G.,** Age-specific features peculiar to the microcirculation system in advanced and senile age, *Kardiologija*, 3, 19, 1976.
91. **Tan, C. Y., Statham, B., Marks, R., and Payne, P. A.,** Skin thickness measured by pulsed ultrasound: its reproducibility, validation and variability, *Br. J. Dermatol.,* 106, 657, 1982.
92. **Gilchrest, B. A., Stoff, J. S., and Soter, N. A.,** Chronologic aging alters the response to ultraviolet-induced inflammation in human skin, *J. Invest. Dermatol.,* 79, 11, 1982.
93. **Merlen, J. F.,** Capillaroscopy at the nail bed in functioning people aged 70 and over, *Int. Angiol.,* 4, 285, 1985.
94. **Haimovici, H., Steinman, C., and Chaplan, L. H.,** Role of arteriovenous anastomoses in vascular diseases of the lower extremity, *Ann. Surg.,* 164, 990, 1966.
95. **Harpuder, K., Stein, I. D., and Byer, J.,** The role of the arteriovenous anastomosis in peripheral vascular disease, *Am. Heart J.,* 20, 539, 1940.
96. **Rubsamen, K. and Hales, J. R. S.,** Role of arteriovenous anastomoses in determining heat transfer across the hindleg skin of sheep, in *Thermal Physiology*, Hales, J. R. S., Ed., Raven Press, New York, 1984, 259.
97. **Holm-Pedersen, P., Nilsson, K., and Branemark, P. I.,** The microvascular system of healing wounds in young and old rats, *Adv. Microcirc.,* 5, 80, 1973.
98. **Yamaura, H. and Matsuzawa, T.,** Decrease in capillary growth during aging, *Exp. Gerontol.,* 15, 145, 1980.
99. **Kreisle, R. A., Stebler, B. A., and Ershler, W. B.,** Effect of host age on tumor-associated angiogenesis in mice, *J. Natl. Cancer. Inst.,* 82, 44, 1990.

100. **Westphal, K. A. and Richardson, D. R.,** Effects of age on cutaneous regional and superficial capillary blood flows during heat stress in the rat, *AGE*, 15, 1, 1992.
101. **Richardson, D. R.,** Functional changes in the cutaneous microcirculation associated with aging, *Proc. 5th World Cong. Microcirc.*, 91, 1991.
102. **Richardson, D., Shepherd, S., and Tyra, J.,** Age-related potentiation of the cutaneous capillary blood flow response to heat stress, *Microcirc. Endoth. Lymph.*, 7, 305, 1991.
103. **Bos, G. M. J., Slaff, D. W., Majoor, G. D., Tangelder, G. J., and Reneman, R. S.,** A model for chronic study of vascular morphology and reactivity of physically intact rat skin microcirculation, *Int. J. Microcirc. Clin. Exp.*, 6, 371, 1983.
104. **Lorincz, A. L.,** Physiology of aging skin, *Il. Med J.*, 107, 59, 1960.
105. **Kligman, A. M.,** Perspectives and problems in cutaneous gerontology, *J. Invest. Dermatol.*, 73, 39, 1979.
106. **Pearce, R. H. and Grimmer, B. J.,** Age and the chemical constitution of normal human dermis, *J. Invest. Dermatol.*, 58, 347, 1972.
107. **Zweifach, B. W. and Intaglietta, M.,** Mechanics of fluid movement across single capillaries in the rabbit, *Microvas. Res.*, 1, 83, 1968.
108. **McClure, W. B. and Aldrich, C. A.,** Time required for disappearance of intradermally injected salt solution, *J. Am. Med. Assoc.*, 81, 293, 1923.
109. **Aschner, B. M.,** Intradermal salt solution test in elderly persons, *Exp. Med. Surg.*, 18, 17, 1960.
110. **Heite, H. J.,** Der functionzusand der kleined gefaesse im Lichte gleichzeitig gemessener quaddel- und fluorescein resorptions geschwindigkeit, *Arch. Klin. Exper. Dermatol.*, 206, 216, 1957.
111. **Christophers, E. and Kligman, A. M.,** Percutaneous absorption in aged skin, in *Advances in Biology of Skin*, Vol. 2, Montagna, W., Ed., Pergamon Press, Oxford, 1965, 163.
112. **Tagami, H.,** Functional characteristics of aged skin, *Acta Dermatol. Kyoto*, 66, 19, 1972.
113. **Roskos, K. V., Maibach, H. I., and Guy, R. H.,** The effect of aging on percutaneous absorption in man, *J. Pharm. Biopharm.*, 17, 617, 1989.
114. **Roskos, K. V., Bircher, A. J., Maibach, H. I., and Guy, R. H.,** Pharmacodynamic measurements of methyl nicotinate percutaneous absorption: the effect of aging on microcirculation, *Br. J. Dermatol.*, 122, 165, 1990.
115. **Goodson, W. H. and Hunt, T. K.,** Wound healing and aging, *J. Invest. Dermatol.*, 73, 88, 1979.
116. **Harutsugu, Y. and Matsuzawa, T.,** Decrease in capillary growth during aging, *Exp. Gerontol.*, 15, 145, 1980.
117. **Kay, M. M. B.,** The thymus: clock for immunologic aging?, *J. Invest. Dermatol.*, 73, 29, 1979.
118. **Ryan, T. J. and Kurban, A. K.,** New vessel growth in the adult skin, *Br. J. Dermatol.*, 82 (Suppl. 5), 92, 1970.
119. **Ingber, D. E.,** Control of capillary growth and differentiation by extracellular matrix: use of a tensegrity (tensional integrity) mechanism for signal processing, *Chest*, 99, 34S, 1991.
120. **Allwood, M. J.,** Blood flow in the foot and calf in the elderly: a comparison with that in young adults, *Clin. Sci.*, 17, 331, 1958.
121. **Oimomi, M., Hatanaka, H., Maeda, Y., Hata, F., Kitamura, Y., Matsumoto, S., and Baba, S.,** Autonomic nervous function determined by changes of periflux blood flow in the aged, *Arch. Gerontol. Geriatr.*, 5, 159, 1986.
122. **Pickering, G. W.,** The peripheral resistance in persistent arterial hypertension, *Clin. Sci.*, 2, 209, 1936.

123. **Ring, G. C., Kurbatov, T., and Shannon, G. J.,** Changes in central pulse and finger plethysmography during aging, *J. Gerontol.,* 14, 189, 1959.
124. **Roth, G. I., Matheny, J. L., Falace, D. A., O'Reilly, J. E., and Norton., J. C.,** Effect of age on the digit blood flow response to sedative concentrations of nitrous oxide, *Anesth. Prog.,* 31, 17, 1984.
125. **Ware, S. K., Bruckner, G., and Richardson, D. R.,** Cutaneous blood flow measurements in clinical studies using laser Doppler flowmetry (LDF) and capillary videomicroscopy (CV), *Proc. 5th World Cong. Microcirc.,* 120, 1991.
126. **Richardson, D. R., Schmitz, M., and Borchers, N.,** Relative effects of static muscle contraction on digital artery and nailfold capillary blood flow velocities, *Microvas. Res.,* 31, 157, 1986.
127. **Schwartz, R. W., Freedman, A. M., Richardson, D. R., Hyde, G. L., Griffen, W. O., Vincent, D. G., and Price, M. A.,** Capillary blood flow: videodensitometry in the atherosclerotic patient, *J. Vas. Surg.,* 1, 800, 1984.
128. **Kravec, T. F., Eggers, G. W. N., and Kettel, L. J.,** Influence of patient age on forearm and systematic vascular response to hypoxemia, *Clin. Sci.,* 42, 555, 1972.
129. **Hellon, R. F., and Lind, A. R.,** The influence of age on peripheral vasodilatation in a hot environment, *J. Physiol.,* 141, 262, 1958.
130. **Sagawa, S., Shiraki, K., Yousef, M. K., and Miki, K.,** Sweating and cardiovascular responses of aged men to heat exposure, *J. Gerontol.,* 43, M1, 1988.
131. **Shiraki, K., Sagawa, S., Yousef, M. K., Konda, N., and Miki, K.,** Physiological responses of aged men to head-up tilt during heat exposure, *J. Appl. Physiol.,* 63, 576, 1987.
132. **Sowers, J. R. and Mohanty, P. K.,** Norepinephrine and forearm vascular resistance responses to tilt and cold pressor test in essential hypertension: effects of aging, *Angiology,* 40, 872, 1989.
133. **Kenney, W. L.,** Control of heat-induced cutaneous vasodilation in relation to age, *Eur. J. Appl. Physiol.,* 57, 120, 1988.
134. **Tankersley, C., Smolander, J., and Fortney, S.,** Skin blood flow (SkBf) responses in young (YM) and older (OM) men during exercise in the heat, *Fed. Proc.,* 46, 1440, 1987.
135. **Johnson, J. M., Brengelmann, G. L., Hales, J. R. S., Vanhoutte, P. M., and Wenger, C. B.,** Regulation of the cutaneous circulation, *Fed. Proc.,* 45, 2841, 1986.
136. **Herbert, R.,** The biology of aging: body temperature regulation, *Geriatr. Nurs. (London),* 6, 16, 1986.
137. **Shock, N. W.,** Systems integration, in *Handbook of the Biology of Aging,* Finch, C. E. and Hayflick, L., Eds., Van Nostrand, New York, 1977, 639.
138. **Drinkwater, B. L. and Horvath, S. M.,** Heat tolerance and aging, *Med. Sci. Sports,* 11, 49, 1979.
139. **Drinkwater, B. L., Bedi, J. F., Loucks, A. B., Roche, S., and Horvath, S. M.,** Sweating sensitivity and capacity of women in relation to age, *J. Appl. Physiol.,* 53, 671, 1982.
140. **Yousef, M. K., Sagawa, S., and Shiraka, K.,** Thermoregulatory responses of the elderly population, *J. Univ. Occup. Environ. Health,* 8, 219, 1986.
141. **Yousef, M. K., Dill, D. B., Vitez, T. S., Hillyard, S. D., and Goldman, A. S.,** Thermoregulatory responses to desert heat: age, race and sex, *J. Gerontol.,* 39, 406, 1984.
142. **Rand, R. P., Burton, A. C., and Ing, T.,** The tail of the rat in temperature regulation and acclimatization, *Can. J. Physiol. Pharmacol.,* 43, 257, 1965.
143. **Young, A. A. and Dawson, N. J.,** Evidence for on-off control of heat dissipation from the tail of the rat, *Can. J. Physiol. Pharm.,* 60, 392, 1982.

144. **Gemmell, R. T. and Hales, J. R. S.,** Cutaneous arteriovenous anastomosis present in the tail but absent from the ear of the rat, *J. Anat.,* 124, 355, 1977.
145. **O'Leary, D. S., Johnson, J. M., and Taylor, W. F.,** Mode of neural control mediating rat tail vasodilation during heating, *J. Appl. Physiol.,* 59, 1533, 1985.
146. **Furuyama, F.,** Strain difference in thermoregulation of rats surviving extreme heat, *J. Appl. Physiol.,* 52, 410, 1982.
147. **Hoffman, H. J.,** Survival distributions for selected laboratory rat strains and stocks, in *Development of the Rodent as a Model System of Aging*, Gibson, D. C., Adelman, R. C., and Finch, C., DHEW Publication NIH79-161 Book II, U.S. Government Printing Office, Washington, DC, 1978, 19.
148. **Blake, J. J., Fargnoli, J., Gershon, D., and Holbrook, N. J.,** Concomitant decline in heat-induced hyperthermia and HSP70 mRNA expression in aged rats, *Am. J. Physiol.,* 260, F663, 1991.
149. **Schubert, V. and Fagrell, B.,** Evaluation of the dynamic cutaneous post-ischaemic hyperaemia and thermal response in elderly subjects and in an area at risk for pressure sores, *Clin. Physiol.,* 11, 169, 1991.
150. **Fox, R. H., Woodward, P. M., Exton-Smith, A. N., Green, M. F., Donnison, D. V., and Wicks, M. H.,** Body temperatures in the elderly: a national study of physiological, social and environmental conditions, *Br. Med. J.,* 1, 200, 1973.
151. **Kolanowski, A. and Gunter, L.,** Hypothermia in the elderly, *Geriatr. Nurs.,* 2, 362, 1981.
152. **Hooi, C. W. M. and Moore, R. E.,** Responses of old and young men to cold exposure, *J. Physiol.,* 293, 78P, 1979.
153. **McDonnald, R. B., Horwitz, B. A., Hamilton, J. S., and Stern, J. S.,** Cold and norepinephrine-induced thermogenesis in younger and older Fischer 344 rats, *Am. J. Physiol.,* 254, R457, 1988.
154. **Owen, T. L., Spencer, R. L., and Duckles, S. P.,** Effect of age on cold acclimation in rats: metabolic and behavioral responses, *Am. J. Physiol.,* 260, R284, 1991.
155. **Rothwell, N. J. and Stock, M. J.,** Effects of age on diet induced thermogenesis and brown adipose tissue metabolism in the rat, *Int. J. Obesity,* 7, 583, 1983.
156. **Collins, K. J., Dore, C., Exton-Smith, A. N., Fox, R. H., MacDonald, I. C., and Woodward, P. C.,** Accidental hypothermia and impaired temperature homeostasis in the elderly, *Br. Med. J.,* 1, 353, 1977.
157. **Fagrell, B., Svedman, P., and Ostergren, J.,** The influence of hydrostatic pressure and contralateral cooling on capillary blood cell velocity and transcutaneous oxygen tension in fingers, *Int. J. Microcirc. Clin. Exp.,* 1, 163, 1982.
158. **Collins, K. J., Exton-Smith, A. N., James, M. H., and Oliver, D. J.,** Functional changes in autonomic nervous responses with ageing, *Age Ageing,* 9, 17, 1980.
159. **Lipsitz, L. A.,** Altered blood pressure homeostasis in advanced age: clinical and research implications, *J. Gerontol.,* 44, M179, 1989.
160. **Roberts, J. and Tumer, N.,** Age-related changes in autonomic function of catecholamines, *Rev. Biol. Res. Aging,* 3, 257, 1987.
161. **Smith, J. J. and Porth, C. J. M.,** Posture and the circulation: the age effect, *Exp. Gerontol.,* 26, 141, 1991.
162. **Robbins, A. S. and Rubenstein, L. Z.,** Postural hypotension in the elderly, *J. Am. Geriatr. Soc.,* 32, 769, 1984.
163. **Lipsitz, L. A., Bui, M., Stiebeling, M., and McArdle, C.,** Forearm blood flow response to posture change in the very old: non-invasive measurement by venous occlusion plethysmography, *J. Am. Geriatr. Soc.,* 39, 53, 1991.
164. **Beiser, G. D., Zelis, R., Epstein, S. E., Mason, D. T., and Braunwald, E.,** The role of skin and muscle resistance vessels in reflexes mediated by the baroreceptor system, *J. Clin. Invest.,* 49, 225, 1970.

165. **Minaker, K. L., Meneilly, G. S., Young, J. B., Landsberg, L., Stoff, J. S., Robertson, G. L., and Rowe, J. W.,** Blood pressure, pulse and neurohumoral responses to nitroprusside-induced hypotension in normotensive aging men, *J. Gerontol.,* 46, M151, 1991.
166. **Hodgson, J. L. and Buskirk, E. R.,** Physical fitness and age, with emphasis on cardiovascular function in the elderly, *J. Am. Geriatr. Soc.,* 25, 385, 1977.
167. **Jokl, E.,** Perspective: physical activity and aging, *Ann. Sport Med.,* 1, 43, 1983.
168. **Posner, J. D., Gorman, K. M., Gitlin, L. N., Sands, L. P., Kleban, M., Windsor, L., and Shaw, C.,** Effects of exercise training in the elderly on the occurrence and time to onset of cardiovascular diagnoses, *J. Am. Geriatr. Soc.,* 38, 205, 1990.
169. **Shephard, R. J.,** Exercise and aging, in *The Biology of Aging*, Bohnke, J. A., Finch, C. E., and Moment, G. B., Eds., Plenum Press, New York, 1978, 131.
170. **Astrand, I., Astrand, P. O., Hallbaeck, I., and Kilbom, A.,** Reduction in maximal oxygen uptake with age, *J. Appl. Physiol.,* 35, 649, 1973.
171. **Dehn, M. and Bruce, R. A.,** Longitudinal variations in maximal oxygen intake with age and activity, *J. Appl. Physiol.,* 33, 805, 1972.
172. **Makrides, L., Heigenhauser, G. J. F., and Jones, N. L.,** High intensity endurance training in 20- to 30- and 60- to 70-yr-old healthy men, *J. Appl. Physiol.,* 69, 1792, 1990.
173. **Guralnik, J. M., Branch, L. G., Cummings, S. R., and Curb, J. D.,** Physical performance measures in aging research, *J. Gerontol.,* 44, M141, 1989.
174. **Christensen, E. H., Nielsen, M., and Hannisdahl, B.,** Investigations of the circulation in the skin at the beginning of muscular work, *Acta Physiol. Scand.,* 4, 162, 1942.
175. **Bevegard, B. D. and Shepherd, J. T.,** Reaction in man of resistance and capacity vessels in forearm and hand to leg exercise, *J. Appl. Physiol.,* 21, 123, 1966.
176. **Blair, D. A., Glover, W. E., and Roddie, I. C.,** Vasomotor responses in the human arm during leg exercise, *Circ. Res.,* 9, 264, 1961.
177. **Johnson, J. M.,** Responses of forearm blood flow to graded leg exercise in man, *J. Appl. Physiol.,* 46, 457, 1979.
178. **Tankersley, C. G., Smolander, J., Kenney, W. L., and Fortney, S. M.,** Sweating and skin blood flow during exercise: effects of age and maximal oxygen uptake, *J. Appl. Physiol.,* 71, 236, 1991.
179. **Florini, J. R.,** Effect of aging on skeletal muscle composition and function, *Rev. Biol. Res. Aging*, 3, 337, 1987.
180. **Wiedeman, M. P.,** Architecture, in *Handbook of Physiology: The Cardiovascular System*, Vol. 4, Sect. 2, Renkin, E. M. and Michell, C. C., Eds., American Physiology Society, Bethesda, MD, 1984, 11.
181. **Eriksson, E. and Myrhage, R.,** Microvascular dimensions and blood flow in skeletal muscle, *Acta Physiol. Scand.,* 86, 211, 1972.
182. **Wiedeman, M. P.,** Patterns of the arteriovenous pathways, in *Handbook of Physiology: Circulation*, Vol. 2, Sect. 2, Hamilton, W. F., Ed., American Physiology Society, Washington, DC, 1963, 891.
183. **Brotzu, G., Carta, M., D'Alia, G., Diaz, G., Montisci, R., and Savona, G.,** Stereomorphological arrangement of capillaries in skeletal muscle in normal and stenosed young and adult rats, *Microvas. Res.,* 27, 286, 1984.
184. **Gray, S. D. and Renkin, E. M.,** Microvascular supply in relation to fiber metabolic type in mixed skeletal muscles of rabbits, *Microvas. Res.,* 16, 406, 1978.
185. **Myrhage, R.,** Capillary supply of the muscle fibre population in hindlimb muscles of the cat, *Acta Physiol. Scand.,* 103, 19, 1978.
186. **Plyley, M. J. and Groom, A. C.,** Geometrical distribution of capillaries in mammalian striated muscle, *Am. J. Physiol.,* 228, 1376, 1975.

187. **Larsson, L.,** Physical training effects on muscle morphology in sedentary males at different ages, *Med. Sci. Sports Exercise*, 14, 203, 1982.
188. **Andersen, P. and Henriksson, J.,** Capillary supply of the quadriceps femoris muscle of man: adaptive response to exercise, *J. Physiol.*, 270, 677, 1977.
189. **Grimby, G., Danneskiold-Samsoe, B., Hvid, K., and Saltin, B.,** Morphology and enzymatic capacity in arm and leg muscles in 78–81 year old men and women, *Acta Physiol. Scand.*, 115, 125, 1982.
190. **Ripoll, E., Sillau, A. H., and Banchero, N.,** Changes in the capillarity of skeletal muscle in the growing rat, *Pflugers Arch.*, 380, 153, 1979.
191. **Brown, M.,** Change in fibre size, not number, in ageing skeletal muscle, *Age Ageing*, 16, 244, 1987.
192. **Young, J. C., Chen, M., and Holloszy, J. O.,** Maintenance of the adaptation of skeletal muscle mitochondria to exercise in old rats, *Med. Sci. Sports Exercise*, 15, 243, 1983.
193. **Gorczynski, R. J., Klitzman, B., and Duling, B. R.,** Interrelation between contracting striated muscle and precapillary microvessels, *Am. J. Physiol.*, 235, H494, 1978.
194. **Hudlicka, O., Zweifach, B. W., and Tyler, K. R.,** Capillary recruitment and flow velocity in skeletal muscle after contractions, *Microvas. Res.*, 23, 201, 1982.
195. **Tyml, K.,** Capillary recruitment and heterogeneity of microvascular flow in skeletal muscle before and after contraction, *Microvas. Res.*, 32, 84, 1986.
196. **Hudlicka, O.,** Growth of capillaries in skeletal and cardiac muscle, *Circ. Res.*, 50, 451, 1982.
197. **Tyml, K. and Mathieu-Costello, O.,** Functional changes in the skeletal muscle microcirculation with aging, *Proc. 5th World Cong. Microcirc.*, 113, 1991.
198. **Tyml, K., Mathieu-Costello, O., and Budreau, C. H.,** Distribution of red blood cell velocity in capillary network, and endothelial ultrastructure, in aged rat skeletal muscle, *Microvas. Res.*, in press.
199. **Amery, A., Bossaert, H., and Verstraete, M.,** Muscle blood flow in normal and hypertensive subjects, *Am. Heart J.*, 78, 211, 1969.
200. **Irion, G. L., Vasthare, U. S., and Tuma, R. F.,** Age-related change in skeletal muscle blood flow in the rat, *J. Gerontol.*, 42, 660, 1987.
201. **Wahren, J., Saltin, B., Jorfeldt, L., and Pernow, B.,** Influence of age on the local circulatory adaptation to leg exercise, *Scand. J. Clin. Lab. Invest.*, 33, 79, 1974.
202. **Martin, W. H., Kohrt, W. M., Malley, M. T., Korte, E., and Stoltz, S.,** Exercise training enhances leg vasodilatory capacity of 65-yr-old men and women, *J. Appl. Physiol.*, 69, 1804, 1990.
203. **Richardson, D. and Shewchuk, R.,** Comparison of calf muscle blood flow responses to rhythmic exercise between mean age 25- and 74-year old men, *Proc. Soc. Exp. Biol. Med.*, 164, 550, 1980.
204. **Hakkila, J.,** Studies on the myocardial capillary concentration in cardiac hypertrophy due to training: an experimental study with guinea pigs, *Ann. Med. Exp. Biol. Fenn.*, 33 (Suppl. 10), 1, 1955.
205. **Tomanek, R. J. and Hovanec, J. M.,** The effects of long-term pressure overload and aging on the myocardium, *J. Mol. Cell. Cardiol.*, 13, 471, 1981.
206. **Tomanek, R. J., Aydelotte, M. R., and Torry, R. J.,** Remodeling of coronary vessels during aging in purebred beagles, *Circ. Res.*, 69, 1068, 1991.
207. **Burch, G. and Giles, T.,** Senile cardiomyopathy, *J. Chron. Dis.*, 24, 1, 1971.
208. **Anversa, P., Hiler, B., Ricci, R., Guideri, G., and Olivetti, G.,** Myocyte cell loss and myocyte hypertrophy in the aging rat heart, *J. Am. Coll. Cardiol.*, 8, 1441, 1986.
209. **Mandache, E., Unge, G., and Ljungqvist, A.,** Myocardial blood capillary reaction in various forms of cardiac hypertrophy: an electron microscopical investigation in the rat, *Virchows Arch. Abt. B. Zellpathol.*, 11, 97, 1972.

210. **Bing, R. J., Hellberg, K., and Wayland, H.,** Microcirculation of the heart, *Adv. Exp. Med. Biol.,* 22, 253, 1972.
211. **Rakusan, K. and Korecky, B.,** The effect of growth and aging on functional capillary supply of the rat heart, *Growth,* 46, 275, 1982.
212. **Friberg, P., Nordlander, M., Lundin, S., and Folkow, B.,** Effects of aging on cardiac performance and coronary flow in spontaneously hypertensive and normotensive rats, *Acta Physiol. Scand.,* 125, 1, 1985.
213. **Hachamovitch, R., Wicker, P., Capasso, J. M., and Anversa, P.,** Alterations of coronary blood flow and reserve with aging in Fischer 344 rats, *Am. J. Physiol.,* 256, H66, 1989.
214. **Isoyama, S., Sato, F., and Takishima, T.,** Effect of age on coronary circulation after imposition of pressure-overload in rats, *Hypertension,* 17, 369, 1991.
215. **Toma, B. S., Wangler, R. D., Dewitt, D. F., and Sparks, H. V.,** Effect of development on coronary vasodilator reserve in the isolated guinea pig heart, *Circ. Res.,* 57, 538, 1985.
216. **Toma, B. S., Wangler, R. D., and Sparks, H. V.,** Metabolic hyperemia is reduced in adult vs. immature guinea pig hearts, *Am. J. Physiol.,* 255, H1460, 1988.
217. **Weisfeldt, M. L., Wright, J. R., Shreiner, D. P., Lakatta, E., and Shock, N. W.,** Coronary flow and oxygen extraction in the perfused heart of senescent male rats, *J. Appl. Physiol.,* 30, 44, 1971.
218. **Vigorito, C., Giordano, A., Casaburi, E., Ferraro, P., Maurelli, B., Rumolo, S., Silvstri, P., and Rengo, F.,** Coronary vascular reserve in elderly subjects, *Bibl. Cardiol.,* 44, 40, 1989.
219. **Lakatta, E. G.,** Heart and circulation, in *Handbook of the Biology of Aging,* Finch, C. E. and Schneider, E. L., Eds., Van Nostrand Reinhold, New York, 1985, 377.
220. **Abu-Erreish, G. M., Neely, J. R., Whitmer, J. T., Whitman, V., and Sanadi, D. R.,** Fatty acid oxidation by isolated perfused working hearts of aged rats, *Am. J. Physiol.,* 232, E258, 1977.
221. **Mikhailishchuk, V. S.,** Age related characteristics of the conjunctival microcirculation in healthy individuals and in patients with hypertension, *Kardiologiia,* 22, 62, 1982.
222. **Davis, E. and Landau, J.,** The small blood vessels of the conjunctiva and nailbed in arteriosclerosis, *Angiology,* 11, 173, 1960.
223. **Curri, S. B. and Curri, S.,** Senile involution of the conjunctival and hypothalamic small blood vessels, *Bibl. Anat.,* 13, 222, 1975.
224. **Donchin, M., Davis, E., Abramson, J. H., Epstein, L. M., and Hopp, C.,** Smoking and conjunctival microaneurysms, *Microcirculation,* 1, 381, 1982.
225. **Merlen, J. F., Coget, J., and Vanderbeken, J. P.,** Capillaroscopic patterns in functioning people aged 70 and over, *Bibl. Anat.,* 11, 325, 1973.
226. **Lee, R. E. and Holze, E. A.,** The peripheral vascular system in the bulbar conjunctiva of young normotensive adults at rest, *J. Clin. Invest.,* 29, 146, 1950.
227. **Wells, R. E. and Edgerton, H.,** Blood flow in the microcirculation of the conjunctival vessels of man, *Angiology,* 18, 699, 1967.
228. **Gillum, R. F.,** Cerebrovascular disease morbidity in the United States, 1970-1983, *Stroke,* 17, 656, 1986.
229. **Tool, J. F.,** Vascular diseases: etiology and pathogenesis, in *Merritt's Textbook of Neurology,* Rowland, L. P., Ed., Lea and Febiger, Philadelphia, PA, 1989, 181.
230. **Heistad, D. D. and Kontos, H. A.,** Cerebral circulation, in *Handbook of Physiology: The Cardiovascular System,* Vol. 3, Sect 2, Shepherd, J. T. and Abboud, F. M., Eds., American Physiology Society, Bethesda, MD, 1983, 137.
231. **Goss, C. M.,** The arteries, in *Gray's Anatomy,* 29th American ed., Lea and Febiger, Philadelphia, PA, 1973, 561.

232. **Klassen, A. C., Sung, J. H., and Stadlan, E. M.,** Histological changes in cerebral arteries with increasing age, *J. Neuropathol. Exp. Neurol.*, 27, 607, 1968.
233. **Baker, A. B.,** Structure of the small cerebral arteries and their changes with age, *Am. J. Pathol.*, 13, 453, 1937.
234. **Sorbara, R.,** Etude comparative du vieillissement des arteres du polygone de Willis, *These Med.*, June, 1972.
235. **Bouissou, H., Emery, M. C., and Sorbara, R.,** Age related changes of the middle cerebral artery and a comparison with the radial and coronary artery, *Angiology*, 26, 257, 1975.
236. **Akima, M., Nonaka, H., Kagesawa, M., and Tanaka, M.,** A study on the microvasculature of the cerebellar cortex: the fundamental architecture of its senile change in the cerebellar hemisphere, *Acta Neuropathol.*, 75, 69, 1987.
237. **Ravens, J. R.,** Vascular changes in the human senile brain, *Adv. Neurol.*, 20, 487, 1978.
238. **Cervos-Navarro, J., Gertz, H. J., and Frydl, V.,** Cerebral blood vessel changes in old people, *Mech. Age. Dev.*, 39, 223, 1987.
239. **Baker, D. M., Santer, R. M., and Blaggan, A. S.,** Morphometric studies on the microvasculature of pre- and paravertebral sympathetic ganglia in the adult and aged rat by light and electron microscopy, *J. Neurocytol.*, 18, 647, 1989.
240. **de Jong, G. I., de Weerd, H., Schuurman, T., Traber, J., and Luiten, P. G. M.,** Microvascular changes in aged rat forebrain. Effects of chronic nimodipine treatment, *Neurobiol. Aging*, 11, 381, 1990.
241. **Knox, C. A., Yates, R. D., Chen, I., and Klara, P. M.,** Effects of aging on the structural and permeability characteristics of cerebrovasculature in normotensive and hypertensive strains of rats, *Acta Neuropathol.*, 51, 1, 1980.
242. **Bell, M. A. and Ball, M. J.,** Morphometric comparison of hippocampal microvasculature in ageing and demented people: diameters and densities, *Acta Neuropathol.*, 53, 299, 1981.
243. **Bell, M. A. and Ball, M. J.,** Neuritic plaques and vessels of visual cortex in aging and Alzheimer's dementia, *Neurobiol. Aging*, 11, 359, 1990.
244. **Anderson, J. M., Hubbard, B. M., Coghill, G. R., and Slidders, W.,** The effect of advanced old age on the neurone content of the cerebral cortex, *J. Neurol. Sci.*, 58, 235, 1983.
245. **Banchero, N.,** Capillary density of skeletal muscle in dogs exposed to simulated altitude, *Proc. Soc. Exp. Biol. Med.*, 148, 435, 1975.
246. **Tayarani, I., Cloez, I., Clement, M., and Bourre, J. M.,** Antioxidant enzymes and related trace elements in aging brain capillaries and choroid plexus, *J. Neurochem.*, 53, 817, 1989.
247. **Miyakawa, T., Shimoji, A., Kuramoto, R., and Higuchi, Y.,** The relationship between senile plaques and cerebral blood vessels in Alzheimer's disease and senile dementia, *Virchows Arch. B. Zellpath.*, 40, 121, 1982.
248. **Naritomi, H., Meyer, J. S., Sakai, F., Yamaguchi, F., and Shaw, T.,** Effects of advancing age on regional cerebral blood flow, *Arch. Neurol.*, 36, 410, 1979.
249. **Martin, A. J., Friston, K. J., Colebatch, J. G., and Frackowiak, R. S. J.,** Decreases in regional cerebral blood flow with normal aging, *J. Cerebral Blood Flow Metabol.*, 11, 684, 1991.
250. **Pantano, P., Baron, J. C., Lebrun-Grandie, P., Duquesnoy, N., Bousser, M. G., and Comar, D.,** Regional cerebral blood flow and oxygen consumption in human aging, *Stroke*, 15, 635, 1984.
251. **Yamaguchi, T., Kanno, I, Uemura, K., Shishido, F., Inugami, A., Ogawa, T., Murakami, M., and Suzuki, K.,** Reduction in regional cerebral metabolic rate of oxygen during human aging, *Stroke*, 17, 1220, 1986.

252. **Fieschi, C., Lenzi, G. L., and Loeb, C. W.,** Preface, in *Effects of Aging on Regulation of Cerebral Blood Flow and Metabolism*, Fieschi, C., Lenzi, G. L., and Loeb, C. W., Eds., Karger, New York, 1984, IX.
253. **Yamamoto, M., Meyer, J. S., Sakai, F., and Yamaguchi, F.,** Aging and cerebral vasodilator responses to hypercarbia: responses in normal aging and in persons with risk factors for stroke, *Arch. Neurol.,* 37, 489, 1980.
254. **Tanahashi, N., Gotoh, F., Tomita, M., Amano, T., Fobari, M., Shinohara, T., and Mihara, B.,** Effect of aging on reactive hyperemia following reopening of occluded middle cerebral artery, *Monogr. Neural Sci.,* 11, 40, 1984.
255. **Mayhan, W. G., Faraci, F. M., Baumbach, G. L., and Heistad, D. D.,** Effects of aging on responses of cerebral arterioles, *Am. J. Physiol.,* 258, H1138, 1990.
256. **Hongo, K., Nakagomi, T., Kassel, N. F., Sasaki, T., Lehman, M., Vollmer, D. G., Tsukahara, T., Ogawa, H., and Torner, J.,** Effects of aging and hypertension on endothelium-dependent vascular relaxation in rat carotid artery, *Stroke*, 19, 892, 1988.
257. **Hatake, K., Kakishita, E., Wakabayashi, I., Sakiyama, N., and Hashida, S.,** Effect of aging on endothelium-dependent vascular relaxation of isolated human basilar artery to thrombin and bradykinin, *Stroke*, 21, 1039, 1990.
258. **Rubanyi, G. and Vanhoutte, P. M.,** Endothelium removal decreased relaxations of canine coronary arteries caused by beta-adrenergic agonists and adenosine, *J. Cardiovas. Res.,* 7, 139, 1985.
259. **Chen, P., Jiang, H., Sobin, S., and Giannotta, S.,** Age related changes in rat brain microcirculation using a new cranial window, *Proc. 5th World Cong. Microcirc.,* 15, 1991.
260. **Mione, M. C., Dhital, K. K., Amenta, F., and Burnstock, G.,** An increase in the expression of neuropeptidergic vasodilator, but not vasoconstrictor, cerebrovascular nerves in aging rats, *Brain Res.,* 460, 103, 1988.
261. **Greenberg, J., Hand, P., Sylvestro, A., and Reivich, M.,** Localized metabolic-flow couple during functional activity, *Acta. Neurol. Scand.,* 60 (Suppl. 72), 12, 1979.
262. **Rogers, R. L., Meyer, J. S., and Mortel, K. F.,** After reaching retirement age physical activity sustains cerebral perfusion and cognition, *J. Am. Geriatr. Soc.,* 38, 123, 1990.
263. **Frackowiak, R. S. J., Wise, R. J. S., Gibbs, J. M., Jones, T., and Leenders, N.,** Oxygen extraction in the aging brain, *Monogr. Neural Sci.,* 11, 118, 1984.
264. **Hunziker, O., Abdel'Al, S., and Schulz, U.,** The aging human cerebral cortex: a stereological characterization of changes in the capillary net, *J. Gerontol.,* 34, 345, 1979.

Chapter 11

Impact of Environmental Factors

Kenneth S. Ramos and Russell C. Bowes III

CONTENTS

0-8493-4547-2/94/$0.00+$.50

I. INTRODUCTION

A. DEFINITIONS

The role of environmental factors in the modulation of vascular cell function and the pathogenesis of vascular disorders has become a subject of increasing interest from a scientific and public perspective. By definition, "environmental factors" are those factors associated with the ambient environment, as well as aspects of the environment under personal control.[1] Ambient environmental factors include physical and chemical contaminants present in air, water, and/or food. These contaminants may be derived from anthropogenic sources, such as automobile exhaust, or may represent natural variations in the environment, such as mycotoxins in food supplies. Whatever the source, ambient factors effect the population at large. In contrast, environmental factors under personal control are those introduced into the body by the individual directly. Examples of personal factors include tobacco smoking, drug use, food selection, and various health habits. Another aspect relevant to this discussion is the whole animal environment. These factors include growth factors and extracellular matrix proteins which can modulate microcirculatory function. Collectively, ambient, personal, and whole animal elements represent environmental factors which can alter microcirculatory physiology.

As previous chapters have documented, the microcirculation consists of a vast array of arterioles, venules, and capillaries which supply all the organs of the body. Subtle changes in the structural and functional integrity of the systemic or regional microcirculation can adversely effect body function. For example, the metabolic deficiency associated with diabetes mellitus leads to disturbances in skin, kidney, lymphatic, and large-vessel microcirculation.[2-4] Cardiopulmonary disorders can also cause alterations in microcirculatory function resulting in progressive tissue hypoxia and/or ischemia.[5] In attempting to understand the etiology of these and other disorders, a number of studies have examined the associated pathologic changes of the microcirculation. Because environmental factors may "target" the microcirculation of specific organ systems, this chapter will focus on the mechanism by which selected environmental factors contribute to organ-specific microcirculatory injury.

B. MECHANISMS OF ENVIRONMENTAL FACTOR-INDUCED INJURY

Environmental factors can damage the microcirculation by a variety of mechanisms. Some factors initiate their effects through free radical-mediated mechanisms while others modulate specific biochemical and/or molecular pathways involved in cellular proliferation. For example, carbon tetrachloride and chloroform can adversely affect microcirculatory function by induction of oxidative stress. These compounds undergo metabolic activation to form free radicals which initiate pro-oxidant states in target cells. Some environmental pollutants such as benzo-[a]-pyrene and 7,12-dimethylbenzanthracene, are formed during the incomplete combustion of facile fuels and have been identified as potent mutagens and atherogens.[6-8] The mechanism by which these chemicals exert many of their biologic effects is dependent upon metabolic conversion by the cytochrome P-450 monooxygenase system to active intermediates which directly interact with cellular macromolecules. 1,3-butadiene is an organic chemical used in the synthesis of rubber.[9-11] This compound causes endothelial-derived hemangiosarcomas in several species.[12-14] Butadiene, like the polycyclic aromatic hydrocarbons, elicits its toxic effects through bioactivation to epoxide intermediates that bind to cellular macromolecules. Compounds such as tetrachlorodibenzo-*p*-dioxin, an aromatic hydrocarbon found in various forms of environmental pollution, interact with a cytosolic receptor that translocates to the nucleus and binds DNA to modulate the transcription of several regulatory genes.[15] Many environmental factors have poorly understood mechanisms of action, particularly with reference to their vascular effects. To date, most research efforts have focused upon the responses of the large vessels to environmental factors.[16-19] For example, monocrotaline is a naturally occurring plant alkaloid which causes cellular hypertrophy and proliferation primarily in the pulmonary arterioles and the right ventricle of the heart, as well as larger vessels. These pulmonary and ventricular changes have been associated with pulmonary hypertension as a result of the monocrotaline-induced hyperplasia of smooth muscle cells.[20] However, the mechanism by which monocrotaline induces cellular proliferation and hyperplasia is not known. A number of environmental factors including high cholesterol diets and toxic vascular insult may contribute to the onset of atherosclerosis. Although atherosclerosis is typically a disease of large and medium-sized vessels, recent evidence suggests that alterations in the microcirculation are present.[21]

II. ROLE OF FREE RADICALS IN MICROVASCULAR INJURY

A growing number of diseases such as arthritis, cancer, cirrhosis, diabetes, and ulcerative colitis are thought to be mediated by free radical formation.[22] Several vascular disorders such as atherosclerosis, hypertension, and heart disease have also been related to alterations in free radical mechanisms.[19] Alterations in free radical mechanisms may be induced by several environmental factors. In fact, the modulatory influence of some of these factors can be used experimentally to promote pro-oxidant states (Table 1). The ability of vitamin E to prevent disseminated intravascular coagulation induced by bacterial endotoxins in the rat suggests that this disorder is related to free radical-mediated mechanisms.[23,24] Free radicals have also been associated with the pathogenesis of hypertensive vascular disease. Acute exposure of rats to angiotensin II results in a hypertensive episode due to irregular constriction patterns and vascular hyperpermeability in small arteries and arterioles.[25] Treatment of hypertensive rats with free radical scavengers inhibited the vascular hyperpermeability and cellular damage associated with angiotensin II-induced hypertension. Because free radical mechanisms play an important role in microcirculatory function, many investigators have examined the effects of free radical-induced damage to the microcirculation using ischemia-reperfusion models.

Normal aerobic respiration results in the formation of reactive oxygen species. Increasing evidence has demonstrated that activated oxygen species are involved in normal biological responses such as cell-mediated immune response and microcirculatory vasodilation.[26-28] Although oxygen radicals can be beneficial, these same radicals can also act as "cellular wrecking" species that effectively destroy cellular macromolecules such as proteins, DNA, RNA, and membrane phospholipids. Superoxide anion (O_2^-) is a free radical formed as a result of the one electron reduction of oxygen. Biochemical agents which directly or indirectly promote superoxide formation include xanthine oxidase, aldehyde oxidase, NADH oxidase, dihydroorotate dehydrogenase, ferric iron, catecholamines, reduced flavins, Q-hydroquinone, and phorbol esters. Hydrogen peroxide (H_2O_2), a powerful oxidant, is formed by the dismutation of two superoxide anions by superoxide

Table 11-1 **Endogenous and exogenous free radical generating compounds**

Oxygen Radical Sources	Mechanism of Action
Xanthine oxidase	An enzyme which reacts with oxygen to produce superoxide radical and hydrogen peroxide
NADPH and NADH oxidases	Enzymes which react with oxygen to yield superoxide radical
Peroxidases	Enzymes that react with peroxide and anions, like chloride to produce hypochlorous acid
Aldehyde oxidases	Enzymes which react with oxygen to form superoxide radical
Fe^{+3}	Metal which reacts with oxygen to produce superoxide radical
Catecholamines	Neurohumoral agents that react with oxygen to produce melanin and superoxide radical
Reduced flavins	Compounds that react with oxygen to yield flavin semiquinone and superoxide radical
Dihydroorotate dehydrogenase	An enzyme which reacts with oxygen to produce superoxide radical
Phorbol esters	Compounds which stimulate superoxide generation in phagocytic cells

dismutase. Decomposition of H_2O_2 results in the generation of hydroxyl radicals. Although hydroxyl radicals are short lived, they can have devastating cellular effects including oxidation of sulfhydryls, denaturation of proteins and nucleotides, and initiation of lipid peroxidation. Lipid peroxyl radicals formed by peroxidation of membrane lipids cause extensive damage to cell membranes leading to loss of fluidity and secretory properties, alterations of ionic gradients, and cell lysis. A final important radical is hypochlorous acid which is formed as a byproduct of the interaction of peroxidases, chloride ion, and hydrogen peroxide. Hydrochlorous acid has a considerably prolonged half life and can chlorinate and/or oxidize amines, sulfhydryl groups, proteins, and nucleic acids.

In order to combat the potentially adverse effects of oxygen radicals, tissues possess a series of free radical scavenger systems (Table 2). As indicated above, superoxide dismutase and catalase are enzymes which work in concert to convert superoxide radicals to hydrogen peroxide, and hydrogen peroxide to oxygen and water, respectively. Vitamin E, along with other isomers of tocopherol, convert superoxide, hydroxyl, and lipid peroxyl radicals to less reactive forms. The glutathione/glutathione peroxidase systems effectively reduce free radical damage by conjugation of glutathione with either hydrogen peroxide or lipid peroxides and subsequent metabolism of the glutathione conjugate to oxidized glutathione and water by glutathione peroxidase. Other important antioxidants include beta-carotene, allopurinol, mannitol, ascorbic acid, and mucin. Collectively these agents protect the cell from aerobic injury. However, under pathologic conditions these mechanisms can be overwhelmed and thus allow free radical-induced cellular damage.

III. INFLUENCES OF ENVIRONMENTAL FACTORS ON SPECIFIC VASCULAR BEDS

A. CARDIAC MICROCIRCULATION

1. Hypoxia

Adequate tissue oxygenation and perfusion is essential to normal tissue function. Under hypoxic or ischemic conditions, the availability of oxygen and/or nutrients is limited and

Table 11-2 **Free radical scavengers**

Scavenger	Mechanism of Action
Superoxide dismutase	Metal-based enzyme which dismutates superoxide to form hydrogen peroxide
Catalase	Heme-based enzyme which converts hydrogen peroxide to oxygen and water
Vitamin E	Compound found in cell membranes which quenches the activity of superoxide, hydroxyl, and lipid peroxyl radicals
Glutathione peroxidase	Glutathione is a nonprotein thiol consisting of three peptides which reduce lipid peroxides to less reactive lipid alcohol radicals
Vitamin C	Ascorbic acid is localized in the cytosol and can act as an antioxidant or, in the presence of transition metals, generate free radicals which may be involved in physiologic responses
Beta-carotene	A lipid soluble compound which has antioxidant capabilities
Allopurinol	A compound which inhibits xanthine oxidase, thus decreasing superoxide and hydroxyl radical formation

thus results in tissue injury. Hypoxic injury to the heart is associated with decreased collateral circulation or interruption of blood flow. The severity of the hypoxic episode associated with tissue injury is a function of the tissue or cell involved, the presence or absence of glycolytic substrates, the duration of the hypoxic episode, and temperature.[29] Because hypoxic injury is directly related to modulation of microcirculatory function, hypoxia has been implicated in microvascular cell injury.

Normal cellular metabolism is dependent upon the balance between energy production and utilization. Adenosine triphosphate (ATP) production is mediated by oxidative phosphorylation of adenosine diphosphate (ADP). Hypoxia reduces oxidative phosphorylation and leads to a compensatory increase in anaerobic glycolysis. Increased anaerobic glycolysis, however, is unable to meet the high energy demands of the cell and results in cellular injury. In general, the events associated with tissue hypoxia include ATP depletion,[30] mitochondrial dysfunction,[31] ionic imbalances,[32,33] changes in Ca^{2+},[34] activation of plasma membrane bound phospholipases,[35] decreased membrane fluidity,[36] formation and rupture of surface blebs,[37] and decreased cytosolic pH.[38] In addition to these changes, hypoxia may result in the formation of reactive oxygen species.[39]

2. Free Radicals

The effects of free radicals on coronary microcirculation have been studied indirectly by the use of radical scavengers.[40] In these studies, an ischemia-reperfusion dog model was employed to promote free radical formation. The effects of two reactive oxygen metabolite scavengers, superoxide dismutase and dimethylthiourea, were tested to evaluate coronary microcirculatory function after 60 min of ischemia followed by 60 min of reperfusion. Superoxide dismutase is predominantly an extracellular agent which reacts with superoxide anions to form hydrogen peroxide.[41] Dimethylthiourea has both intra- and extracellular effects, primarily reacting with hydroxyl radicals and hydrogen peroxide.[42] These studies assessed changes of microvascular permeability using the double radioisotope protein leak index (PLI) method. In untreated dogs, ischemia-reperfusion increased PLI more than three-fold relative to nonischemic tissue. The increase in PLI was proportional to the regional severity of ischemic blood flow. Superoxide dismutase or dimethylthiourea treatment decreased PLI by 45 and 66%, respectively. These treatments also reduced protein leakage at all levels of regional ischemic blood flow, but did not increase blood flow to ischemic regions. These results indicate that free radical scavengers decrease functional coronary microvascular injury due to ischemia-reperfusion and suggest that regional microcirculatory ischemic-reperfusion injury involves free radical formation.

A similar study has investigated the role of superoxide dismutase and catalase treatment in isolated rat heart after short-term ischemia and reperfusion.[43] Superoxide dismutase and catalase improved cardiac function as assessed by measurements of cardiac output and dP/dT during reperfusion of ischemic hearts. These compounds had no effect during the preischemic or ischemic periods, but improved heart function during reperfusion. Using indirect-fluorescent antibodies against exogenous superoxide dismutase and catalase, it was suggested that exogenous superoxide dismutase can gain access to the cytoplasm of myocytes via the coronary microcirculation. This proposal is consistent with other studies showing that superoxide dismutase and catalase can pass from coronary capillary endothelium into myocytes.[44] Thus, superoxide dismutase and catalase may exert their protective effects within cardiac myocytes.

3. Atherogenic Stimuli

Recent studies have emerged examining the effects of atherosclerosis on the microvasculature. Atherosclerosis is a form of arteriosclerosis in which plaques containing cholesterol, lipoid material, and lipophages are deposited within the intima of arteries. Initial vascular lesions are associated with smooth muscle cell proliferation and migration into the vessel lumen. These events, along with enhanced calcification and altered lipid metabolism, result in progression of the disease. The study of atherosclerosis as a pathologic process serves to exemplify the influence of the environment on blood vessels because this disease is modulated by diet and personality, as well as toxic insult.[7] The microvasculature of atherosclerotic animals does not exhibit the morphologic lesions observed in larger vessels.[45] However, evidence has begun to accumulate suggesting that atherosclerosis modulates microvasculature physiology. Recent studies by Chilian et al.[21] have evaluated the effects of atherosclerosis on coronary microvascular constriction. Several potent vasoconstrictors, phenylephrine, serotonin, and ergonovine, were given to control and atherosclerotic monkeys. Microvascular resistance was then assessed by measurements of coronary microvascular pressure. Serotonin (50 μg/min) decreased microvascular resistance in normal animals, but increased resistance in atherosclerotic animals. Phenylephrine (50 μg/kg/min) increased microvascular resistance in atherosclerotic animals, but did not alter resistance in controls animals. Ergonovine (10 μg/kg/min) increased microvascular resistance in both normal and atherosclerotic monkeys. Collectively, these results indicate that atherosclerosis alters normal microvascular physiology although no morphologic lesions are present. Over the last several decades, the pathogenesis of atherosclerosis has focused mainly on intimal filtration of lipoproteins as the primary cause for large vessel alterations. However, there is evidence that abnormalities of the arterial microcirculation may contribute to the etiology of atherosclerosis.[46] The arterial microcirculation normally penetrates the adventitia and outer third of the media. However, the arterial microvasculature penetrates completely into the media and partially into the intima in early atherosclerotic lesions consisting of a thickened intimal layer without atheroma.[47] These studies suggest that atherosclerosis may be associated with alterations in both arterial and cardiac microcirculation and that these alterations may contribute to the etiology of the disease.

4. Nitro Compounds

Certain organic chemicals, such as nitroglycerin, have profound effects on the systemic, as well as the cardiac microcirculation. Nitroglycerin has been frequently used in the treatment of angina pectoris and ischemia, and in the production of explosives. This compound, as well as other nitrates, has vasodilator actions which are mediated by stimulation of soluble guanylate cyclase within vascular smooth muscle cells.[48] Recent studies have investigated the vasodilator effects of nitroglycerin and metabolites on porcine coronary microvessels of different sizes.[49] The microvascular response of vessels preconstricted with acetylcholine was assessed using a video-imaging apparatus. Nitroglycerin caused enhanced microvascular dilation as the size of the vessel increased. S-nitrosocysteine and nitric oxide also caused vessel dilation in a size-dependent manner. Interestingly, LY 83583, a depletor of vascular guanylate cyclase, reduced microvessel responses to all nitro compounds confirming that vasodilator effects are mediated by guanylate cyclase. Ambient exposure of industrial workers to nitroglycerin or other nitrates may result in modulated microcirculatory physiology.[50]

5. Ethanol

Over consumption of ethanol is associated with various tissue disorders including liver and brain tissue degeneration as well as vascular vasodilation and microcirculatory proliferation. Ethanol has been shown to effect myocardial capillary density.[51] Studies by Mall et al.[52] investigated ethanol-induced capillary proliferation as assessed by capillary density, capillary diameter, and endothelial cell nuclei in rats. After 3 weeks of ethanol administration, capillary density and diameter remained constant, but capillary endothelial cell nuclei increased. After 5 months of ethanol exposure there was increased density of myocardial capillaries with a decrease in capillary diameter. Because ethanol and its metabolite acetaldehyde have been reported to increase myocardial blood flow,[53,54] it has been suggested that capillary proliferation is secondary to enhanced myocardial blood flow. Studies investigating this possibility used dipyridamole, a coronary vasodilator, to determine whether increased blood flow correlates with capillary proliferation.[55] After 4 weeks of dipyridamole treatment, the capillary endothelial cell nuclei increased in number, while no changes in capillary density or diameter were observed. These findings correspond to changes seen in rats dosed with ethanol for 3 weeks, suggesting a possible correlation between increased blood flow and capillary endothelial proliferation. Studies by Tornling et al.[56] also showed the dipyridamole increased thymidine incorporation in capillary endothelial cells relative to controls. Obviously, long-term studies are needed to further characterize chemically induced capillary proliferation via enhanced blood flow.

6. Dietary Factors

Dietary factors are important in the pathogenesis of microvascular disorders. Selenium-vitamin E deficiency in swine is a prime example of how dietary insufficiency can adversely effect the cardiac microcirculation. Clinical illness, tissue lesions, and death in pigs fed diets low in selenium and vitamin E have been widely reported.[57-59] Pathologic studies of pig hearts have shown disseminated foci of fiber necrosis and extensive damage in myocardial arterioles and blood capillaries. Other systemic lesions include mineralization of cardiocytes, liver necrosis, and skeletal muscle myopathy.[60,61] Pigs fed selenium- and vitamin E-deficient diets for 21 days showed thrombosis of arterioles and accumulation of fibrinoid in the arteriolar walls.[62] The thrombosed arterioles contained disrupted endothelial cells and luminal accumulation of hyaline. Nonthrombosed arterioles exhibited thickened endothelial cells loosely attached to each other, extensive fibrin deposits, and damaged smooth muscle cells. However, no detectable lesions were observed in cardiac capillaries. Collectively, these results suggest that the primary site of microcirculatory damage is the arteriolar endothelial cells. Vitamin E and selenium-dependent glutathione peroxidase are involved in quenching lipid peroxidation present in the cell membrane. Consequently, cofactor depletion would likely allow for increased lipid peroxidation. Tocopherol supplementation of selenium and vitamin E deficient weaned pigs showed no signs of disease suggesting that free radicals are involved in the development of this disease.[60] Several studies have shown a link between calcium overload and the resulting necrosis of cardiac myocytes and free radical-induced injury.[41,63,64] This phenomena is blocked by antagonistic action of magnesium or the antioxidant effects of vitamin E. Studies by Korpela further investigated the pathogenesis of mulberry heart disease by evaluating tissue calcium/magnesium levels in diseased and control pigs.[65] Pigs diagnosed with mulberry heart disease exhibit increased calcium and decreased magnesium levels in both heart and liver compared to control animals. The significance of these findings may be related to oxidative damage to cellular membranes and the subsequent influx of calcium. Thus the altered calcium/magnesium concentrations seem to reflect disturbed electrolyte homeostasis related to oxidant damage of cardiac and microcirculatory constituents. Further investigations will facilitate a better understanding of the pathogenesis of this and other free radical-mediated cardiovascular disorders.

7. Exercise

Just as dietary components have grown in importance so have health habits such as exercise. In 1969, Tomanek conducted studies to compare capillary numbers in rats that were exercised for 0 or 12 weeks using pelikan ink infusion.[66] Capillary/muscle fiber ratios and capillaries/mm^2 were higher in the exercised relative to unexercised group. Thus exercise appears to stimulate cardiac capillary growth. Mechanisms related to increased vasodilation as described for ethanol-induced capillary expansion may be involved.

B. CEREBRAL MICROCIRCULATION

1. Ethanol

The brain microvasculature is the most important anatomical and physiological component of the blood-brain barrier. Brain capillary endothelial cells are responsible for the formation of the blood-brain barrier and are accessible to potentially harmful circulating compounds. Alterations in microvascular integrity can be precipitated by cerebral injuries, brain hypoxia, chronic alcohol exposure, and aging. For instance, chronic alcohol exposure induces oxygen imbalance, cortical and subcortical vascular constriction, and decreased blood flow in rats. Studies by Altura and Altura have examined the effects of ethanol (10 to 500 mg/dl) on *in situ* rat microcirculation using a TV-image intensification microscope.[67] These doses parallel those needed for graded euphoria, mental-haziness, muscular incoordination, stupor, and coma in humans. Alcohol administration over a period of 30 min resulted in a dose-dependent vasoconstriction of rat cortical arterioles. Doses above 300 mg/dl causes arteriolar spasms that were irreversible and usually resulted in vessel rupture. Mg^{2+} as well as several other Ca^{2+} antagonists such as verapamil, minodipine, nitreindipine, and nisoldipine, completely reversed or prevented spasms. Because chronic ethanol exposure is associated with cerebral stroke,[68] these data suggest that alcohol-induced vasoconstriction, spasm, and rupture of arterioles contributes to stroke etiology. Studies by De Witte et al.[69] have examined the effects of chronic alcohol exposure on the density of the rat cortical vascular network. These studies showed that rats exposed to alcohol for 2 and 4 weeks exhibited a more developed cortical microvascularization than controls. This increase was similar to that observed after surgical cortical injury in control animals. When rats were exposed to alcohol and Sabeluzole, a benzothiazol derivative which has antihypoxic/antiischemic effects,[70] the alcohol-induced cortical hypervascularization was significantly reduced. These findings suggest that chronic alcohol consumption results in systemic hypoxia to the brain and the increased density of cortical microvasculature may represent a compensatory response. Lieber et al.[71] have shown that chronic alcohol consumption activates the cytochrome P-450 ethanol oxidizing system, and thus increases oxygen consumption. In fact, higher cytochrome P-450 activity has been identified in brain microvessel homogenates relative to brain mitochondria and microsomal homogenates in the rat.[72] The production of free radicals arising from these reoxygenization processes could then induce brain cell damage and compensatory vascularization.

2. Heavy Metals

Lead is extremely deleterious to brain, as well as other tissues. Acute lead exposure in suckling rats causes brain tissue swelling, edema, hemorrhage, necrosis, and altered capillary permeability.[73-76] At the biochemical level, lead initiates its toxic effect on cell mitochondria by disturbing heme synthesis, oxidative phosphorylation, and intracellular calcium metabolism as shown in Figure 1. Because acute lead exposure has become of lesser importance in recent years, most studies have focused on the microcirculatory alterations associated with chronic lead toxicity. Autoradiographic studies in developing rats have shown that brain capillary endothelial cells are a major site of lead accumulation.[77] Maxwell et al.[78] have investigated the effect of lead in cultured cerebral microvessel endothelial cell division and glucose uptake. Reduced cell number have been observed after 4 days of lead exposure at doses toxic to humans (10^{-4} *M*). Exposure of cultured endothelial cells to lead for 2 days resulted in a 71% inhibition of [^{3}H]-thymidine incorporation. Glucose specific and nonspecific carrier-mediated uptakes were also inhib-

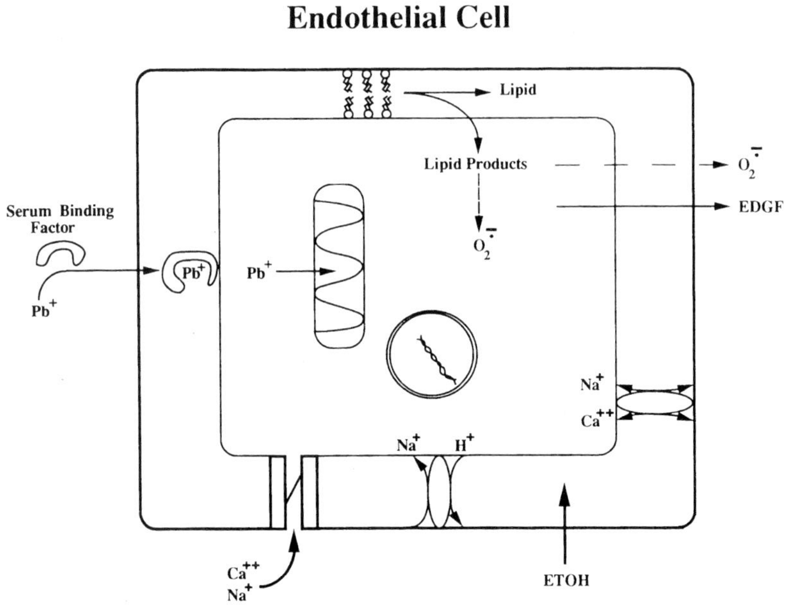

Figure 11-1 Environmental factors which potentially modulate microvascular endothelial function such as lead, alcohol, and dietary lipids. Lead accumulates within endothelial mitochondria resulting in disrupted heme synthesis, reduced oxidative phoshorylation, and altered Ca^{2+} metabolism. Ethanol causes membrane perturbations which may eventually lead to significant disruption of functional and/or structural integrity. Dietary lipids are incorporated into the cellular lipid pool and metabolized by oxygenases to yield biologically active compounds. Subsequent metabolism of lipid by-products may result in enhanced oxygen-derived free radical formation.

ited by lead exposure. In addition, lead toxicity only occurred when serum was present in the media suggesting that serum contains a factor which aids the transport of lead into the cell. Studies by Gebhart and Goldstein have examined the effects of low-level lead exposure in cultured adrenal endothelial cells and rat brain astrocytes.[79] The co-culture of adrenal endothelial cells and brain astrocytes results in the expression of brain capillary endothelial cell markers in the adrenal cell line.[80] This co-culture system also results in cellular interactions similar to those observed in the normal *in vivo* blood-brain barrier. Reduced cellular proliferation was observed when astrocyte cells were cultured in media containing lead (10 μM). In contrast, endothelial cells exhibited enhanced mitogenic activity in the presence of lead. In co-culture, astrocytes were less sensitive to the cytotoxic effects of lead than astrocytes cultured in the absence of endothelial cells. This was attributed to induced maturation of astrocytes by endothelial cell interactions. Studies by Tiffany et al.[81] have reported decreased cell numbers when astrocytes from immature Wistar rats were cultured in the presence of 1 μM lead. However, mature Sprague-Dawley rat astrocytes were resistant to low concentrations of lead. This finding is in accord with studies which showed that adult rats are more resistant to lead toxicity.[82] The observed resistance was associated with sequestering of lead by mature astrocytes away from target mitochondria to nontoxic sites. These studies collectively suggest that lead toxicity may disturb the programmed growth and differentiation of the blood-brain barrier in immature brain tissue.

3. Dietary Factors

a. Linoleic Acid (LA)

Many dietary components consist of compounds that can ultimately affect the brain and its microcirculation. Linoleic acid (LA) is an essential fatty acid found in plants. When ingested by mammals, LA can be converted into arachidonic acid (AA), as well as other biologically important fatty acids. *In vitro* studies using cerebromicrovascular endothelial cells have shown that these cells are important in the elongation and desaturation of essential fatty acids.[83] Thus, microvascular endothelial cells can process essential polyunsaturated fatty acids to form AA and/or other biologically active lipids. AA is readily metabolized by brain cytochrome P-450 monooxygenase, cyclooxygenase, and lipooxygenase systems.[84] The products of AA metabolism include prostaglandins, thromboxane, leukotrienes, hydroxyeicosatetraenoic acids, and epoxyeicosatrienoic acids (EETs). Prostaglandins, thromboxanes, and leukotrienes are derived from the oxidation of AA by cyclooxygenase and lipooxygenase and have been shown to have vasoactive effects on cerebral arterioles in various species.[85-88] However, prostaglandins do not regulate cerebral circulation during hypercapnia.[89] The mechanisms by which these arachidonate metabolites initiate the observed vasoactive effects are currently under investigation. Studies by Rosenblum have demonstrated that arteriolar vasodilation by bradykinin is mediated by hydroxyl free radicals.[28] Superoxide dismutase and desferoxamine, an iron scavenger, inhibit the bradykinin-induced vasodilation by blocking iron catalyzed formation of hydroxyl radicals. Kontos et al.[26] have shown that both the arachidonate- and bradykinin-mediated arteriolar dilation are associated with oxygen free radical formation. Thus, normal physiological responses to circulating hormones may be mediated by free radical generation. One might suggest that steady state substrate levels would facilitate proper free-radical formation to physiological responses. However, at times of excess substrate availability or increased cellular metabolism, the cell may undergo a pathogenic response.

b. Epoxyeicosatrienoic Acid (EET)

EETs are another product of AA. These compounds are formed by the cytochrome P-450-dependent epoxygenase pathway.[90] The cytochrome P-450 isozymes are extremely important in the regulation of cellular metabolism and cerebral microvascular endothelial cells have the highest P-450 activity relative to other cell types in the brain. EETs are found in various tissues including endothelial cells and may be important in microcirculatory regulation.[91] In fact, studies have suggested that these eicosanoids may be important in the pathology of atherosclerosis.[92] Ellis et al.[93] have investigated the ability of EETs and AA to dilate cerebral arterioles upon perfusion into the cranial window of rabbits and cats. A brief dose-dependent dilation was produced by 5,6-EET in both species, whereas other EETs had no effect. However, AA induced cerebral dilation to a greater extent than 5,6-EET. Indomethacin, a cyclooxygenase inhibitor, or superoxide dismutase plus catalase, prevented the dilation induced by 5,6-EET or AA, suggesting that this fatty acid metabolite produces vasodilation via cyclooxygenase and associated free radical-mediated pathways.

c. Eicosapentaenoic Acid (EPA)

Studies examining the effects of dietary fish oils containing the omega-3 polyunsaturated fatty acid, eicosapentaenoic acid (EPA) in rabbits, showed similar results to EET and AA with respect to arterial dilation.[94] Normal EPA concentration is low in the brain but can be increased by dietary supplementation. These fatty acids are known to incorporate into the phospholipid pool and inversely alter AA concentrations. Using the cranial window technique, it was demonstrated that EPA caused a dose-dependent increase of arteriolar diameter. Again, indomethacin or catalase plus superoxide dismutase decreased the dilator response of EPA. These studies, as well as others,[26,28,95] indicate that the formation of oxygen free radicals results in dilation of the cerebral microvasculature, which in turn could contribute to the pathophysiology of various cerebral disorders.

To further characterize the role of AA in microvascular pathophysiology, Villacara et al.[96] conducted experiments to evaluate the effects of free AA on permeability, membrane fluidity, and lipid peroxidation in cultured cerebromicrovascular endothelial cells. AA induced a reversible alteration of endothelial permeability as reflected by trypan blue albumin exclusion. Indomethacin pretreatment did not modulate the effects of AA, suggesting that cyclooxygenase is not involved in these alterations. Fluorescence anisotropy studies showed that AA increases membrane fluidity in endothelial cells. When endothelial cells were exposed to AA and H_2O_2, membrane permeability increased irreversibly. This alteration was associated with enhanced formation of malondialdehyde, a product of lipid peroxidation, and was prevented by catalase suggesting that release of AA from cell membranes under certain conditions may alter the function of the blood-brain barrier.

4. Free Radicals

As indicated previously, oxygen free radicals mediate the vasodilator effects of several hormones. However, prolonged vascular exposure to H_2O_2 and superoxide anion has deleterious effects under certain conditions. For example, cat cerebral endothelial and vascular smooth muscle cells from both small (<100 μm) and large (>100 μm) arterioles exposed to free radicals for 15 min develop lesions and cellular abnormalities.[27] Superoxide dismutase or catalase eliminated the free radical-induced effects suggesting that the superoxide anion and H_2O_2 cause endothelial and smooth muscle cell alterations.

Elevated oxygen tension can result in free-radical formation. Studies using an *in vitro* model system have evaluated the elevated oxygen tension, on the proliferation, morphology, and integrity of microvasculature.[97] Hamsters exposed to 85% oxygen for 7 days showed a reversible reduction in central nervous system capillaries as a result of endothelial cell degeneration. Recovery of animals under normoxic conditions for 7 days, increased the number of capillaries. This phenomenon has been further characterized using cultured endothelial cells and smooth muscle-derived pericytes.[98] These cells were cultivated at oxygen concentrations of 21% (normoxia) and 40% (hyperoxia). Under normal aerobic conditions, a small percentage of oxygen escapes aerobic glycolysis and undergoes univalent reduction. An excess of free oxygen would be expected to enhance free radical formation. These studies showed that proliferation of endothelial cells was significantly inhibited under hyperoxic conditions. In contrast, pericyte proliferation was similar in both groups indicating that endothelial cells are more sensitive to hyperoxic conditions than pericytes. Endothelial cell recovery from 1, 3, or 5 days of hyperoxia and 1 day normoxia was proportional to the duration of hyperoxic conditions. Endothelial cell damage was attributed to lipid peroxidation because both lysosome and mitochondrial membranes in endothelial cells were altered as a function of hyperoxia. Thus, the over production and/or over exposure of free radicals may adversely affect the cellular components of the cerebral microcirculation.

C. GASTROINTESTINAL MICROCIRCULATION

The gastrointestinal system is the principle site of nutrient intake and absorption. Several types of epithelial cells in the gastrointestinal tract perform a variety of functions including uptake of compounds, secretion of digestive enzymes, and mechanical breakdown of food stuffs. Beneath the epithelial cell layers consists a vast array of connective tissue components, capillaries, and smooth muscle cells. The smooth muscle cell layer, called the muscularis mucosa, provides contractile activity while the capillaries provide nutrients and oxygen and carry absorbed substrates from the gastrointestinal tract to the liver.

1. Platelet-Activating Factor

The gastric mucosa is dependent upon endogenous signaling compounds to direct its function. Endogenous mediators stimulate gastric mucus secretion, HCl production, and gastric contraction. However, platelet-activating factor (PAF), which is an endogenous pro-inflammatory phospholipid, induces extensive vasocongestion and hemorrhagic damage in rat gastric mucosa and histologically appears to be a potent ulcerogen.[99-101] Studies by Pique et al.[102] have investigated the effects of morphine and capsaicin pretreatment followed by intravenous injection of PAF on the microcirculation of neonatal rats. Morphine is a commonly used narcotic which inhibits peripheral sensory neurons, while capsaicin is an ingredient of red peppers which disrupts afferent neurons. Treatment of neonates with PAF resulted in microcirculatory damage as assessed by a decrease in mucosal blood flow. Pretreatment of neonates with capsaicin or morphine further decreased PAF-induced alterations in mucosal blood flow and was associated with enhanced vasocongestion, hemorrhagic damage, glandular disruption, and epithelial damage. An opioid antagonist was found to reverse the morphine-induced enhancement in gastric damage, thus implicating opioid receptors in this response. These findings indicate that the combination of endogenous and exogenous substances may alter gastric microcirculatory function.

2. Burn Injury

Kitajima et al.[103] have investigated the role of gastric microcirculation in the development of acute gastric mucosal lesions by using the burn-stressed rat model. In these studies, rat dorsi were exposed to boiling water for 15 sec to initiate burn stress and examined at 2, 5, and 24 h to assess microcirculatory alterations. All burn-stressed rats had decreased gastric mucosal blood flow, as determined by hydrogen gas or Xe-133 clearance, which was associated with enhanced gastric ulceration, decreased acid production, and increased pepsin output. Studies by Kitajima and Itoh showed that burn-stressed rats had reduced energy metabolism of the mucosa, diminished mitochondrial ATP synthesis, decreased aerobic metabolism, and increased anaerobic metabolism.[104] Thus, alterations in gastric mucosa microcirculation may lead to the formation of acute gastric mucosal lesions.

3. Ethanol

As stated previously, alcohol has profound effects on the terminal arterioles and muscular venules in splanchnic vascular beds. *In situ* studies by Altura et al.[105] have evaluated the effects of ethanol on rat splanchnic terminal arterioles and muscular venules. Administration of ethanol resulted in a dose-dependent dilation of arterioles and venules. Ethanol also inhibited epinephrine-, angiotensin II-, and vasopressin-induced arteriolar and venular vasoconstriction in a dose-dependent fashion. The administration of propranolol, a beta-adrenergic blocker which normally acts as a vasodilator antagonist, in conjunction with ethanol enhanced the vasodilator effects of ethanol. In subsequent studies, Altura and Gebrewold investigated the effects of the metabolites of ethanol, acetaldehyde, or acetate on rat mesenteric arterioles and muscular venules.[106] Administration of acetaldehyde or acetate caused a dose-dependent vasoconstriction of arterioles and venules. These findings indicate that ethanol exerts direct effects on splanchnic microvascular smooth muscle. Ethanol administration to isolated arteries and veins has been shown to reduce calcium concentrations, suggesting that ethanol interferes with the mobility of Ca^{2+} across vascular membranes.[107] Thus, ethanol may elicit its vasodilatory effects by perturbation of Ca^{2+} mobility.

D. HEPATIC MICROCIRCULATION

The liver is the primary organ involved in the detoxification of exogenous and endogenous chemicals. Detoxification of substrates is accomplished by a series of enzyme systems located primarily in parenchymal cells. The most notable enzyme system is the mixed function oxidases or microsomal monooxygenase systems. Cytochrome P-450 isozymes, the terminal oxidase of the monooxygenase system, constitute the majority of the phase I enzymes involved in oxidative reactions. Cytochrome P-450 isozymes exhibit some degree of substrate specificity and can be "induced" by a variety of compounds. In phase II metabolism, synthetic enzymes further metabolize compounds that have undergone phase I metabolism. Phase II enzymes include epoxide hydrolase, which converts reactive epoxides to less reactive diols, and glutathione, glucuronyl, and sulfo-transferases, which are involved in conjugation reactions. The action of Phase I and II enzyme systems generally results in detoxification and excretion of chemicals. However, certain chemicals, such as benzo[a]pyrene and carbon tetrachloride, can form chemical species which are more toxic than the parent compound. These types of reactions are referred to as metabolic activation of the parent compound and often result in extensive liver damage and release of toxic species into the general circulation.

1. Ethanol

Anatomically, the liver is a conglomeration of several cell types, including hepatocytes and Kupffer cells along with an extensive vascular network composed of endothelial and smooth muscle cells. One of the most common hepatotoxins in humans is alcohol. Ethanol can be metabolized by cytochrome P-450IIE to yield acetaldehyde, a toxic metabolite. Acute exposure of humans to alcohol results in depressed reticuloendothelial function, as well as alterations in the immune response. Elevated levels of circulating endotoxin have been observed in humans intoxicated with alcohol and during alcohol-related liver disease.[108,109] Interestingly, rats given endotoxin in the absence of alcohol exhibited no signs of hepatic damage, while rats given both endotoxin and alcohol had extensive hepatic damage.[110] The increase in circulating endotoxin in alcoholics has been attributed to a spill-over of gut-derived endotoxin which is no longer cleared by depressed Kupffer cells. Kupffer cells remove circulating endotoxin from the blood stream by active endocytosis.[111] During the process of endotoxin clearance from the blood, Kupffer cells release pro-inflammatory cellular mediators which include tumor necrosis factor, interleukin-1, eicosanoids, and reactive free radicals. Chronic exposure to alcohol results in liver fibrosis, cirrhosis, and hepatitis. Recent studies have investigated the acute effects of alcohol on the hepatic microvasculature in mice.[112] Ethanol given at a dose of 4 gm/kg elicited hepatocellular damage as evidenced by the formation of vacuoles and/or swollen organelles, vascular endothelial cellular swelling, and transient plugging of sinusoidal blood flow by leukocytes. These events parallel intravascular events seen in sepsis and/or upon administration of tumor necrosis factor.[113,114] Thus, dysfunction of Kupffer cells appears to result in the release of endotoxin and/or mediators which alter microcirculatory function.

2. Carbon Tetrachloride

Cirrhosis of the liver is the fourth leading cause of death among American adults.[115] This disease is characterized by loss of the normal lobular architecture and enhanced fibrosis and nodular regeneration of liver parenchyma. This disorder has several etiologies including chronic inflammation, chronic alcohol abuse, cardiac disease, and toxicity. Carbon tetrachloride is used in the production of several organic chemicals, with an estimated 60,000 metric tons released into the environment each year.[116] Inhalation or administration of carbon tetrachloride causes extensive liver necrosis and cirrhosis in experimental animals.[117] The toxicity of carbon tetrachloride is mediated by cytochrome P-450 reduction of the parent compound to the trichloromethyl free radical as shown in Figure 2. The trichloromethyl radical can then effectively initiate membrane lipoperoxidation events which lead to endoplasmic reticular, lysosomal, and mitochondrial membrane damage.[118,119] Varin and Huet performed comparative microcirculation studies in noncirrhotic and chemically-induced cirrhotic rats.[120] Alterations in the hepatic microcirculation were assessed by monitoring the ability of radiolabeled albumin, sucrose, and water, compounds which gain access to extravascular spaces, to pass from sinusoids into hepatocytes. These values were compared to outflow of labeled erythrocytes, which are confined to the vascular space. In addition, the outflow recovery studies of lidocaine, a substance that penetrates liver cells, was performed. In cirrhotic livers, the sinusoidal vascular space exhibited a reduction in the diffusion of albumin into the extravascular space, relative to noncirrhotic livers. When lidocaine was administered to cirrhotic livers, compound penetration into liver cells was reduced and a substantial portion of the lidocaine appeared in the outflow corresponding to the erythrocytes. This phenomena was also observed for water and sucrose suggesting poor hepatocyte permeability. These findings indicated the development of small channels with poorly permeable walls. Upon microscopic examination of cirrhotic livers, most of the hepatic sinusoids remained structurally intact, however, the space between the microvascular endothelial cells and the hepatocytes was widened and filled with collagen. In addition, cirrhotic livers contained occasional capillary channels, similar in diameter to vascular sinusoids, which were located in fibrotic bands invading the parenchymal nodules. These findings demonstrate that carbon tetrachloride-induced cirrhotic livers contain microvascular alterations which lead to progressive loss of macromolecule penetration into liver parenchyma. To elucidate hepatic microcirculatory function in fibrotic and/or cirrhotic livers, recent studies have employed methods such as intravital, epifluorescent TV microscopy which measures red blood cell velocities in microvessels, vascular diameters, and acinar dimensions on the liver surface. Sherman et al.[121] have examined rat hepatic microvascular changes associated with the hepatic injury induced by carbon tetrachloride or dietary insufficiency of choline. Carbon tetrachloride (CCl_4) undergoes cytochrome P-450-mediated metabolic activation to form a free radical that causes peroxidation and endoplasmic reticular damage. Histological findings showed that fibrotic lesions which occasionally formed bridges between terminal venules were observed in both CCl_4-treated and choline-deficient animals. Cirrhotic animals contained extensive deposits of fibrous tissue, some regenerative nodules, and focal areas of necrosis. Changes were also observed in microvascular morphology in both fibrotic and cirrhotic animals relative to

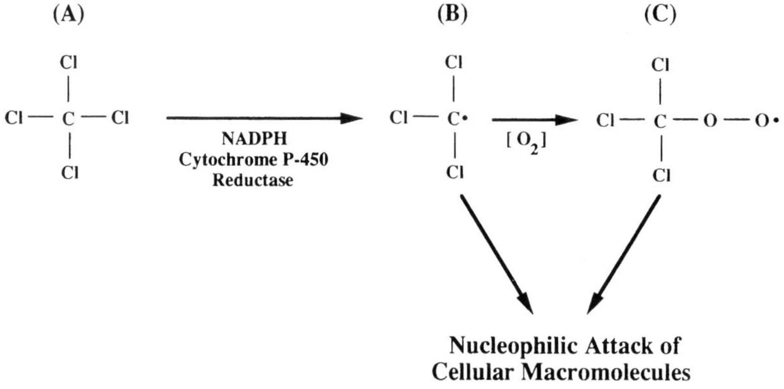

Figure 11-2 The metabolic activation scheme of carbon tetrachloride (A) by microsomal NADPH-cytochrome P-450 reductase in microvascular endothelium and/or liver parenchymal cells. Reduction of the parent molecule results in the formation of the tetrachloromethyl radical (B). Subsequent oxygenation of the radical yields a second radical (C). Both radicals primarily target nucleophilic rich centers within the endoplasmic reticulum, mitochondria, and lysosomes.

controls. The diameter of terminal hepatic venules in the fibrotic and cirrhotic livers was increased relative to controls. The increased diameter of hepatic venules was associated with increased red blood cell velocities suggesting that carbon tetrachloride and choline-induce liver degeneration is associated with changes in hepatic microcirculation.

E. INTEGUMENTARY MICROCIRCULATION

The integumentary system, which includes the epidermal, dermal, and subcutaneous layers, is the primary organ responsible for protecting the body from the adverse effects of the environment. The epidermis is a series of squamous epithelial cell layers which rest on a basement membrane. The dermis lies beneath the epidermis and contains glandular epithelial cells, fibrous connective tissue, nerve endings, and cutaneous capillaries. The subcutaneous layer lies under the dermis and is composed of loosely arranged fibrous connective tissue and subcutaneous capillaries, arterioles, and venules. As dictated by its location, the integumentary system is continually exposed to ambient factors which directly modulate cutaneous microcirculation.

1. Temperature

Studies by Song et al.[122] have shown that heating the skin to 40°C causes an overall increase of cutaneous blood flow. Cooling of the skin to 5°C resulted in a momentary decrease followed by an increase in blood flow. Prolonged cooling, however, resulted in a gradual and sustained decrease of cutaneous blood flow. Studies by Stojanov and Proctor have investigated the influence of adenosine, norepinephrine, and angiotensin II in temperature-induced alterations of cutaneous blood flow in hamsters.[123] Nanomolar concentrations of adenosine evoked vasoconstrictor responses which were potentiated when the skin temperature was elevated. The A_1 receptor antagonist, 8-phenyltheophylline, attenuated adenosine-induced vasoconstriction. In contrast to adenosine, norepinephrine-induced vasoconstriction was reduced at low temperatures, but unaffected at high temperatures. These results are consistent with studies by Flavahan et al.[124] showing that responses mediated by alpha-adrenergic receptors are sensitive to changes in temperature. Studies examining the effects of thermal injury have characterized a series of pathophysiologic phenomena which lead to both local and distant tissue injury.[125] The first thermal-induced effect occurs distal to the burn injury and involves intravascular hemolysis and acute lung injury attributed to complement activation and intravascular stimulation of neutrophils. These responses result in oxygen radical production and subsequent injury to red blood cells and pulmonary vascular endothelium. The second thermal-induced event occurs at the site of cutaneous burn injury and leads to enhanced vascular permeability and edema formation. The initial response to the local skin injury involved a phasic increase of vascular permeability followed by a sustained phase of enhanced permeability. Mediators involved in these vascular changes may include histamine, bradykinin, serotonin, prostaglandins, and leukotrienes.[126-128] In addition to these mediators, free radical involvement has been implicated in thermally induced cutaneous injury.[129] In other studies, Till et al.[130] examined microcirculatory blood flow, vascular permeability, and xanthine oxidase levels upon incubation of rat dorsal skin in 70°C water for 30 sec to initiate thermal injury. Under these conditions, increased plasma levels of xanthine oxidase decreased capillary blood flow and enhanced vascular permeability. Administration of allopurinol and lodoxamide, xanthine oxidase inhibitors, prevented changes in permeability and edema formation, but did not alter blood flow. The vascular permeability changes were attenuated by catalase, superoxide dismutase, DMSO, and dimethylthiourea. These findings suggest that changes in cutaneous microcirculation induced by thermal injury are mediated by xanthine oxidase-mediated formation of superoxide, hydrogen peroxide, and hydroxyl radicals.

2. Atherogenic Stimuli

Studies by Schwartz et al.[131] have investigated alterations in the cutaneous microcirculation in atherosclerotic smokers, atherosclerotic nonsmokers, and healthy nonsmokers. To assess differences in cutaneous microcirculation, the capillary blood velocity of hallux nail fold capillaries was measured at rest and following 1 min of ankle cuff occlusion. Atherosclerotic patients had lower capillary blood velocities as compared to nonatherosclerotic patients. The capillary blood velocity increased in all groups following occlusion and was not different between any of the groups. These studies demonstrate that atherosclerosis, but not smoking, directly alters capillary blood flow. Additional studies by Schwartz et al.[132] have investigated alterations in the precapillary sphincter in superficial cutaneous capillaries of atherosclerotic smokers, atherosclerotic nonsmokers, and healthy nonsmokers. Atherosclerotic patients exhibited reduced precapillary sphincter vasoconstriction of individual microvessels as compared to smokers and nonsmokers. Kyrle et al.[133] have investigated microvascular alterations in the generation of thromboxane A_2 and prostacyclin in atherosclerotic patients. These studies measured thromboxane A_2, a platelet aggregating and vasoconstrictor substance generated in platelets, and prostacyclin, an antiaggregatory and vasodilatory agent mainly synthesized by vascular endothelial cells, from a cutaneous microvascular injury. Prostacyclin levels were lower in atherosclerotic patients as compared to control patients, while no differences in thromboxane levels were observed between the two groups. Collectively, these findings suggest that atherosclerosis alters both the physiological and biochemical behavior of the cutaneous microcirculation.

F. PULMONARY MICROCIRCULATION

The pulmonary microcirculation is particularly interesting in light of the variety of cell types which participate in the gas exchange mechanism. These cell types include alveolar type I, alveolar type II, and capillary endothelial cells. The alveolar type I and capillary endothelial cells comprise the gas exchange segment, whereas the alveolar type II cells secrete surfactant, a phospholipid compound which reduces the surface tension of pulmonary fluids. From a physiological standpoint, the pulmonary microcirculation behaves differently from the systemic microcirculation.

1. Hypoxia

Under hypoxic conditions the systemic circulation undergoes vasodilation to maintain adequate tissue perfusion. In contrast, the pulmonary vasculature vasoconstricts during hypoxia, a response which may help decrease perfusion to poorly ventilated segments and minimize ventilation/perfusion deficiencies.[134] The major site of the pulmonary vascular response to alveolar hypoxia appears to be precapillary. Parker et al.[135] have evaluated the isogravimetric capillary pressure and pre- and postcapillary pulmonary vascular resistance in dog lungs under normal and hypoxic conditions. These investigations have shown that hypoxia causes a decrease in capillary pressure and an increase in precapillary, but not postcapillary, vascular resistance. A similar study by Nagasaka et al.[136] showed that the lung microvascular pressure was enhanced to a greater extent in arterioles as compared to venules during hypoxia in cats. Additional studies by Cope et al.[137] using 100% nitrogen infusion into intact dog lungs, have shown that hypoxic conditions results in precapillary vasoconstriction.

2. Paraquat

The pulmonary circulation is extremely sensitive to environmental influences. In recent years several studies have focused on paraquat-induced pulmonary microvascular injury. Paraquat, a quaternary dipyridylium compound used widely as a herbicide, causes extensive lung damage in humans and animals.[138] Pulmonary injury is characterized by exudative pulmonary edema, followed by intraalveolar and interstitial fibrosis.[139] Type II alveolar epithelial cells actively accumulate paraquat and exhibit extensive morphological damage. Pulmonary endothelial cells also show ultrastructural evidence of damage after paraquat administration. The toxic effects of paraquat are related to its ability to generate free radicals (Figure 3). In the absence of oxygen, paraquat can undergo a one-electron reduction by NADPH to form free radicals. Upon reoxygenation, these radicals immediately reoxidize to the divalent cation form with a concomitant production of reactive oxygen species. The redox cycling of paraquat results in continuous release of oxygen free radicals which can cause peroxidative injury to membranes. Giri et al.[140] have found that intraperitoneal administration of paraquat to mice increases pulmonary vascular permeability and causes pulmonary edema. Interestingly, superoxide dismutase did not alter the toxicity of acute paraquat exposure suggesting that the toxic effects of paraquat are mediated through free radical species other than superoxide. Studies by Shibamoto et al.[141] have investigated the dose- and time-dependent changes of microvascular endothelial permeability and microvascular pressure upon exposure to paraquat. In these experiments, an initial loss in lobe weight and a dose-dependent increase of microvascular permeability was observed after paraquat infusion. Capillary filtration was found to increase, while isogravimetric capillary pressure decreased in a dose- and time-dependent fashion. Three hours of hyperoxia exacerbated the increased capillary filtration and decreased capillary pressure induced by paraquat. In contrast to these results, under hypoxic conditions paraquat administration resulted in capillary filtration and capillary pressure rates comparable to normoxic conditions. Additional studies have shown that a hypoxic environment increased survival time in paraquat-treated mice,[142] but not rats.[143] Collectively, these findings suggests that the toxicity of paraquat is mediated by reactive oxygen species, other than superoxide, in a species-dependent fashion.

3. Free Radicals

To further characterize the role of free radicals in pulmonary microcirculatory toxicity, Crapo et al.[144] have investigated oxygen free radical-induced damage in rats exposed to high oxygen tension. Rats exposed to 100% oxygen sustained injury to the pulmonary capillary endothelium. Decreased capillary surface area and capillary lumen volume were also observed. In contrast, exposure of animals to 85% oxygen resulted in proliferation

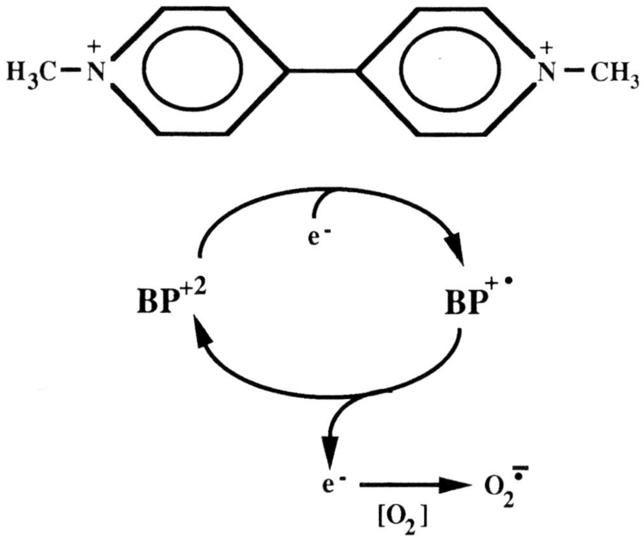

Figure 11-3 Paraquat, a bipyridyl herbicide, undergoes a one electron reduction by cytochrome P-450 to form an unstable intermediate. This intermediate quickly redox cycles to the divalent cation yielding a free electron which may in turn react with oxygen to generate free radicals.

of alveolar Type II epithelial cells and capillary endothelial cell death. This toxic response was associated with compensatory hypertrophy of the surviving endothelial cells. Recent studies by He et al.[145] have investigated lung damage in several rat strains exposed to oxygen free radicals. These studies were designed to determine if increased susceptibility to oxidant injury is related to differences in lung antioxidant capability. The microcirculation of perfused Fisher or Sprague-Dawley rat lungs was evaluated by measurements of microvascular pressure and permeability. Under hyperoxic conditions, microvascular permeability was increased in Fisher, but not Sprague-Dawley rats, while the microvascular pressure was similar in both strains. In Fisher rats, catalase was found to prevent hyperoxia-induced increased permeability, while neither superoxide dismutase nor allopurinol afforded any protection. In other studies, the effects of reactive oxygen metabolites in perfused Wistar rat lungs were investigated.[146] These studies examined the antioxidant role of plasma in free radical-induced pulmonary microvascular injury by measuring fluid filtration rates. Reactive oxygen species were generated by the addition of xanthine oxidase and hypoxanthine into the perfusate. Under these conditions, a time-dependent increase of fluid filtration rate was observed. When new plasma perfusate was introduced, fluid filtration rates decreased relative to pre-existing levels. The addition of catalase into the initial perfusate prevented the alterations in capillary permeability induced by xanthine oxidase/hypoxanthine. These findings are in agreement with studies by Tate et al.[147] which showed that xanthine oxidase increased alveolar-capillary membrane permeability.

4. Dietary Factors

Oleic acid is an unsaturated fatty acid present in corn and soy oil, grass, butter, lard, and eggs. In various species this fatty acid causes hemorrhagic pulmonary edema independent of complement, eicosanoids, blood components, and oxygen radicals.[148,149] Studies by

Townsley et al.[150] have examined the role of lipid peroxidation in oleic acid toxicity in canine lungs. Pretreatment with the antioxidants, promethazine, and diphenyl-*p*-phenylenediamine, reversed or attenuated oleic acid-induced increase in microvascular permeability suggesting that oleic acid mediates its toxic effects by lipid peroxidation of cellular components.

5. Monocrotaline

As stated previously, monocrotaline is a carcinogenic alkaloid derived from the seeds of *Crotalaria spectabilis*. Monocrotaline causes medial thickening of pulmonary arteries/arterioles and pulmonary hypertension.[151,152] ^{3}H-thymidine labeling studies have demonstrated that monocrotaline-induced thickening of medial and advential layers was associated with enhanced labeling of rat pulmonary arterial smooth muscle, fibroblasts, and endothelial cells.[153] Enhanced thymidine uptake is also observed in endothelial cells from alveolar capillaries. Vascular endothelial cells appear to be the primary site of cellular damage both *in vivo* and in lung slices.[154] Studies by Olson et al.[155] have examined alterations in lung ornithine decarboxylase, the initial rate-limiting enzyme involved in polyamine biosynthesis, in rats treated with monocrotaline. A single dose of monocrotaline enhanced lung ornithine decarboxylase for 7 days. Suppression of polyamine synthesis prevented monocrotaline-induced arterial medial thickening.[156] These results suggest that monocrotaline-mediated effects involve alterations in cellular proliferation. Cast corrosion studies have investigated the morphologic changes induced by monocrotaline in rats.[157] Monocrotaline-treated animals exhibited decreased vascular density and focal capillary loss. Thrombosis of capillaries was considered the main cause of decreased vascular density. Further studies by Schraufnagel have shown that monocrotaline treatments were associated with capillary growth on the pleural surface of the lung which is supplied by bronchial vessels.[158] However, the pulmonary bed did not contain evidence of new capillary growth. These differences may be accounted for by differences in extracellular matrix deposition around capillaries. Bronchial capillaries are surrounded by more fibroblasts and pericytes than alveolar capillaries. These cells contain a variety of enzymes, such as elastase and collagenase, and basement membrane components, including collagen, laminin, and proteoglycans, which are essential for endothelial migration. Thus, the angiogenic and proliferative effects induced by monocrotaline may depend on extracellular matrix components.

G. RENAL MICROCIRCULATION

The kidney performs important detoxifying functions by filtering and eliminating metabolic byproducts in the urine. Another important function of the kidney is the maintenance of proper ionic and osmotic balance. These functions require intact operation of the renal glomerulus. Anatomically, the glomerulus is a meshwork of capillaries, which consist of the fenestrated capillary endothelium, endothelial-derived podocytes, the mesenchymal-derived mesangial cells and parietal epithelium of Bowman's capsule. Blood travels through renal arterioles into the glomerular capillary loops resulting in high hydrostatic pressures in the glomerulus. This increase in pressure potentiates the filtering ability of the glomerulus and allows substrate passage into other parts of the kidney.

1. Heavy Metals

Recent studies have examined the cytotoxic effects of divalent metals, cobalt, nickel, manganese, zinc, copper, cadmium, and mercury, on glomerular function.[159] Mesangial cells are known to produce an extracellular matrix known as mesangium. This matrix contains various components which include collagen, fibronectin, and dermatan sulphate proteoglycans, as well as other proteoglycans. Studies using isolated rat glomeruli assessed protein and proteoglycan synthesis by [^{3}H]-leucine and [^{35}S]-sulphate incorporation upon exposure to these metals. At concentrations which inhibit 50% of the incorporation of [^{3}H]-leucine into protein, mercury and cadmium preferentially decreased dermatan sulfate proteoglycan synthesis suggesting that these metals alter matrix synthesis in mesangial cells.

2. Free Radicals

Acute glomerulonephritis is characterized by proteinuria, edema, hematuria, renal failure, and hypertension. One or more of these phenomena may involve free radical formation. Damage to glomerular endothelial cells has been attributed to neutrophilic release of oxygen species. Thus, acute glomerular damage appears to mainly involve phagocytic cells.[160] In contrast, chronic glomerular nephritis and glomerular sclerosis are characterized by the slow progressive glomerular nephritis caused by various etiologies ultimately leading to irreversible renal failure. These disorders are often associated with mesangial cell proliferation and/or IgA deposition in mesangial areas. Many studies have implicated hypercholesterolemia in the initiation and progression of glomerular sclerosis. Hypercholesterolemia causes glomerular hypertension and compromised renal function. These effects include microvascular endothelial cell injury, with release of vasoactive factors, vascular lipid deposition, intracapillary thrombosis; mesangial injury with accumulation of lipoproteins, increased matrix production, macrophage accumulation and cellular proliferation; and epithelial cell injury with proteinuria and decreased water permeability.[161]

3. Cholesterol

Several mechanisms by which high cholesterol levels are thought to induce glomerular injury include enhanced mesangial deposition of lipoproteins, hyperlipidemia-induced mesangial cell proliferation, enhanced glomerular macrophage activity, and alterations in the glomerular basement membrane. High serum cholesterol levels have been associated with increased renal vascular resistance in isolated kidneys.[162] Studies by Kasiske et al.[163] have investigated the role of cholesterol in the spontaneous development of glomerular injury in hyperlipidemic rats. These studies employed the use of mevinolin, a cholesterol synthesis inhibitor, and clofibric acid, a compound which blocks hepatic release of lipoproteins, inhibits cholesterol biosynthesis, and enhances lipoprotein lipase activity. Rats treated with these agents exhibited reduced mesangial matrix expansion and cellularity. These findings were associated with a reduction in the percent of glomeruli exhibiting focal sclerosis. Since mevinolin and clofibric acid did not alter glomerular hemodynamic function, these results suggest that abnormal lipid metabolism may be important in the pathogenesis of glomerular sclerosis. Moorhead et al.[164] have shown that cultured rat mesangial cells incubated in low-density lipoprotein at twice rat serum concentrations (250 μg/ml) exhibited morphologic changes and cellular detachment. These changes were associated with a decrease in [^{3}H]-thymidine incorporation and enhanced [^{51}Cr] release, a marker of cellular damage, suggesting that low-density lipoproteins may alter mesangial cell function.

4. Extracellular Matrix

As stated previously, mesangial cells synthesize extracellular matrix proteins which are released into the mesangium. Alterations in collagen synthesis have been associated with glomerular disease in humans.[165] Haralson et al.[166] have evaluated the relative amounts and molecular forms of collagen synthesized by normal cultured rat mesangial cells. The secreted and cell-associated fractions contained collagen types I, III, IV, and V. However, type I collagen comprised 95% of the total collagen synthesized. Studies by Yoshioka et al.[167] have investigated type I and type III collagen deposition in normal and diseased human renal tissue. Normal kidneys exhibited immunofluorescence of type I and type III collagen in the renal interstitium, but not in intra-glomerular structures. In contrast, immunofluorescence of collagen type I and III was localized in the glomeruli of kidneys with various types of glomerular nephritis. Collagen type III staining was greater in amount and frequency, as compared to type I collagen staining. Type I collagen was localized in the sclerosed glomeruli and infrequently in glomerular mesangium. Mesangial staining for type I collagen was present particularly when mesangial matrix was increased. These findings suggest that chronic glomerular disorders are associated with differential synthesis of collagens.

5. Carbon Tetrachloride

Chronic administration of carbon tetrachloride causes glomerular injury in rats.[168] Glomerular sclerosis as well as tubular and interstitial damage are characteristic of CCl_4 administration. Ohyama et al.[169] dosed rats with CCl_4 for 20 weeks, homogenized the kidneys, and isolated a 5-kDa protein from treated animals. Cultured mesangial cells were then incubated in the presence of this protein and pro-collagen synthesis was evaluated. The 5-kDa protein stimulated cultured mesangial cell synthesis of pro-collagen I and IV. The observed increase was associated with enhanced mRNA expression for pro-collagen type I and IV. These results are in accord with similar studies by Hatahara and Seyer which isolated a hepatic fibrogenic factor from rats chronically dosed with CCl_4.[170] This hepatic fibrogenic factor was found to stimulate the synthesis of collagen types I, III, and V. These findings again suggest that alterations in mesangial cell synthesis and deposition of collagen are associated with glomerular disease. Extracellular matrix proteins are known to be important in cellular proliferation.[171] Thus, the enhanced proliferative behavior of mesangial cells which occurs in chronic kidney diseases may be related to alterations in extracellular matrix environment. Other extracellular environmental factors which are altered in glomerular disease include fibronectins and proteoglycans. For example, Okuda et al.[172] have examined expression of proteoglycans, fibronectin, and TGF-beta, a growth factor found in various cell types, in antithymocyte-induced glomerular nephritis. Cultured nephritic glomeruli had increased proteoglycan and fibronectin synthesis and TGF-beta mRNA expression as compared to normal glomeruli. When the media from the cultured nephritic glomeruli was added to normal cultured mesangial cells, there was enhanced proteoglycan synthesis. Both glomeruli and mesangial proteoglycan synthesis was reduced when anti-serum against TGF-beta was added to the media suggesting that TGF-beta is involved in extracellular matrix deposition. Other growth factors such as interleukin-1, PDGF, and tissue necrosis factor cause mesangial cell proliferation without altering extracellular matrix proteins.[173,174]

6. Extracellular Substances

In addition, substances found extracellularly, such as prostaglandins and endothelium-derived relaxing factor (EDRF), do not enhance mesangial cell proliferation or matrix production, but can modulate mesangial function.[175] Shultz et al.[176] have examined the effects of EDRF derived from cultured bovine endothelial cells on cGMP levels in co-cultured rat mesangial cells. EDRF caused increased cGMP levels in mesangial cells which were associated with relaxation of vascular smooth muscle. Studies by Frieman et al.[177] have shown that atherosclerosis impairs EDRF-dependent vascular relaxation by acetylcholine and thrombin.

7. Dietary Factors

Dietary lipids can directly modulate renal function. For example, Kelley et al.[178] have shown that a fish oil diet rich in eicosapentaenoic acid reduces cyclooxygenase metabolites and suppresses lupus nephritic mice. The dietary intake of fatty acids and their subsequent metabolism into various eicosanoids modulates glomerular function.[179] Studies by Takahashi et al.[180] have investigated the primary metabolites of arachidonic acid in rat cortical and medullary microsomal fractions. The cytochrome P-450-derived epoxyeicosatrienoic acids (EETs) accounted for over 50% of the total products in the cortex. The vascular effects of epoxyeicosatrienoic acids was evaluated by administering 5,6-EET to rats. Equimolar doses of 5,6-EET resulted in a dose-dependent renal vasoconstriction and a reduced glomerular filtration rate. These effects were reversed by ibuprofen, a cyclooxygenase inhibitor, suggesting that 5,6-EET mediates its effects through cyclooxygenase metabolism. Harris et al.[181] have investigated the role of EET in rat mesangial cell proliferation. One-day administration of 8,9- or 14,15-EET increased cell proliferation, [^{3}H]-thymidine incorporation, and Na^+/H^+ exchange. However, the cyclooxygenase inhibitor, indomethacin, did not alter this response. Over 90% of the radioactivity was incorporated into cellular lipids 24 h after addition of [^{14}C] 14,15-EET. Thus epoxyeicosatrienoic acids have differential mechanisms by which they exert their biologic effects. Studies by Badr et al.[182] have examined the proliferative effects of leukotriene D_4 on cultured mesangial cells. Leukotriene D_4 induced a time- and concentration-dependent increase in phosphoinositide hydrolysis, [^{3}H]-thymidine incorporation, and mitogenesis. While certain arachidonic metabolites such as EET and the leukotrienes have been shown to enhance mesangial cell proliferation, other metabolites, such as prostaglandin E_2 appear to have antiproliferative effects. Studies by Stahl et al.[183] investigated a possible role of prostaglandin E_2 (PGE_2) in interleukin-1 mediated mesangial cell proliferation. Cultured rat mesangial cells exposed to interleukin-1 exhibited a dose-dependent increase in [^{3}H]-thymidine uptake and PGE_2 formation. When PGE_2 formation was inhibited by indomethacin, interleukin-1-induced cell proliferation increased an additional seven-fold. Thus, arachidonic acid metabolites can modulate the proliferative behavior of mesangial cells, as well as alter physiologic behavior of the kidney.

8. Ethanol

Alcohol has been shown to cause nephropathy in humans.[184] This disorder is associated with intense IgA accumulation in mesangial cells.[185] Smith et al.[186] have investigated the effects of chronic alcohol administration on glomerular morphology in rats. After 6 weeks of ethanol administration, rats developed lesions which resemble IgA nephropathy. Morphologically, alcohol-induced glomerular alterations included mesangial IgA and IgM deposition, increased deposition of mesangial matrix, increased mesangial cell proliferation, and podocyte foot effacement. Further studies are needed to fully understand the changes seen in alcohol-induced nephropathy.

9. T-2 Toxin

T-2 toxin, a trichothecene mycotoxin produced by various species of *Fusarium*, is a natural contaminant of foods and animal feeds.[187] Siren and Feuerstein have investigated the acute effects of T-2 toxin on local blood flow and vascular resistance in renal, hindquarter, and mesenteric vascular beds by laser Doppler.[188] Administration of a single bolus of T-2 toxin (1 mg/kg) resulted in reduced blood flow and increased vascular resistance in all blood vessels studied, with no effects on arterial pressure or heart rate. These changes were associated with increased plasma renin, particularly at the time of reduced renal blood flow. Thompson and Wannemacher have shown that a lethal dose of T-2 toxin causes a rapid decrease in protein synthesis, in kidney, muscle, intestine, spleen, liver, and heart rat tissues within 3 h with partial recovery by 9 h.[189] The decrease in protein synthesis was followed by decreased DNA synthesis in all tissues suggesting that disruption of protein synthesis precedes the alterations in DNA synthesis. These studies, as well as studies by Borison et al.[190] suggest that T-2 toxin inhibits protein synthesis of microvessels. This phenomena in turn may lead to cellular damage, loss of plasma from the vasculature, decreased cardiac output, and circulatory shock.

H. SKELETAL MUSCLE

1. Free Radicals

Skeletal muscle, like cardiac muscle, utilizes large amounts of oxygen and nutrients to support contractile function. The high rate of oxidative phosphorylation required to maintain adequate energy levels leads to the formation and release of various oxygen-derived free radicals. A growing amount of evidence has indicated that free radicals play an important role as mediators of skeletal muscle damage during strenuous physical activity.[191] Many of the biochemical alterations associated with intense physical activity resemble those observed during ischemic-reperfusion injury. Within this context, the microvasculature of exercised animals after ischemia and reperfusion has been examined by Sexton et al.[192] The skeletal muscle microcirculation of isolated perfused rat hindquarters was assessed by changes in capillary permeability, total vascular resistance, and regional blood distribution. Pre-ischemic data showed that exercise trained hindquarters had decreased total and precapillary vascular resistance, increased flow rates, and increased capillary filtration coefficients relative to controls. After ischemia-reperfusion, isogravimetric flow rates were greater in exercised trained muscle. However, no differences were observed in total vascular resistance or capillary filtration suggesting that exercise does not significantly alter free radical-induced damage in skeletal muscle.

2. Temperature

Local tissue cooling has been shown to affect microvascular smooth muscle cells.[193] Intravital microscopy has been used to measure the diameter of arterioles and venules from the rat cremaster muscle. At a temperature of 34°C, the addition of norepinephrine caused a reduction in vessel diameter. Cooling the tissue to 26°C caused an additional constriction of arterioles and venules. The terminal arterioles exhibited the most pronounced inhibition of rhythmic vasomotion. However, cooling-induced constriction was only evident after adrenergic stimulation by norepinephrine in response to cooling. The loss of adrenergic tone upon exposure to phentolamine, an $alpha_1$- and $alpha_2$-adrenergic antagonist, resulted in abolition of cooling-induced vasoconstriction. The mechanism by which cooling augmented adrenergic constriction was evaluated by the use of yohimbine, a postjunctional $alpha_2$-adrenoreceptor inhibitor, or prazosin, a $alpha_1$-adrenoreceptor inhibitor. Yohimbine abolished vessel constriction, while prazosin had no effect on cooling-induced constriction. These results suggest that cooling augments adrenergic tone in microvessels by increasing $alpha_2$-dependent vasoconstriction.

3. Ethanol

Ethanol can modulate microcirculatory function in skeletal muscle. Chronic ingestion of alcohol is associated with chronic muscle myopathy and hypertension.[194,195] Ethanol administration exerts vasodilatory effects in the peripheral circulation, irrespective of the route of administration.[196] The vasodilatory effect observed in splanchnic and cutaneous circulation is associated with increased systemic blood pressure. However, some studies have found that ethanol causes constriction of certain peripheral blood vessels, particularly microvessels located in skeletal muscle.[197] *In situ* microscopic studies of skeletal (cremaster) muscle were performed after acute administration of ethanol, acetaldehyde, and acetate.[198] Administration of ethanol resulted in a concentration-dependent vasoconstriction of arterioles and venules. The metabolites of ethanol, acetaldehyde, and acetate produced a concentration-dependent vasodilation in these same vessels. Cyclooxygenase inhibitors could not inhibit the ethanol, acetaldehyde, and acetate-induced response. Also, blockade of serotoninergic, histaminergic, cholinergic, or opiate receptors did not attenuate the effects induced by these agents. These results suggest that metabolism of ethanol is not involved in the vasoconstrictor response. Collectively, these data suggest that ethanol, acetaldehyde, and acetate elicit direct responses in skeletal muscle.

4. Cholesterol

Hypercholesterolemia has been shown to affect skeletal muscle microcirculation. In recent studies by Schuschke et al.,[199] the vasoconstrictive response of norepinephrine in both arterioles and venules from the cremaster muscle was evaluated in rats fed diets high in cholesterol for 3 and 5 weeks. An attenuated vasoconstrictor response to norepinephrine was relative to control rats fed the high cholesterol diet. No histological changes were observed in the aorta, vasa vasorum, or periaortic microvasculature. Studies by Yamamoto et al.[200] have investigated the effects of several vasodilators in atherosclerotic rabbits with high serum cholesterol. The administration of acetylcholine to the cremaster muscle reduced the cholinergic arteriolar dilation in atherosclerotic rabbits relative to controls. When the rabbit cremaster was dosed with nitroprusside, an endothelium-independent vasodilator, the vasodilatory response was similar in both atherosclerotic and control animals. High cholesterol loading has been associated with alterations in vascular adrenergic receptor affinity.[201] Thus, cholesterol may modulate skeletal microvasculature by altering cellular receptor function.

5. Dietary Factors

Copper deficiency causes numerous abnormalities including structural and functional defects of the vascular system, hypercholesterolemia, and anemia.[202-204] Angiogenesis is also a copper-dependent process.[205] Various enzymes are affected by the lack of copper including lysyl oxidase, superoxide dismutase, and ceruloplasmin.[206] Schuschke et al.[207] have evaluated the effects of copper over supplementation or deficiency on the rat cremaster muscle microcirculation. In these studies, rats were fed copper supplemented or deficient diets for 5 weeks and endogenous histamine and platelet thrombi formation were assessed. These studies showed that copper deficiency increased blood cholesterol and decreased the hematocrit. Platelet aggregation induced by photoactivation of fluorescent-labeled albumin in copper-supplemented rats was enhanced. In contrast, photoactivation in copper-deficient skeletal muscle only yielded mild aggregation which did not compromise tissue perfusion. Platelet aggregometry studies did not demonstrate reduced platelet aggregation in the copper-deficient group. These findings suggest that copper deficiency alters the microvascular endothelium by inhibiting the adhesion of platelets to the endothelial cell surface.

IV. CONCLUSION

The work summarized in this chapter serves to illustrate the profound impact of environmental factors upon the general microcirculation. Table 3 lists these factors with their putative biological effects. Our approach has emphasized the target-organ specificity associated with some forms of environmental insult. Although in retrospect the potential influence of environmental factors in the microcirculation seems obvious, to date only a limited number of studies have been conducted to examine such responses in a rigorous fashion. The heterogeneous nature which characterizes environmental factors represents a significant obstacle to continued progress in this area. A number of ubiquitous chemical agents which potentially alter microcirculatory function have yet to be examined. Future advances in this field of research would require dynamic exchange among various biomedical disciplines. Recent breakthroughs in cell and molecular biology should afford us the opportunity to reevaluate the influence of environmental factors on the physiology and pathophysiology of the microcirculation. New doors have yet to be opened!

Table 11-3 **Environmental factors implicated in microcirculatory dysfunction**

Environmental Factor	Mechanism of Action
Alcohol	Increases cardiac capillary density and decreases capillary diameter. Decreases the ability of liver Kupffer cells to metabolize endotoxins which result in endothelial swelling and sinusoidal plugging. Induces cerebral arteriolar vasoconstrictions, vascular spasms, and rupture. Prolonged exposure leads to cortical microvascularization. Initiates arteriolar and venular vasoconstriction in skeletal muscle and inducing vasodilation of splanchnic and skin microvessels. Interfers with catacholamine, angiotensin, and vasopressin mediated vasoconstriction of splanchnic microvessels by perturbing Ca mobility.
Hypercholesterolemia	Results in renal microvascular endothelial and mesangial cell injury. Attenuates the vasoconstrictor response of norepinephrine in skeletal muscle arterioles and venules, while reducing the vasodilatory effects of acetylcholine in arterioles.
Selenium-vitamin E deficiency	Accumulation of fibrinoid in cardiovascular arteriolar walls and disruption of microvascular endothelial cells.
Exercise	Increased cardiac capillary growth.
Chemicals	
Carbon tetrachloride	Collagen deposition between microvascular endothelial cells and hepatocytes. Hepatic capillary proliferation into fibrous tissue. Increased diameter of hepatic venules. Alterations in mesangial cell synthesis and deposition of collagen.
Cytokins	TGF-β decreases mesangial proteoglycan synthesis. Interleukin 1 increases mesangial cell proliferation.
Metals	Accumulation of lead occurs in capillary endothelial cells resulting in decreased glucose uptake. Cultured endothelial cells exhibit enhanced mitogenic activity. Cd and Hg — decrease mesangial cell proteoglycan synthesis. Cu deficiency alters skeletal muscle microvascular endothelium resulting in platelet nonadherence.
Monocrotaline	Pulmonary arteriolar thickening. Enhanced thymidine uptake in capillary endothelial cells. Capillary growth in the pleural surface of the lung.
PAF-morphine and capsaicin	Decreases gastric mucosal blood flow resulting in vasocongestion and hemorrhagic damage to the mucosa.
Paraquat	Free radical-related ultrastructural damage to pulmonary microvascular endothelial cells.
T-2 Toxin	Decreases renal microvascular blood flow and increases vascular resistance. Decreases protein synthesis in renal tissue.
Dietary	
Arachidonic acid	Dose-dependent dilation of cerebral arterioles and enhanced endothelial permeability.
Choline deficiency	Increased diameter of hepatic venules and accumulation of fibrin in sinusoids.

Table 11-3 **Environmental factors implicated in microcirculatory dysfunction (*Continued*)**

Environmental Factor	Mechanism of Action
Epoxyeicosatrienioc acids	5,6-EET causes a dose-dependent dilation of cerebral arterioles. 14,15-EET increases mesangial cell proliferation, thymidine incorporation, and Na^+/H^+ exchange.
Fish oil (Eicosapentanoic Acid)	Dose-dependent increase in the diameter of cerebral arterioles.
Oleic acid	Increased pulmonary microvascular permeability which is associated with increased lipid peroxidation.
Hyperoxia	Injuried pulmonary capillary endothelial cells with a compensatory increase in proliferation. Reduction in central nervous system capillaries which is associated with endothelial cell degeneration. Decreased proliferation in cultured cerebral endothelial cells which is associated with lipid peroxidation of lysosome and mitochondrial membranes.
Temperature	Cooling enhances skeletal muscle α-2-adrenergic vasocontrictive response of norepinephrine in arterioles. Heating increases cutaneous blood flow while cooling decreases blood flow. Adenosine potentiates the skin microvessel vasoconstrictor response to heat, while the norephinephrine-induced vasoconstrictor response decreases during cooling.
Burn stress	Decreases gastric blood flow resulting in mucosal damage. Microvascular permeability increases and appears to be mediated through free radical mechanisms.

REFERENCES

1. **Harlan, W. R., Sharrett A. R., Weill H., Turino G. M., Borhani N. O., and Resnekov L.,** Impact of the environment on cardiovascular disease. Report of the American Heart Association Task Force on environment and the cardiovascular system, *Circulation*, 63(1), 243A, 1981.
2. **Mogensen, C. E.,** Renal functional changes in diabetes, *Diabetes,* 24, 872, 1976.
3. **Meurer, M. and Szeimies, R. M.,** Diabetes mellitus and skin diseases, *Curr. Probl. Dermatol.,* 20, 11, 1991.
4. **Pinter, G. G. and Atkins J. L.,** Role of postglomerular microvessels in pathophysiology of diabetic nephropathy. Assessment and hypothesis, *Diabetes*, 40(7), 791, 1991.
5. **Epstein, S. E., Cannon, R. O., and Bonow, R. O.,** Exercise testing inpatients with microvascular angina, *Circulation*, 83 (Suppl. 5), III73, 1991.
6. **Fujiki, H., Suganuma, M., Yoshizawa, S., Kanazawa, H., Sugimura, T., Manam, S., Kahn, S. M., Jiang, W., Hoshina, S., and Weinstein, I. B.,** Codon 61 mutations in the c-Harvey-ras gene in mouse skin tumors induced by 7, 12-dimethylbenz[a] anthracene plus okadaic acid class tumor promoters, *Mol. Carcinogen.*, 2(4), 184, 1989.
7. **Ramos, K.,** Cellular and molecular basis of xenobiotic-induced cardiovascular toxicity: application of cell culture systems, in *Cellular and Molecular Toxicology and In Vitro Toxicology*, Acosta, D., Ed., CRC Press, Boca Raton, FL, 1990, chap. 6.

8. **Albert, R. E., Miller, M. L., Cody T. E., Barkley, W., and Shukla R.,** Cell kinetics and benzo[a]pyrene-DNA adducts in mouse skin tumorigenesis, in *Chemically Induced Cell Proliferation Implications of Risk Assessment*, Vol. 369, Butterworth, B. E., Slaga, T. J., Farland, W., and McClain, M., Eds., Wiley-Liss, New York, 1991, 115.
9. **Mullins, J. A.,** Industrial emissions of 1, 3-butadiene, *Environ. Health Persp.*, 86, 9, 1990.
10. **Landrigan, P. J.,** Critical assessment of epidemiologic studies on the human carcinogenicity of 1, 3-butadiene, *Environ. Health Persp.*, 86, 143, 1990.
11. **Acquavella, J. F.,** Future directions in epidemiologic studies of 1,3-butadiene-exposed workers, *Environ. Health Persp.*, 86, 129, 1990.
12. **Miller, R. A., Melnick, R. L., and Boorman, G. A.,** Neoplastic lesions induced by 1,3-butadiene in B6C3F$_1$ mice, *Exp. Pathol.*, 37, 136, 1989.
13. **Miller, R. A. and Boorman, G. A.,** Morphology of neoplastic lesions induced by 1,3-butadiene in B6C3F$_1$ mice, *Environ. Health Persp.*, 86, 37, 1990.
14. **Melnick, R. L., Huff, J., Chou, B. J., and Miller, R. A.,** Carcinogenicity of 1,3-butadiene in C57BL/6 × C3H F$_1$ mice at low exposure concentrations, *Cancer Res.*, 50, 6592, 1990.
15. **Safe, S. H., Gasiewicz, T., and Whitlock, J. P., Jr.,** Mechanisms working group, in, *Environmental Toxin Series*, Vol. 3, Safe, S., Hutzinger, O., and Hill, T. A., Eds., Springer-Verlag, Berlin, 1990, chap. 2.
16. **Ramos, K. and Cox, L.,** Primary cultures of rat aortic endothelial smooth muscle cells: I. An in vitro model to study xenobiotic-induced vascular cytotoxicity, *In Vitro Cell. & Develop. Biol.*, 23, 288, 1987.
17. **Cox, L. R., Murphy, S. K., and Ramos, K.,** Modulation of phosphoinositide metabolism in aortic smooth muscle cells by allylamine, *Exp. Mol. Pathol.*, 53, 52, 1990.
18. **Ramos, K. S., McMahon, K. K., Alipui, C., and Demick, D.,** Modulation of DNA synthesis in aortic smooth muscle cells by dinitrotoluenes, *Cell Biol. Toxicol.*, 7, 111, 1991.
19. **Ramos, K.,** Vascular toxicology: a cellular and molecular perspective, in *Cardiovasc. Toxicol.*, Acosta, D., Ed., Raven Press, New York, in press.
20. **Huxtable, R. J.,** New aspects of the toxicology and pharmacology of pyrrolizidine alkaloids, *Gen. Pharmacol.*, 10(3), 159, 1979.
21. **Chilian, W. M., Dellsperger, K. C., Layne, S. M., Eastham, C. L., Armstrong, M. A., Marcus, M. L., and Heistad, D. D.,** Effects of atherosclerosis on the coronary microcirculation, *Am. J. Physiol.*, 258, H529, 1990.
22. **Hooper, C.,** Free radicals: research on biochemical bad boys comes of age, *J. NIH Res.*, 1, 101, 1989.
23. **Beller, F. K., Graeff, H., and Gorstein, F.,** Disseminated intravascular coagulation during the continuous infusion of endotoxin in rabbits. Morphologic and physiologic studies, *Am. J. Obstet. Gynecol.*, 103(4), 544, 1969.
24. **Yoshikawa, T., Furukawa, Y., Murakami, M., Watanabe, K., and Kondo, M.,** Effect of vitamin E on endotoxin-induced disseminated intravascular coagulation in rats, *Thrombosis Haemostas*, 48(2), 235, 1982.
25. **Wilson, S. K.,** Role of oxygen-derived free radicals in acute angiotensin. II. Induced hypertensive vascular disease in the rat, *Circ. Res.*, 66, 722, 1990.
26. **Kontos, H. A., Wei, E. P., Povlishock, J. T., and Christman, C. W.,** Oxygen radicals mediate the cerebral arteriolar dilation from arachidonate and bradykinin in cats, *Circ. Res.*, 55, 295, 1984.
27. **Wei, E. P., Kontos, H. A., Christman, C. W., DeWitt, D. S., and Povlishock, J. T.,** Superoxide generation and reversal of acetylcholine induced cerebral vasodilation after acute hypertension, *Circ. Res.*, 57, 781, 1985.
28. **Rosenblum, W. I.,** Hydroxyl radical mediates the endothelium-dependent relaxation produced by Bradykinin in mouse cerebral arterioles, *Circ. Res.*, 61, 601, 1987.

29. **Kehrer, J. P., Jones, D. P., Lemasters, J. L., Farber, J. L., and Jaeschke, H.,** Mechanisms of hypoxic cell injury, *Toxicol. Appl. Pharmacol.*, 106, 165, 1990.
30. **Kane, A. B., Petrovich, D. R., Stern, R. O., and Farber, J. L.,** ATP depletion and the loss of cell integrity in anoxic hepatocytes and silica-treated P388D_1 macrophages, *Am. J. Physiol.*, 248, C256, 1985.
31. **Aw, T. Y., Andersson, B. S., and Jones, D. P.,** Suppression of mitochondrial respiratory function after short-term anoxia, *Am. J. Physiol.*, 252, C362, 1987b.
32. **Acosta, D., Ramos, K., and Li-Goldman, C.,** Cell injury of cultured rat myocardial cells after reoxygenation of hypoxic cultures in the presence and absence of calcium, *In Vitro*, 20, 642, 1984.
33. **Andersson, B. S., Aw, T. Y., and Jones, D. P.,** Mitochondrial transmembrane potential and pH gradient during anoxia, *Am. J. Physiol.*, 252, C349, 1987.
34. **Steenbergen, C., Murphy, E., Watts, W. A., and London, R. E.,** Correlation between cytosolic free calcium, contracture, ATP, and irreversible ischemic injury in perfused rat heart, *Circ. Res.*, 66, 135, 1990.
35. **Farber, J. L., Martin, J. T., and Young, E. E.,** Accelerated phospholipid degradation in anoxic rat hepatocytes, *Arch. Biochem. Biophys.*, 211, 312, 1981.
36. **Chein, K. R., Abrams, J., Serroni, A., Martin, J. T., and Farber, J. L.,** Accelerated turnover and associated membrane dysfunction in irreversible ischemic liver cell injury, *J. Biol. Chem.*, 253, 4809, 1978.
37. **Lemasters, J. J., DiGuiseppi, J., Nieminen, A. L., and Herman, B.,** Blebbing, free Ca^{++} and mitochondrial membrane potential preceding cell death in hepatocytes, *Nature (London)*, 325, 78, 1987.
38. **Bond, J. M., Gores, G. J., Herman, B., and Lemasters, J. J.,** Reversal of hypercontraction, protection by acidic pH, and change of cytosolic pH during "chemical hypoxia" and anoxia in cardiac myocytes, in *Optical Microscopy for Biology*, Herman, B. and Jacobson, K. A., Eds., Alan R. Liss, New York, 1990, 295.
39. **Maupoil, V. and Rochette, L.,** Evaluation of free radical and lipid peroxide formation during global ischemia and reperfusion in isolated perfused rat heart, *Cardiovasc. Drug Ther.*, 2, 615, 1988.
40. **Dauber, I. M., Lesnefsky, E. J., VanBenthuysen, K. M., Weil, J. V., and Horwitz, L. D.,** Reactive oxygen metabolite scavengers decrease functional coronary microvascular injury due to ischemia-reperfusion, *Am. J. Physiol.*, 260, H42, 1991.
41. **Hess, M. L. and Manson, N. H.,** Molecular oxygen: friend and foe. The role of oxygen radical system in the calcium paradox, the oxygen paradox and ischemia/reperfusion injury, *J. Mol. Cell. Cardiol.*, 16, 69, 1984.
42. **Fox, R. B.,** Prevention of granulocyte-mediated oxidant lung injury in rats by a hydroxyl radical scavenger, dimethylthiourea, *J. Clin. Invest.*, 74, 1456, 1984.
43. **Koke, J. R., Christodoulides, N. J., Chudej, L. L., and Bittar, N.,** Exogenous superoxide dismutase and catalase promote recovery of function in isolated rat heart after regional ischemia and may be transported from capillaries into myocytes, *Mol. Cell. Biochem.*, 96, 97, 1990.
44. **Chudej, L., Christodoulides, N., Koke, J., and Bittar, N.,** Superoxide dismutase and catalase prevent reperfusion injury and are transported in the myocytes of dog hearts, *FASEB J.*, 3(4), A2298, 1989.
45. **Debakey, M. E.,** Patterns of atherosclerosis and rates of progression, in *Atherosclerosis Reviews*, Vol. 3, Paoletti, R. and Gotto, A. M., Jr., Eds., Raven Press, New York, 1978, 1.
46. **Groszek, E. and Grundy, S. M.,** The possible role of the arterial microcirculation in the pathogenesis of atherosclerosis, *J. Chronic Dis.*, 33, 679, 1980.
47. **Geiringer, E.,** Intimal vascularization and atherosclerosis, *J. Pathol. Bacteriol.*, LXIII, 201, 1951.

48. **Winbury, M. M., Howe, B. B., and Hefner, M. A.,** Effect of nitrates and other coronary dilators on large and small coronary vessels: an hypothesis for the mechanism of action of nitrates, *J. Pharmacol. Exp. Therap.*, 168, 70, 1969.
49. **Sellke, F. W., Myers, P. R., Bates, J. N., and Harrison, D. G.,** Influence of vessel size on the sensitivity of porcine coronary microvessels to nitroglycerin, *Am. J. Physiol.*, 258, H515, 1990.
50. **Kurppa, K., Hietanen, E., Klockars, M., Partinen, M., Rantanen, J., Ronnemaa T., and Vikar, J.,** Chemical exposures at work and cardiovascular morbidity. Atherosclerosis, ischemic heart disease, hypertension, cardiomyopathy, and arrhythmias, *Scand. J. Work Environ. Health*, 10, 381, 1984.
51. **Mall, G., Mattfeldt, T., Rieger, P., Volk, B., and Frolov, V. A.,** Morphometric analysis of the rabbit myocardium after chronic ethanol feeding-early capillary changes, *Basic Res. Cardiol.*, 77, 57, 1982.
52. **Mall, G., Mattfeldt, T., and Volk, B.,** Ultrastructural morphometric study on the rat heart after chronic ethanol feeding, *Virch. Arch. A, Pathol. Anat. Histol.*, 389, 59, 1980.
53. **Friedman, H. S., Matsuzaki, S., Choe, S., Fernando, H. A., Celis, A., Zaman, Q., and Lieber, C.,** Demonstration of dissimilar acute hemodynamic effects of ethanol and acetaldehyde, *Cardiovasc. Res.*, 13, 477, 1979.
54. **Abel, F. L.,** Direct effects of ethanol on myocardial performance and coronary resistance, *J. Pharmacol. Exp. Therap.*, 212, 28, 1980.
55. **Mattfeldt, T. and Mall, G.,** Dipyridamole-induced capillary endothelial cell proliferation in the rat heart — A morphometric investigation, *Cardiovasc. Res.*, 17, 229, 1983.
56. **Tornling, G., Unge, G., Skoog, L., Ljungqvist, A., Carlsson, S., and Adolfsson, J.,** Proliferative activity of myocardial capillary wall cells in dipyridamole-treated rats, *Cardiovasc. Res.*, 12, 692, 1978.
57. **Trapp, A. L., Keahey, K. K., Whitenack, D. L., and Whitehair, C. K.,** Vitamin E-selenium deficiency in swine: differential diagnosis and nature of field problem, *J. Am. Vet. Med. Assoc.*, 157(3), 289, 1970.
58. **Piper, R. C., Froseth, J. A., McDowell, L. R., Kroening, G. H., and Dyer, I. A.,** Selenium-vitamin E deficiency in swine fed peas (*Pisum sativum*), *Am. J. Vet. Res.*, 36(3), 273, 1975.
59. **McDowell, L. R., Froseth, J. A., Piper, R. C., Dyer, I. A., and Kroening, G. H.,** Tissue selenium and serum tocopherol concentrations in selenium-vitamin E deficient pigs fed peas (*Pisum sativum*), *J. Anim. Sci.*, 45, 1326, 1977.
60. **Bengtsson, G., Hakarainen, J., Jonsson, L., Lannek, N., and Lindberg, P.,** Requirement for selenium (as selenite) and vitamin E (as alpha-tocopherol) in weaned pigs. I. The effect of varying alpha-tocopherol levels in a selenium deficient diet on the development of the VESD syndrome, *J. Anim. Sci.*, 46(1), 143, 1978.
61. **Rice, D. A. and Kennedy, S.,** Vitamin E, selenium, polyunsaturated fatty acid concentrations and glutathione peroxidase activity in tissues from pigs with dietetic microangiopathy (Mulberry Heart Disease), *Am. J. Vet. Res.*, 50(12), 2101, 1989.
62. **Van Vleet, J. F., Carlton, W., and Olander, H. J.,** Hepatosis dietetica and Mulberry Heart Disease associated with selenium deficiency in Indiana swine, *J. Am. Vet. Med. Assoc.*, 157, 1208, 1970.
63. **Ashraf, M.,** Oxygen derived radicals related injury in the heart during calcium paradox, *Virchows Arch. B*, 54, 27, 1987.
64. **Pascoe, G. A. and Reed, D. J.,** Cell calcium, vitamin E, and the thiol redox system in cytotoxicity, *Free Rad. Biol. Med.*, 6, 209, 1989.
65. **Korpela, H.,** Hypothesis: increased calcium and decreased magnesium in heart muscle and liver of pigs dying suddenly of microangiopathy (Mulberry Heart Disease): an animal model for study of oxidative damage, *J. Am. Coll. Nutr.*, 10(2), 127, 1991.

66. **Tomanek, R. J.,** Effects of age and exercise on the extent of the myocardial capillary bed, *Anat. Rec.,* 167, 55, 1969.
67. **Altura, B. M. and Altura, B. T.,** Alcohol, the cerebral circulation and strokes, *Alcohol,* 1, 325, 1984.
68. **Altura, B. M., Altura, B. T., and Gebrewold, A.,** Alcohol-induced spasms of cerebral blood vessels: relation to cerebrovascular accidents and sudden death, *Science,* 220, 331, 1983.
69. **De Witte, Ph., Gewiss, M., and Heidbreder, Ch.,** Cortical microvascular changes in chronological aging, cortical insults and chronic alcohol intoxication in rats. Effects of antihypoxic drugs on these phenomena, *Alcohol,* 6(6), 423, 1989.
70. **Wauquier, A., Clincke, G., Ashton, D., De Ryck, M., Fransen, J., and Van Clemen, G.,** R58735: A new antihypoxic drug with anticonvulsant properties and possible effects on cognitive functions, *Drug Devel. Res.,* 8, 373, 1986.
71. **Lieber, C. S., DeCarli, L. M., Feinman, L., Hasumura, Y., Korsten, M., and Teschke, R.,** Effect of chronic alcohol consumption on ethanol and acetaldehyde metabolism, in *Alcohol Intoxication and Withdrawal,* Vol. 2, Gross, M. M., Ed., Plenum Press, New York, 1975, 185.
72. **Perrin, R., Minn, A., Ghersi-Egea, J.-F., Grassiot, M.-C., and Siest, G.,** Distribution of cytochrome P-450 activities towards alkoxyresorufin derivatives in rat brain regions, subcellular fractions and isolated cerebral microvessels, *Biochem. Pharmacol.,* 40(9), 2145, 1990.
73. **Pentschew, A. and Garro, F.,** Lead encephalo-myelopathy of the suckling rat and its implications on the porphyrinopathic nervous diseases. With special reference to the permeability disorders of the nervous system's capillaries, *Acta Neuropathol.,* 6, 266, 1966.
74. **Clasen, R. A., Hartmann, J. F., Starr, A. J., Coogan, P. A., Pandolfi, S., Laing, I., Becker, R., and Hass, G. M.,** Electron microscopic and chemical studies of vascular changes and edema of lead encephalopathy, *Am. J. Pathol.,* 74, 215, 1974.
75. **Goldstein, G. W., Asbury, A. K., and Diamond, I.,** Pathogenesis of lead encephalopathy, *Arch. Neurol.,* 31, 382, 1974.
76. **Lefauconnier, J. M., Lavielle, E., Terrien, N., Bernard, G., and Fournier, E.,** Effect of various lead doses on some cerebral capillary funcions in the suckling rat, *Toxicol. Appl. Pharmacol.,* 55, 467, 1980.
77. **Thomas, J. A., Dallenbach, F. D., and Thomas, M.,** The distribution of radioactive lead (^{210}Pb) in the cerebellum of developing rats, *J. Pathol.,* 109, 45, 1973.
78. **Maxwell, K., Vinters, H., Berliner, J., Bready, J., and Cancilla, P.,** Effect of inorganic lead on some functions of the cerebral microvessel endothelium, *Toxicol. Appl. Pharmacol.,* 84, 389, 1986.
79. **Gebhart, A. M. and Goldstein, G. W.,** Use of an in vitro system to study the effects of lead on astrocyte-endothelial cell interactions: a model for studying toxic injury to the blood-brain barrier, *Toxicol. Appl. Pharmacol.,* 94, 191, 1988.
80. **De Bault, L. E. and Cancilla, P. A.,** Some properties of isolated endothelial cells in culture, in *The Cerebral Microvasculature,* Vol. 131, Eisenberg, H. M. and Suddith, R. L., Eds., Plenum Press, New York, 1980, 69.
81. **Tiffany-Castiglioni, E., Zmudzki, J., Wu, J., and Bratton, G.,** Effects of lead treatment on intracellular iron and copper concentrations in cultured astroglia, *Metab. Brain Dis.* 2, 61, 1987.
82. **Holtzman, D., Devries, C., Nguyen, H., Olson, J., and Bensch, K.,** Maturation of resistance to lead encephalopathy: cellular and subcellular mechanisms, *Neurotoxicology,* 5, 97, 1984.
83. **Moore, S. A., Yoder, E., and Spector, A. A.,** Role of the blood-brain barrier in the formation of long-chain omega-3 and omega-6 fatty acids from essential fatty acid precursors, *J. Neurochem.,* 55(2), 391, 1990.

84. **Moncado, S. and Vane, J. R.,** Arachidonic acid metabolites and the interactions between platelets and blood-vessel walls, *N. Engl. J. Med.*, 300, 1142, 1979.
85. **Rosenblum, W. I.,** Constriction of pial arterioles by prostaglandin $F_{2\text{-alpha}}$, *Stroke*, 6, 293, 1975.
86. **Ellis, E. F., Wei, E. P., and Kontos, H. A.,** Vasodilation of cat cerebral arterioles by prostaglandins D_2, E_2, G_2, I_2, *Am. J. Physiol.*, 237, H381, 1979.
87. **Kontos, H. A., Wei, E. P., Povlishock, J. T., Dietrich, W. D., Magiera, C. J., and Ellis, E. F.,** Cerebral arteriolar damage by arachidonic acid and prostaglandin G_2, *Science*, 209, 1242, 1980.
88. **Rosenblum, W. I.,** Constricting effect of leukotrienes on cerebral arterioles in mice, *Stroke*, 16, 262, 1985.
89. **Busija, D. W.,** Role of prostaglandins in the response of the cerebral circulation to carbon dioxide in conscious rabbits, *J. Cerebr. Blood Flow Metab.*, 3, 376, 1983.
90. **Fitzpatrick, F. A. and Murphy, R. C.,** Cytochrome P-450 metabolism of arachidonic acid: formation and biological actions of "epoxygenase"-derived eicosanoids, *Pharmacol. Rev.*, 40, 229, 1989.
91. **Revtyak, G. E., Jognson, A. R., and Campbell, W. B.,** Cultured bovine coronary arterial endothelial cells synthesize HETEs and prostacyclin, *Am. J. Physiol.*, 254, C8, 1988.
92. **Abraham, N. G., Pinto, A., Mullane, K. M., Levere, R. D., and Spokas, E.,** Presence of cytochrome P-450-dependent monooxygenase in intimal cells of the hog aorta, *Hypertension*, 7(6), 899, 1985.
93. **Ellis, E. F., Police, R. J., Yancey, L., McKinney, J. S., and Amruthesh, S. C.,** Dilation of cerebral arterioles by cytochrome P-450 metabolites of arachidonic acid, *Am. J. Physiol.*, 259, H1171, 1990.
94. **Ellis, E. F., Police, R. J., Yancey, L. M., GrabeeL, M. N., Heizer, M. L., and Holt, S. A.,** Effect of fish oil n-3 fatty acids on cerebral microcirculation, *Am. J. Physiol.*, 258, H1780, 1990.
95. **Kamitani, T., Little, M. H., and Ellis, E. F.,** Evidence for a possible role of the brain kallikrein-kinin system in the modulation of the cerebral circulation, *Circ. Res.*, 57, 545, 1985.
96. **Villacara, A., Spatz, M., Dodson, R. F., Corn, C., and Bembry, J.,** Effect of arachidonic acid on cultured cerebromicrovascular endothelium: permeability, lipid peroxidation, and membrane "fluidity," *Acta Neuropathol.*, 78, 310, 1989.
97. **Hannah, R. S. and Hannah, K. J.,** Hyperoxia: effects on the vascularization of the developing central nervous system, *Acta Neuropathol.*, 51, 141, 1980.
98. **D'Amore, P. A. and Sweet, E.,** Effects of hyperoxia on microvascular cells in vitro, *In Vitro Cell. Develop. Biol.*, 23(2), 123, 1987.
99. **Whittle, B. J. R., Morishita, T., Ohya, Y., Leung, F. W., and Guth, P. H.,** Microvascular actions of platelet-activating factor on rat gastric mucosa and submucosa, *Am. J. Physiol.*, 251, G772, 1986.
100. **Esplunges, J. V. and Whittle, B. J. R.,** Gastric mucosal damage induced by local intra-arterial administration of Paf in the rat, *Br. J. Pharmacol.*, 93, 222, 1988.
101. **Rosam, A. C, Wallace, J. L., and Whittle, B. J. R.,** Potent ulcerogenic actions of platelet-activating factor on the stomach, *Nature*, 319, 54, 1986.
102. **Pique, J. M., Esplugues, J. V., and Whittle, B. J. R.,** Influence of morphine or capsaicin pretreatment on rat gastric microcirculatory response to PAF, *Am. J. Physiol.*, 258, G352, 1990.
103. **Kitajima, M., Shimizu, A., Torii, H., Ikeda, Y., and Oshima, A.,** Gastric microcirculatory change and development of acute gastric mucosal lesions (stress ulcer), *Acta Physiol. Hung.*, 73(2-3), 137, 1989.
104. **Kitajima, M. and Itoh, H.,** Gastric mucosal blood flow and energy metabolism in stress, *Microcirculation Annual 1985*, Tsuchiya, M., Ed., Excerpta Medica, Amsterdam, 1985, 243.

105. **Altura, B. M., Ogunkoya, A., Gebrewold, A., and Altura, B.,** Effects of ethanol on terminal arterioles and muscular venules: direct observations on the microcirculation, *J. Cardiovasc. Pharmacol.*, 1, 97, 1979.
106. **Altura, B. M. and Gebrewold, A.,** Failure of acetaldehyde or acetate to mimic the splanchnic arteriolar or venular dilator actions of ethanol: direct *in situ* studies on the microcirculation, *Br. J. Pharmacol.*, 73, 580, 1981.
107. **Altura, B. M., Altura, B. T., Carella, A., and Turlapaty, P. D.,** Ca^{2+} coupling in vascular smooth muscle: Mg^{2+} and buffer effects on contractility and membrane Ca^{2+} movements, *Can. J. Physiol. Pharmacol.*, 60(4), 459, 1982.
108. **Bode, C., Kugler, V., and Bode, J. C.,** Endotoxemia in patients with alcoholic and non-alcoholic cirrhosis and in subjects with no evidence of chronic liver disease following acute alcohol excess, *J. Hepatol.*, 4, 8, 1987.
109. **Nolan, J. P.,** Alcohol as a factor in the illness of University service patients, *Am. J. Med. Sci.*, 249, 135, 1965.
110. **Bhagwandeen, B. S., Apte, M., Manwarring, L., and Dickeson, J.,** Endotoxin induced hepatic necrosis in rats on an alcohol diet, *J. Pathol.*, 152, 47, 1987.
111. **McCuskey, R. S., Urbaschek, R., McCuskey, P. A., and Urbaschek, B.,** In vivo microscopic observations of the responses of Kupffer cells and the hepatic microcirculation to *Mycobacterium bovis* BCG alone and in combination with endotoxin, *Infect. Immun.*, 42, 362, 1983.
112. **McCuskey, R. S.,** In vivo microscopy of the liver following acute administration of ethanol, *Progr. Clin. Biol. Res.*, 325, 341, 1990.
113. **McCuskey, R. S., McCuskey, P. A., Urbaschek, R., and Urbaschek, B.,** Hepatic microvascular alterations during sepsis, *Circ. Shock*, 13, 88, 1984a.
114. **McCuskey, R. S., Urbaschek, R., McCuskey P. A., and Urbaschek, B.,** Microvascular responses to tumor necrosis factor, *FASEB*, J 2, A1873, 1988.
115. **Procter, E. and Chatamra, K.,** High yield micronodular cirrhosis in rat, *Gastroenterology*, 83, 1183, 1982.
116. **Recknagel, R. O., Glende, E. A., Jr., Dolak, J. A., and Waller, R. L.,** Mechanisms of carbon tetrachloride toxicity, *Pharmacol. Ther.*, 43, 139, 1989
117. **Zimmerman, H. J.,** *Hepatotoxicity: The Adverse Effects of Drugs and Other Chemicals on the Liver*, Appleton-Century-Crofts, New York, 1978.
118. **Recknagel, R. O., Glende, E. A., Jr., and Hruszkewycz, A. M.,** Chemical mechanisms in carbon tetrachloride toxicity, in *Free Radicals in Biology*, Vol. 3, Pryor, W. A., Ed., Academic Press, New York, 1977, 97.
119. **Brattin, W. J., Glende, E. A., Jr., and Recknagel, R. O.,** Pathological mechanisms in carbon tetrachloride hepatotoxicity, *J. Free Rad. Biol. Med.*, 1, 17, 1985.
120. **Varin, F. and Huet, P. M.,** Hepatic microcirculation in the perfused cirrhotic rat liver, *J. Clin. Invest.*, 76, 1904, 1985.
121. **Sherman, I. A., Pappas, S. C., and Fisher, M. M.,** Hepatic microvascular changes associated with development of liver fibrosis and cirrhosis, *Am. J. Physiol.*, 258, H460, 1990.
122. **Song, C. W., Chelstrom, L. M., Levitt, S. H., and Haumschild, D. J.,** Effects of temperature on blood circulation measured with the laser doppler method, *Int. J. Rad. Oncol. Biol. Phys.*, 17, 1041, 1989.
123. **Stojanov, I. and Proctor, K. G.,** Temperature-sensitive adenosine-mediated vasoconstriction in the skin microcirculation, *J. Pharmacol. Exp. Ther.*, 253(3), 1083, 1989.
124. **Flavahan, N. A., Lindblad, L.-E., Verbeuren, T. J., Shepherd, J. T., and Vanhoutte, P. M.,** Cooling and $alpha_1$- and $alpha_2$-adrenergic responses in cutaneous veins: role of receptor reserve, *Am. J. Physiol.*, 249, H950, 1985.

125. **Ward, P. A. and Till, G. O.,** Pathophysiologic events related to thermal injury of skin, *J. Trauma*, 30(12), 1990.

126. **Carvajal, H. F., Brouhard, B. H., and Linares, H. A.,** Effect of antihistamine — antiserotonin and ganglionic blocking agents upon increased capillary permeability following burn trauma, *J. Trauma*, 15(11), 1975.

127. **Alexander, F., Mathieson, M., Teoh, K. H. T., Huval, W. H., Lelcuk, S., Valeri, R., Shepro, D., and Hechtman, H. B.,** Arachidonic acid metabolites mediate early burn edema, *J. Trauma*, 24(8), 709, 1984.

128. **Hambrecht, G. S. and Hilton, J. G.,** The effect of catalase, indomethacin and FPL 55712 on vascular permeability in the hamster cheek pouch following scald injury, *Prostagland. Leuk. Med.*, 14, 297, 1984.

129. **Nishigaki, I., Hagihara, M., Hiramatsu, M., Izawa Y., and Yagi, K.,** Effect of thermal injury on lipid peroxidation levels of rat, *Biochem. Med.*, 24, 185, 1980.

130. **Till, G. O., Hatherill J. R., Tourtellotte, W. W., Lutz, M. J., and Ward, P. A.,** Lipid peroxidation and acute lung injury after thermal trauma to skin, evidence of a role for hydroxyl radical, *Am. J. Pathol.*, 119, 185, 1980.

131. **Schwartz, R. W., Fu, H. Q., Logan, N. M., Richardson, D. R., and Hyde, G. L.,** Effects of atherosclerosis on the cutaneous regional and microcirculatory response to ischemia, *Arch. Surg.*, 125, 485, 1990.

132. **Schwartz, R. W., Hu, Q. F., Logan, N. M., Richardson, D. R., and Hyde, G. L.,** Effects of atherosclerosis and chronic smoking on the regional arterial and microcirculatory response to gravity, in *Proceedings of the Southern Assocation for Vascular Surgery*, Key West, FL, 1989.

133. **Kyrle, P. A., Minar, E., Brenner, B., Eichler, H. G., Heistinger, M., Marosi, L., and Lechner, K.,** Thromboxane A2 and prostacyclin generation in the microvasculature of patients with atherosclerosis-effect of low dose aspirin, *Thromb. Haemostasis*, 61(3), 374, 1989.

134. **Von Euler, U. S. and Liljestrand, G.,** Observation on the pulmonary arterial blood pressure in the cat, *Acta Physiol. Scand.*, 12, 301, 1946.

135. **Parker, R. E., Granger, D. N., and Taylor, A. E.,** Estimates of isogravimetric capillary pressures during alveolar hypoxia, *Am. J. Physiol.*, 241, H732, 1981.

136. **Nagasaka, Y., Bhattacharya, J., Nanjo, S., Gropper, M. A., and Staub, N. C.,** Micropuncture measurement of lung microvascular pressure profile during hypoxia in cats, *Circ. Res.*, 54(1), 90, 1984.

137. **Cope, D. K., Parker, J. C., Taylor, M. D., Houston, M., and Taylor, A. E.,** Pulmonary capillary pressures during hypoxia and hypoxemia: experimental and clinical studies, *Crit. Care Med.*, 17, 853, 1989.

138. **Rannels, D. E., Pegg, A. E., Clark, R. S., and Addison, J. L.,** Interaction of paraquat and amine uptake by rat lungs perfused in situ, *Am. J. Physiol.*, 249, E506, 1985.

139. **Fisher, H. K., Clements, J. A., and Wright, R. R.,** Enhancement of oxygen toxicity by the herbicide paraquat, *Am. Rev. Resp. Dis.*, 107, 246, 1973.

140. **Giri, S. N., Hollinger, M. A., and Schiedt, M. J.,** The effects of paraquat and superoxide dismutase on pulmonary vascular permeability and edema in mice, *Arch. Environ. Health*, 36, 149, 1981.

141. **Shibamoto, T., Taylor, A. E., and Parker, J. C.,** PO_2 modulation of paraquat-induced microvascular injury in isolated dog lungs, *J. Appl. Physiol.*, 68(5), 2119, 1990.

142. **Rhodes, M. L., Zavala, D. C., and Brown, D.,** Hypoxic protection in paraquat poisoning, *Lab. Invest.*, 35, 496, 1976.

143. **Warden, J. A. and Rhodes, M. L.,** Failure of hypoxia to protect against paraquat toxicity in rats, *Am. Rev. Resp. Dis. Suppl.*, 117, 265, 1978.

144. **Crapo, J. D., Barry, B. E., Foscue, H. A., and Shelburne, J.,** Structural and biochemical change in rat lungs occurring during exposures to lethal and adaptive doses of oxygen, *Am. Rev. Resp. Dis.,* 122, 123, 1980.
145. **He, L., Chang, S. W., Ortiz de Montellano, P., Burke, T. J., and Voelkel, N. F.,** Lung injury in Fisher but not Sprague-Dawley rats after short-term hyperoxia, *Am. J. Physiol.*, 259, L451, 1990.
146. **Kjaeve, J., Vaage, J., and Bjertnaes, L.,** Increased microvascular permeability caused by toxic oxygen metabolites is partly reversed by exchanging the perfusate in isolated rat lungs, *Acta Anaesthesiol. Scand.*, 33, 605, 1989.
147. **Tate, T. M., VanBenthuysen, K. M., Shasby, D. M., McMurtry, E. F., and Repine, J. E.,** Oxygen-radical-mediated permeability edema and vasoconstriction in isolated perfused rabbit lungs, *Am. Rev. Resp. Dis.*, 126, 802, 1982.
148. **Dickey, B. F., Thrall, R. S., McCormick, J. R., and Ward, P. A.,** Oleic acid-induced lung injury in the rat, *Am. J. Physiol.*, 103(3), 376, 1981.
149. **Eiermann, G. J., Dickey, B. F., and Thrall, R. S.,** Polymorphonuclear leukocyte participation in acute oleic-acid-induced lung injury, *Am. Rev. Resp. Dis.*, 128, 845, 1983.
150. **Townsley, M. I., Taylor, G. E., Korthuis, R. J., and Taylor, A. E.,** Promethazine of DPPD pretreatment attenuates oleic acid-induced injury in isolated canine lungs, *J. Appl. Physiol.*, 59, 39, 1985.
151. **Meyrick, B., Gamble, W., and Reid, L.,** Development of *Crotalaria* pulmonary hypertension: hemodynamic and structural study, *Am. J. Physiol.*, 239, H693, 1980.
152. **Roth, R. A. and Reindel, J. F.,** Lung vascular injury from monocrotaline pyrrole, a putative hepatic metabolite, *Adv. Exp. Med. Biol.*, 283, 477, 1991.
153. **Meyrick, B. O. and Reid, L. M.,** Crotalaria-induced pulmonary hypertension, *Am. J. Pathol.*, 106, 84, 1982.
154. **Hilliker, K. S., Garcia, C. M., and Roth, R. A.,** Effects of monocrotaline and monocrotaline pyrrole on 5-hydroxytryptamine and paraquat uptake by lung slices, *Res. Comm. Chem. Pathol. Pharmacol.*, 40(2), 179, 1983.
155. **Olson, J. W., Altiere, R. J., and Gillespie, M. N.,** Prolonged activation of rat lung ornithine decarboxylase in monocrotaline-induced pulmonary hypertension, *Biochem. Pharmacol.*, 33(22), 3633, 1984.
156. **Olson, J. W., Atkinson, J. E., Hacker, A. D., Altiere, R. J., and Gillespie, M. N.,** Suppression of polyamine biosynthesis prevents monocrotaline-induced pulmonary edema and arterial medial thickening, *Toxicol. Appl. Pharmacol.*, 81, 91, 1985.
157. **Schraufnagel, D. E. and Schmid, A.,** Pulmonary capillary density in rats given monocrotaline, *Am. Rev. Resp. Dis.*, 140, 1405, 1989.
158. **Schraufnagal, D. E.,** Monocrotaline-induced angiogenesis. Differences in the bronchial and pulmonary vasculature, *Am. J. Pathol.*, 137(5), 1083, 1990.
159. **Templeton, D. M. and Chaitu, N.,** Effects of divalent metals on the isolated rat glomerulus, *Toxicology*, 61, 119, 1990.
160. **Ward, P. A., Johnson, K. J., and Till, G. O.,** Oxygen radicals and microvascular injury of lungs and kidney, *Acta Physiol. Scand.*, 548, 79, 1986.
161. **Anderson, S., King, A. J., and Brenner, B. M.,** Hyperlipidemia and glomerular sclerosis: an alternative viewpoint, *Am. J. Med.*, 87, 5-34N, 1989.
162. **Kasiske, B. L., O'Donnell, M. P., Cleary, M. P., and Keane, W. F.,** Treatment of hyperlipidemia reduces glomerular injury in obese Zucker rats, *Kidney Int.,* 33, 667, 1988.
163. **Kasiske, B. L., Cleary, M. P., O'Donnell, M. P., and Keane, W. F.,** Effects of genetic obesity on renal structure and function in the Zucker rat, *J. Lab. Clin. Med.*, 106, 598, 1985.

164. **Moorehead, J. F., Wheeler, D. C., Fernando, R., Sweny, P., and Varghese, Z.,** Injury to rat mesangial cells in culture by low density lipoproteins, *Kidney Int.,* 35, 433, 1989.

165. **Yoshioka, K., Takemura, T., Matsubara, K., Miyamoto, H., Akano, N., and Maki, S.,** Immunohistochemical studies of reflux nephropathy. The role of extracellular matrix, membrane attack complex, and immune cells in glomerular sclerosis, *Am. J. Pathol.,* 129(2), 223, 1987.

166. **Haralson, M. A., Jacobson, H. R., and Hoover, R. L.,** Collagen polymorphism in cultured rat kidney mesangial cells, *Lab. Invest.,* 57(5), 513, 1987.

167. **Yoshioka, K., Tohda, M., Takemura, T., Akano, N., Matsubara, K., Ooshima, A., and Maki, S.,** Distribution of type I collagen in human kidney diseases in comparison with type III collagen, *J. Pathol.,* 162, 141, 1990.

168. **Zimmerman, S. W., Norback, D. H., and Powers, K.,** Carbon tetrachloride nephrotoxicity in rats with reduced renal mass, *Arch. Pathol. Lab. Med.,* 107, 264, 1983.

169. **Ohyama, K., Seyer, J. M., Raghow, R., and Kang, A. H.,** A factor from damaged rat kidney stimulates collagen biosynthesis by mesangial cells, *Biochim. Biophys. Acta,* 1053, 173, 1990.

170. **Hatahara, T. and Seyer, J. M.,** Isolation and characterization of a fibrogenic factor from CCL*4*-damaged rat liver, *Biochim. Biophys. Acta,* 716, 377, 1982.

171. **Furcht, L. T.,** Critical factor controlling angiogenesis: cell products, cell matrix, and growth factors, *Lab. Invest.,* 55(5), 505, 1986.

172. **Okuda, S., Languino, L. R., Ruoslahti, E., and Border, W. A.,** Elevated expression of transforming growth factor-beta and proteoglycan production in experimental glomerulonephritis, *J. Clin. Invest.,* 86, 453, 1990.

173. **Lovett, D. H., Ryan, J. L., and Sterzel, R. B.,** Stimulation of rat mesangial cell proliferation by macrophage interleukin 1^1, *J. Immunol.,* 131(6), 2830, 1983.

174. **Border, W. A., Okuda, S., Languino, L. R., and Ruoslahti, E.,** Transforming growth factor-beta regulates production of proteoglycans by mesangial cells, *Kidney Int.,* 37, 689, 1990.

175. **Schlondorff, D.,** The glomerular mesangial cell: an expanding role for a specialized pericyte, *FASEB J,* 1, 272, 1987.

176. **Shultz, P. J., Schorer, A. E., and Raij, L.,** Effects of endothelium-derived relaxing factor and nitric oxide on rat mesangial cells, *Am. J. Physiol.,* 258, F162, 1990.

177. **Frieman, P. C., Mitchell, G. G., Heistad, D. D., Armstrong, M. L., and Harrison, D. G.,** Atherosclerosis impairs endothelium-dependent vascular relaxation to acetylcholine and thrombin in primates, *Circ. Res.,* 58, 783, 1986.

178. **Kelley, V. E., Ferretti, A., Izui, S., and Strom, T. B.,** A fish oil diet rich in eicosapentaenoic acid reduces cyclooxygenase metabolites and suppresses lupus in MRL-lpr mice, *J. Immunol.,* 134, 1914, 1985.

179. **Stahl, R. A. K. and Thaiss, F.,** Eicosanoids: biosynthesis and function in the glomerulus, *Renal Physiol.,* 10, 1, 1987.

180. **Takahashi, K., Capdevila, J., Karara, A., Falck, J. R., Jacobson, H. R., and Badr, K. F.,** Cytochrome P-450 arachidonate metabolites in rat kidney: characterization and hemodynamic responses, *Am. J. Physiol.,* 258, F781, 1990.

181. **Harris, R. C., Homma, T., Jacobson, H. R., and Capdevila, J.,** Epoxyeicosatrienoic acids activate Na^+/H^+ exchange and are mitogenic in cultured rat glomerular mesangial cells, *J. Cell. Physiol.,* 144, 429, 1990.

182. **Badr, K. F., Mong, S., Hoover, R. L., Schwartzberg, M., Ebert, J., Jacobson, H. R., and Harris, R. C.,** Leukotriene D_4 binding and signal transduction in rat glomerular mesangial cells, *Am. J. Physiol.,* 257, F280, 1989.

183. **Stahl, R. A., Thaiss, F., Haberstroh, U., Kahf, S., Shaw, A., and Schoeppe, W.,** Cyclooxygenase inhibition enhances rat interleukin 1 beta-induced growth of rat mesangial cells in culture, *Am. J. Physiol.*, 259, F419, 1990.
184. **Smith, S. M. and Hoy, W. E.,** Frequent association of mesangial glomerulonephritis and alcohol abuse: a study of 3 ethnic groups, *Mod. Pathol.*, 2(2), 138, 1989.
185. **Bene, M. C., Korwin, J. D., Hurault de Ligny, B., Aymard, B., Kessler, M., and Faure, G. C.,** IgA nephropathy and alcoholic liver cirrhosis, *Am. J. Clin. Pathol.*, 89, 769, 1989.
186. **Smith, S. M., Yu, G. S. M., and Tsukamoto, H.,** IgA nephropathy in alcohol abuse an animal model, *Lab. Invest.*, 62(2), 179, 1990.
187. **Creasia, D. A., Thurman, J. D., Wannemacher, R. W., Jr., and Bunner, D. L.,** Acute inhalation toxicity of T-2 mycotoxin in the rat and guinea pig, *Fund. Appl. Toxicol.*, 14, 54, 1990.
188. **Siren, A. and Feuerstein, G.,** Effect of T-2 toxin on regional blood flow and vascular resistance in the conscious rat, *Toxicol. Appl. Pharmacol.*, 83, 438, 1986.
189. **Thompson, W. L. and Wannemacher, R. W., Jr.,** In vivo effects of T-2 mycotoxin on synthesis of proteins and DNA in rat tissues, *Toxicol. Appl. Pharmacol.*, 105, 483, 1990.
190. **Borison, H. L., Goodhear, M. L., and Thut, D. C.,** Hypovolemic shock in acute lethal T-2 mycotoxicosis, *Toxicol. Appl. Pharmacol.*, 108, 107, 1991.
191. **Sjodin, B., Westing, Y. H., and Apple, F. S.,** Biochemical mechanisms for oxygen free radical formation during exercise, *Sports Med.*, 10(4), 236, 1990.
192. **Sexton, W. L., Korthuis, R. J., and Laughlin, M. H.,** Microvascular injury after ischemia and reperfusion in skeletal muscle of exercise-trained rats, *J. Appl. Physiol.*, 68(6), 2329, 1990.
193. **Faber, J. E.,** Effect of local tissue cooling on microvascular smooth muscle and postjunctional alpha2-adrenoreceptors, *Am. J. Physiol.*, 255, H121, 1988.
194. **Beevers, D. G.,** Alcohol and hypertension, *Lancet*, 2, 14, 1977.
195. **Ashley, M. J. and Rankin, J. G.,** Hazardous alcohol consumption and diseases of the circulatory system, *J. Stud. Alcohol*, 41, 1040, 1980.
196. **Altura, B. M.,** Pharmacology of venular smooth muscle: new insights, *Microvasc. Res.*, 16, 91, 1978.
197. **Altura, B. M. and Altura, B. T.,** Peripheral vascular actions of ethanol and its interaction with neurohumoral substances, *Neurobehav. Toxicol. Teratol.*, 5, 211, 1983.
198. **Altura, B. M., Altura, B. T., and Gebrewold, A.,** Comparative effects of ethanol, acetaldehyde and acetate on arterioles and venules in skeletal muscle: direct in situ studies on the microcirculation and their possible relationship to alcoholic myopathy, *Microcirc. Endothel. Lymph.*, 6, 107, 1990.
199. **Schuschke, D. A., Saari, J. T., Ackermann, D. M., and Miller, F. N.,** Progressive microcirculatory changes caused by hypercholesterolemia in rats, *Am. J. Physiol.*, 258, H1464, 1990.
200. **Yamamoto, H., Bossaller, C., Cartwright, J., Jr., and Henry, P. D.,** Videomicroscopic demonstration of defective cholinergic arteriolar vasodilation in atherosclerotic rabbit, *J. Clin. Invest.*, 81, 1752, 1988.
201. **Tsutsumi, S., Tsuji, K., Ogawa, K., Ito, T., and Satake, T.,** Effect of dietary salt and cholesterol loading on vascular adrenergic receptors, *Blood Vessels*, 25, 209, 1988.
202. **Kitano, S.,** Membrane and contractile properties of rat vascular tissue in copper-deficient conditions, *Circ. Res.*, 46, 681, 1980.
203. **Lei, K. Y.,** Cholesterol metabolism in copper-deficient rats, *Nutr. Rep. Int.*, 15, 597, 1977.

204. **Lee, G. R., Williams, D. M., and Cartwright, G. E.,** Role of copper and iron in metabolism and heme biosynthesis, in *Trace Elements of Human Health and Disease*, Prasad, A. S. and Oberleas, D., Eds., Academic Press, New York, 1976, 373.
205. **Folkman, J. and Klagsbrun, M.,** Angiogenic factors, *Science Washington DC,* 235, 442, 1987.
206. **Owen, C. A.,** *Biochemical Aspects of Copper. Copper Proteins, Ceruloplasmin, and Copper Protein Binding*, Noyes Publishing, Park Ridge, NJ, 1982, 9.
207. **Schuschke, D. A., Saari, J. T., Ackermann, D. M., and Miller, F. N.,** Microvascular responses in copper-deficient rats, *Am. J. Physiol.*, 257, H1607, 1989.

INDEX

A

D

E

F

G

H

I

J

K

L

M

N

O

P

Q

R

S

T

U

V